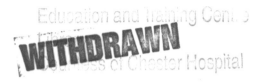
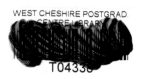

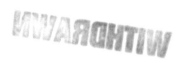

the**clinics**.com

ENDOCRINOLOGY AND METABOLISM CLINICS OF NORTH AMERICA

Endocrinopathies of Transplant Medicine

GUEST EDITOR
Tracy L. Breen, MD

CONSULTING EDITOR
Derek LeRoith, MD, PhD

December 2007 • Volume 36 • Number 4

SAUNDERS

An Imprint of Elsevier, Inc.
PHILADELPHIA   LONDON   TORONTO   MONTREAL   SYDNEY   TOKYO

W.B. SAUNDERS COMPANY
A Division of Elsevier Inc.

1600 John F. Kennedy Boulevard • Suite 1800 • Philadelphia, Pennsylvania 19103-2899

http://www.theclinics.com

ENDOCRINOLOGY AND METABOLISM	Volume 36, Number 4
CLINICS OF NORTH AMERICA	ISSN 0889-8529
December 2007	ISBN-13: 978-1-4160-5067-4
Editor: Rachel Glover	ISBN-10: 1-4160-5067-1

The ideas and opinions expressed in *Endocrinology and Metabolism Clinics of North America* do not necessarily reflect those of the Publisher. The Publisher does not assume any responsibility for any injury and/or damage to persons or property arising out of or related to any use of the material contained in this periodical. The reader is advised to check the appropriate medical literature and the product information currently provided by the manufacturer of each drug to be administered to verify the dosage, the method and duration of administration, or contraindications. It is the responsibility of the treating physician or other health care professional, relying on independent experience and knowledge of the patient, to determine drug dosages and the best treatment for the patient. Mention of any product in this issue should not be construed as endorsement by the contributors, editors, or the Publisher of the product or manufacturers' claims.

Endocrinology and Metabolism Clinics of North America (ISSN 0889-8529) is published quarterly by Elsevier Inc., 360 Park Avenue South, New York, NY 10010-1710. Months of publication are March, June, September, and December. Business and editorial offices: 1600 John F. Kennedy Boulevard, Suite 1800, Philadelphia, PA 19103-2899. Customer Service Office: 6277 Sea Harbor Drive, Orlando, FL 32887-4800. Periodicals postage paid at New York, NY and additional mailing offices. Subscription prices are USD 220 per year for US individuals, USD 364 per year for US institutions, USD 113 per year for US students and residents, USD 276 per year for Canadian individuals, USD 437 per year for Canadian institutions, USD 301 per year for international individuals, USD 437 per year for international institutions and USD 157 per year for Canadian and foreign students/residents. To receive student/resident rate, orders must be accompanied by name of affiliated institution, date of term, and the *signature* of program/residency coordinator on institution letterhead. Orders will be billed at individual rate until proof of status is received. Foreign air speed delivery is included in all *Clinics* subscription prices. All prices are subject to change without notice. POSTMASTER: Send address changes to *Endocrinology and Metabolism Clinics of North America*, Elsevier Periodicals Customer Service, 6277 Sea Harbor Drive, Orlando, FL 32887-4800. **Customer Service: (+1) 800-654-2452 (US). From outside of the US, call (+1) 407-345-4000; e-mail: hhspcs@harcourt.com.**

Reprints. For copies of 100 or more, of articles in this publication, please contact the Commercial Rights Department, Elsevier Inc., 360 Park Avenue South, New York, NY 10010-1710; phone: (+1) 212-633-3813; fax: (+1) 212-462-1935; e-mail: reprints@elsevier.com.

Endocrinology and Metabolism Clinics of North America is covered ... Index Medicus, EMBASE/Excerpta Medica, Current Contents/Clinical Medicine, Current Contents/Life Sciences, Science Citation Index, ISI/BIOMED, BIOSIS, and Chemical Abstracts.

Printed in the United States of America.

CONSULTING EDITOR

DEREK LEROITH, MD, PhD, Chief, Division of Endocrinology, Metabolism, and Bone Diseases, Mount Sinai School of Medicine, New York, New York

GUEST EDITOR

TRACY L. BREEN, MD, Division of Endocrinology, Metabolism, and Bone Diseases, Mount Sinai School of Medicine, New York, New York

CONTRIBUTORS

ENVER AKALIN, MD, Renal Division; and Recanati/Miller Transplantation Institute, Mount Sinai School of Medicine, New York, New York

NAGAKO AKENO, PhD, Research Instructor, Division of Endocrinology, University of Cincinnati College of Medicine, Cincinnati, Ohio

JASON T. BLACKARD, PhD, Research Assistant Professor, Division of Digestive Diseases, University of Cincinnati College of Medicine, Cincinnati, Ohio

NAGA CHALASANI, MD, Associate Professor of Medicine and Director, Division of Gastroenterology and Hepatology, Indiana University School of Medicine, Indianapolis, Indiana

WASSIM CHEMAITILLY, MD, Department of Pediatrics, Schneider Children's Hospital, New Hyde Park, New York

RAJANI DINAVAHI, MD, Renal Division; and Recanati/Miller Transplantation Institute, Mount Sinai School of Medicine, New York, New York

PETER EBELING, MD, Chair of Medicine and Head of Endocrinology, The Royal Melbourne Hospital; and Department of Medicine, Western Hospital, University of Melbourne, Victoria, Australia

PAOLO FIORINA, MD, PhD, Instructor, Transplantation Research Center, Children's Hospital–Brigham and Women's Hospital, Harvard Medical School; and Harvard Stem Cell Institute, Boston, Massachusetts; Associate Physician, Transplantation Medicine, San Raffaele Scientific Institute, Milan, Italy

PHILIP A. GOLDBERG, MD, Clinical Assistant Professor, Department of Internal Medicine, Section of Endocrinology and Metabolism, Yale University School of Medicine, New Haven, Connecticut

NAVEEN A.T. HAMDY, MD, Associate Professor of Medicine and Head, Clinic Section, Department of Endocrinology and Metabolic Diseases, Leiden University Medical Center, Leiden, the Netherlands

MOUEN KHASHAB, MD, Fellow in Gastroenterology and Hepatology, Division of Gastroenterology and Hepatology, Indiana University School of Medicine, Indianapolis, Indiana

GERALD S. LIPSHUTZ, MD, MS, FACS, Assistant Professor of Surgery, Kidney and Pancreas Transplantation Program, Departments of Surgery and Oncology, University of California Los Angeles, David Geffen School of Medicine, Los Angeles, California

PHUONG-CHI T. PHAM, MD, Associate Professor of Medicine, Division of Nephrology, Department of Medicine, University of California Los Angeles, David Geffen School of Medicine, Los Angeles; and Olive View-UCLA Medical Center, Sylmar, California

PHUONG-THU T. PHAM, MD, Assistant Professor of Medicine, Division of Nephrology; Director of Outpatient Services; and Kidney and Pancreas Transplantation, Department of Medicine, University of California Los Angeles, David Geffen School of Medicine, Los Angeles, California

LUCIANO POTENA, MD, PhD, Institute of Cardiology, University of Bologna, Bologna, Italy

CHARLES A. SKLAR, MD, Department of Pediatrics, Memorial Sloan-Kettering Cancer Center, New York, New York

ANTONIO SECCHI, MD, Associate Professor of Medicine, Universita' Vita-Salute; and Head, Transplant Unit, San Raffaele Scientific Institute, Milan, Italy

ELIZABETH SHANE, MD, Professor of Medicine, Division of Endocrinology, Department of Medicine, College of Physicians and Surgeons, Columbia University, New York, New York

EMILY STEIN, MD, Instructor of Medicine, Division of Endocrinology, Department of Medicine, College of Physicians and Surgeons, Columbia University, New York, New York

SAVITHA SUBRAMANIAN, MD, Instructor of Medicine, Division of Metabolism, Endocrinology, and Nutrition, University of Washington, Seattle, Washington

YARON TOMER, MD, Professor of Medicine, Division of Endocrinology, Cincinnati VA Medical Center; and Division of Endocrinology, University of Cincinnati College of Medicine, Cincinnati, Ohio

DACE L. TRENCE, MD, Associate Professor of Medicine, Division of Metabolism, Endocrinology, and Nutrition, University of Washington; and Director, Diabetes Care Center, University of Washington Medical Center, Seattle, Washington

HANNAH A. VALANTINE, MD, MRCP, FACC, Senior Associate Dean and Professor of Medicine, Cardiovascular Medicine, Stanford University School of Medicine, Stanford, California

ALAN H. WILKINSON, MD, FRCP, Professor of Medicine, Division of Nephrology; and Director of Kidney and Pancreas Transplantation, Department of Medicine, University of California Los Angeles, David Geffen School of Medicine, Los Angeles, California

CONTENTS

Cardiac Allograft Vasculopathy and Insulin Resistance—Hope for New Therapeutic Targets

Luciano Potena and Hannah A. Valantine

Cardiac allograft vasculopathy (CAV) is a major cause of death in patients surviving more than 1 year after heart transplantation. An important cluster of CAV risk factors occurs as a consequence of insulin resistance and manifests as part of the metabolic syndrome. This article summarizes the pathologic features of CAV and reviews the contribution of the major components of insulin resistance in CAV development and progression. It focuses on the few studies that have analyzed the impact of the individual metabolic abnormalities and inflammation and on therapeutic strategies to minimize the clinical manifestation of insulin resistance after heart transplantation.

Endocrine Complications of Hematopoietic Stem Cell Transplantation

Wassim Chemaitilly and Charles A. Sklar

Advances in hematopoietic stem cell transplantation (HSCT) have resulted in broader indications for this therapeutic modality in both malignant diseases and nonmalignant conditions. This article focuses on the late endocrine abnormalities that are most commonly observed following successful HSCT, with a special emphasis on pediatric HSCT recipients, for whom long-term follow-up data are increasingly available.

Pancreatic Islet Cell Transplant for Treatment of Diabetes

Paolo Fiorina and Antonio Secchi

Islet cell transplantation recently has emerged as one the most promising therapeutic approaches to improving glycometabolic control in type 1 diabetic patients, and, in many cases, to obtaining insulin independence. Islet cell transplantation requires a relatively short hospital stay and has the advantage of being a relatively noninvasive procedure. The rate of insulin independence 1 year after islet cell transplantation has improved significantly in recent years (60% at 1 year after transplantation compared to the 15% in the past years). Data from a recent international trial confirmed that islet cell transplantation potentially can be a cure for type 1 diabetes. Recent data indicate that insulin independence after islet cell transplantation is associated with an improvement in glucose metabolism and quality of life and with a reduction in hypoglycemic episodes. Islet cell transplantation is still in its initial stages, and many obstacles still need to be overcome. Once clinical islet transplantation has been established, this treatment could be offered to diabetic patients long before the onset of diabetic complications or to patients with life-threatening hypoglycemic unawareness and brittle diabetes.

complications of thyroid disease such as cardiac arrhythmias. This article reviews the epidemiology and clinical manifestations of IIT and the mechanisms causing IIT, focusing on the role of HCV.

This article briefly discusses nonalcoholic fatty liver disease (NAFLD) and its association with the metabolic syndrome, its pathogenesis and natural history. It then presents a detailed discussion on the efficacy and safety of different insulin sensitizers in patients who have NASH.

FORTHCOMING ISSUES

RECENT ISSUES

Endocrinol Metab Clin N Am
36 (2007) xiii–xvi

ENDOCRINOLOGY
AND METABOLISM
CLINICS
OF NORTH AMERICA

Foreword

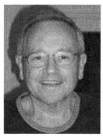

Derek LeRoith, MD, PhD
Consulting Editor

The issue opens with a discussion on the development of diabetes after solid organ transplant by Drs. P-T and P-C Pham, Lipshutz, and Wilkinson. This form of diabetes is now called "new onset diabetes after transplantation" (NODAT). Obviously, individuals who are prone to diabetes are at higher risk. However, the appearance of NODAT is precipitated by the use of certain agents commonly used as immunosuppressants. Corticosteroids and calcineurin inhibitors such as cyclosporine and tacrolimus are culprits, with tacrolimus causing more diabetes compared with cyclosporine, especially in hepatitis C virus–positive patients. Although corticosteroids worsen insulin resistance, all three agents may affect beta cell function. Cytomegalovirus-positive patients are also prone to diabetes, possibly due to the release of inflammatory cytokines that could affect beta cell function. The development of diabetes also adversely affects the long-term results of solid organ transplantation; early and effective therapy is highly recommended. Certain oral agents, such as the meglitinides, are metabolized by cytochrome p450 enzymes that may be affected by the immunosuppressant agents. Otherwise, the treatment of NODAT is routine use of all agents available. Probably the most critical suggestion made by the authors is pretransplantation work-up for prediabetes to anticipate NODAT.

Drs. Subramanian and Trence discuss the effects of immunosuppressant agents on glucose and lipid metabolism in more detail. Glucocorticoids have numerous effects on glucose metabolism, including increased gluconeogenesis, glycogenolysis, and effects on beta cell function. Interestingly, the appearance of diabetes is also associated with patients demonstrating

0889-8529/07/$ - see front matter © 2007 Elsevier Inc. All rights reserved.
doi:10.1016/j.ecl.2007.08.002

endo.theclinics.com

histocompatible leukocyte antigens (HLA) types A30, B27, and Bw42. Hyperlipidemia is also found with corticosteroid use, due to multiple effects on fat metabolism pathways. When tapering off the steroids, morning cortisol and adenocorticotropic hormone stimulation tests can aid in determining adrenal reserve. In contrast to corticosteroids, cyclcosporine has a greater effect on beta cell function. Simlar to steroids, cyclosporine causes hyperlipidemia. Although tacrolimus affects glucose metabolism more than cyclosporine, it affects lipid metabolism less. Mycophenolate mofetil, on the other hand, is extremely useful, as it has very little effect on glucose and lipid metabolism. Sirolimus or rapamycin probably has beneficial effects on beta cell function, but a major problem is the hyperlipidemia associated with its use.

A critical aspect of post-transplantation diabetes is management of the hyperglycemia. Recently, intensive insulin therapy has become widely accepted, as the standard of care for patients in the intensive care unit would include the immediate post-transplant period. Once in the step-down situation, basal-bolus with correction regimens is used, and then finally patients are followed up in the outpatient setting, at which stage they may be treated with oral agents. Philip Goldberg presents a very practical approach to all of these settings and also stresses the importance of managing the hyperlipidemia, since the combination of uncontrolled glucose and lipids will undoubtedly lead to worse cardiovascular outcomes.

The chronic effects of end stage renal disease on calcium and bone metabolism are discussed by Neveen Hamdy. The chronic renal disease causes retention of phosphate, reduced 1,25-hydrocy vitamin D synthesis, and hypocalcemia with secondary hyperparathyroidism, which, with time, results in significant bone disease. A mixed osteodystrophy is commonly seen with elements of osteoporosis, osteomalacia, and osteitis fibrosa cystica. These conditions need urgent attention and therapy to reduce the hyperparathyroidism as well as to avoid post-transplantation problems, such as hypophosphatemia secondary to the hyperparathyroidism and normal renal function. Post-transplantation hyperparathyroidism may persist for some time, but hypercalcemia is indicative of autonomous "tertiary" hyperparathyroidism and may require parathyroidectomy. Post-transplant osteoporosis is aggrevated or induced by immunosuppressant agents such as glucocorticoids and calcineurin inhibitors.

A very common disorder post-transplant is osteoporosis. As discussed by Drs. Shane, Ebeling, and Stein, alterations in bone morphology probably begins even pre-transplant because of the chronic disorder that has led to the transplantation. For example, end-stage renal disease is associated with osteodystrophy, end-stage liver disease patients have low testosteroneand 1,25 vitamin D levels, and patients awaiting lung and bone marrow transplantation have similar problems. Post-transplantation use of corticosteroids and cyclosporine, for example, worsens the bone disorder through multiple mechanisms. The most important therapy is prevention (ie, pre-transplantation evaluation and vigilance) in the early post-transplantation period when the greatest amount of bone loss occurs. The various agents available for treating osteoporosis should be considered in these patients.

Cardiac transplant patients may develop an allograft vasculopathy. Current opinion, as discussed by Drs. Potena and Valantine, suggests that insulin resistance and associated factors, including inflammation, may be the primary cause. In their article, they describe the known pathophysiology of the disorder and propose that the insulin resistance that is enhanced by the immunosuppressant agents may be the major culprit and could be helped by the use of thiazolidinediones (TZDs) or metformin.

The article by Chemaitilly and Sklar discusses the endocrine-related complications following hematopoietic stem cell transplantation. Virtually every hormonal axis is affected, including growth hormone deficiency, thyroid, ACTH, gonadotropins, and bone. The exact cause of these hormonal dysfunctions is only partially known and relates to the therapy that includes whole body irradiation and chemotherapeutic agents, though causes have not been ruled out. Nevertheless, the effects on the endocrine systems require careful evaluation and therapy.

Islet cell transplantation for patients who have type 1 diabetes has been the "holy grail" for many decades. Recently, the Edmonton group made major strides in improving the process. Improvements in islet cell isolation, a more appropriate immunosuppressant regimen, and multiple transplantations in an individual patient certainly explained the recent successes. Drs. Fiorina and Secchi discuss the multinational study that demonstrated the improved outcomes of islet cell transplantation. Many patients were initially insulin-free for a number of years. Unfortunately, the percent of patients insulin-free dropped to 15% at 5 years. In addition, there were numerous side effects from the immunosuppression, and we are left with a situation where more research is needed to perfect this technique.

In their article, Lipshutz and Wilkinson present the reasoning for pancreas–kidney transplantation in patients who have type 1 diabetes and end-stage renal disease. Given the situation wherein immunosuppressant agents are needed for a kidney transplant, a simultaneous pancreas transplant, or even a kidney followed later by a pancreas, makes control of the diabetes both simpler and often as close to perfect as one can hope for. This situation could lead to a marked reduction in diabetic complications including damage to the transplanted pancreas. The authors also develop the theme that the pancreas alone in certain cases of type 1 diabetes should also be considered, although this scenario remains highly controversial and not widely accepted.

Drs. Dinavahi and Akalin present data and an argument that preemptive kidney transplantation, and even preemptive kidney/pancreas transplantation, results in improved outcomes in patients who have end-stage renal disease. Commonly, patients are treated with chronic dialysis while waiting for a transplant, and this process, as well as the ongoing disorder, often leads to severe deterioration of the patients overall condition, to the point that the patients do poorly after the transplant. They contend that early referral of the patient to a nephrologist as renal function deteriorates may allow for a preemptive transplant with a much better overall outcome.

As discussed by Drs. Tomer, Blackard, and Akeno, an important side effect of interferon use is the development of thyroid disease. Many patients with hepatitis C who are being considered for liver transplantation also undergo treatment with interferon alpha. The effects of INFα may be by way of immune modulatory effects with the appearance of thyroid antibodies or direct toxic effects to the thyroid gland. The thyroid autoimmune processes include Hashimotos thyroiditis and Graves' disease, whereas the non-immune process presents as a destructive thyroiditis. Although the development of thyroid antibodies occurs quite often in individuals treated with INFα, the incidence of thyroid disease is much lower.

Non-alcoholic fatty liver disease (NAFLD) and non-alcoholic steatohepatitis (NASH) are very common disorders, and NASH is a significant cause of liver failure, leading to transplantation. Both NAFLD and NASH are secondary to the metabolic syndrome commonly seen with obesity and type 2 diabetes, in which insulin resistance is the common pathophysiologic disorder. Although NAFLD is more benign with simple steatosis, NASH leads to fibrosis, cirrhosis, and eventually liver transplantation. Khashab and Chalasani describe the results of small trials that test the use of thiazolidinediones and metformin trials in cases of NAFLD and NASH with significant success. Although the TZDs seem more potent in this effect, metformin is not associated with weight increase and bone effects that are known to occur with TZDs.

With the increase in solid in organ transplantation, endocrine disorders have become more commonly recognized, many due to iatrogenic causes. Both the academic and practicing endocrinologist will find the articles in this issue extremely valuable. Dr. Tracy Breen has indeed excelled in bringing together this important issue.

Derek LeRoith, MD, PhD
*Division of Endocrinology
Metabolism, and Bone Diseases
Mount Sinai School of Medicine
One Gustave L. Levy Place
Box 1055
New York, NY 10029, USA*

E-mail address: derek.leroith@mssm.edu

ELSEVIER
SAUNDERS

Endocrinol Metab Clin N Am
36 (2007) xvii–xviii

ENDOCRINOLOGY
AND METABOLISM
CLINICS
OF NORTH AMERICA

Preface

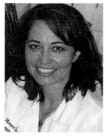

Tracy L. Breen, MD
Guest Editor

In 1954, the first successful kidney transplantation heralded a revolution in the treatment of end-stage organ failure. With the use of cyclosporine in the 1970s and the development of more advanced immunosuppressive regimens, transplantation success rates steadily improved, leading to a progressive increase in the number of organ transplants performed across the world.

Almost 30,000 solid organ transplants were performed in the United States in 2005; during that same year, there were over 150,000 individuals living with a functioning transplant. As the number of transplant procedures has grown, so has our awareness and understanding of the significant peri-transplant morbidity and long-term sequelae facing these patients. Endocrine disorders, such as insulin resistance and diabetes mellitus, metabolic bone disease, and thyroid dysfunction, are increasingly recognized as common ailments facing the transplant population.

In this issue of the *Endocrinology and Metabolism Clinics of North America*, scholars from multiple disciplines review the current knowledge of endocrine disorders that both precede and develop after organ transplantation. A major objective of this issue is to highlight common peri-transplant endocrinopathies by reviewing the effects that both transplantation and immunosuppression have upon the various endocrine systems. In addition to comprehensive discussions of the unique mechanisms of transplant-induced

doi:10.1016/j.ecl.2007.08.001   *endo.theclinics.com*

disorders, practical clinical recommendations are presented to assist the diverse team of specialists and clinicians caring for this complex and unique group of individuals.

Tracy L. Breen, MD
Division of Endocrinology, Metabolism, and Bone Diseases
Mount Sinai School of Medicine
One Gustave L. Levy Place
Box 1055
New York, NY 10029, USA

E-mail address: tracy.breen@mountsinai.org

ELSEVIER
SAUNDERS

Endocrinol Metab Clin N Am
36 (2007) 873–890

ENDOCRINOLOGY
AND METABOLISM
CLINICS
OF NORTH AMERICA

New Onset Diabetes Mellitus After Solid Organ Transplantation

Phuong-Thu T. Pham, MD[a],
Phuong-Chi T. Pham, MD[a,b],
Gerald S. Lipshutz, MD, MS, FACS[c],
Alan H. Wilkinson, MD, FRCP[a],*

[a]Kidney and Pancreas Transplantation, Department of Medicine, University of California,
Los Angeles, David Geffen School of Medicine, Peter Morton Building, 200 UCLA
Medical Plaza, Suite 365, Los Angeles, CA 90095-1693, USA
[b]Olive View-UCLA Medical Center, 14445 Olive View Drive,
Nephrology Division, 2B-182, Sylmar, CA 93142, USA
[c]Departments of Surgery and Urology, University of California, Los Angeles,
David Geffen School of Medicine, Los Angeles, CA 90095, USA

New onset diabetes mellitus after transplantation (NODAT) is a well-known complication following solid organ transplantation and has been reported to occur in 4% to 25% of renal transplant recipients, 2.5% to 25% of liver transplant recipients, and 2% to 53% of all solid organ transplants [1–3]. The variation in the reported incidence may be due in part to the lack of a universal agreement on the definition of NODAT, the duration of follow-up, and the presence of modifiable and non-modifiable risks factors. Over the last decade, hepatitis C virus (HCV) infection has increasingly been recognized as a risk factor for NODAT. In HCV-infected liver recipients, the prevalence of post-transplant diabetes ranges between 40% and 60% [3–5]. Similar to the findings in non-transplant settings, diabetes mellitus developing after transplantation has been shown to be associated with an increased risk of cardiovascular disease and infectious complications. Furthermore, reduced patient survival and accelerated graft loss have been reported [6]. This article presents an overview of the literature on the current diagnostic criteria for NODAT and discusses suggested risk factors for the development of NODAT, its potential pathogenic mechanisms, and its impact on post-transplant outcomes after solid organ transplantation.

* Corresponding author.
E-mail address: awilkinson@mednt.ucla.edu (A.H. Wilkinson).

0889-8529/07/$ - see front matter © 2007 Elsevier Inc. All rights reserved.
doi:10.1016/j.ecl.2007.07.007

Suggested guidelines for early identification and management of NODAT are also discussed.

Definition and diagnosis of new onset diabetes mellitus after transplantation

Over the years, the precise incidence of NODAT has been difficult to determine due to the lack of a standard definition of the condition. Historically, post-transplant diabetes has variably been defined as a random glucose level greater than 200 mg/dL or a fasting glucose level greater than 140 mg/dL or the need for insulin therapy in the post-transplant period. In 2003, the International Expert Panel consisting of experts from the transplant and diabetes field set forth International Consensus Guidelines for the diagnosis and management of NODAT [1,7]. It is recommended that the definition and diagnosis of NODAT should be based on the definition of diabetes mellitus and impaired glucose tolerance (IGT) as described by the World Health Organization (WHO) [7]. Diabetes mellitus is defined as a fasting plasma glucose (FPG) level of ≥ 126 mg/dL (7.0 mmol/L) or a plasma glucose level of ≥ 200 mg/dL (11.1 mmol/L) 2 hours after a 75-g oral glucose challenge (oral glucose tolerance test) confirmed by repeat testing on a different day. FPG values between 110 and 125 mg/dL (6.1–6.9 mmol/L) are defined as impaired fasting glucose (IFG), and 2-hour plasma glucose values between 140 and 199 mg/dL (7.8–11.1 mmol/L) are defined as IGT. The diabetes guidelines acknowledge that both IFG and IGT are important predictive factors for the progression to overt diabetes and are well-established risk factors for microvascular and cardiovascular disease [8]. The current WHO and American Diabetes Association (ADA) guidelines for the diagnosis of pre-diabetic states (IFG and IGT) and diabetes mellitus are provided in Box 1 [1].

Risk factors for new onset diabetes mellitus after transplantation

Although the risk factors for developing diabetes after transplantation may vary among studies, commonly reported predisposing factors include African American and Hispanic ethnicity, obesity defined as a body mass index ≥ 30 kg/m^2, age older than 40 years, a family history of diabetes among first-degree relatives, IGT before transplantation or the presence of other components of the metabolic syndrome (eg, hypertriglyceridemia, low high-density lipoprotein [HDL] defined as HDL <40 g/dL in men and <50 g/dL in women, hypertension, and hyperuricemia), recipients of deceased donor kidneys, HCV infection, and immunosuppressive therapy including corticosteroids and the calcineurin inhibitors tacrolimus and, to a lesser extent, cyclosporine [9]. The antimetabolites azathioprine and mycophenolate mofetil have not been shown to be diabetogenic. In fact, the concomitant use of mycophenolate mofetil has been suggested to

---

Box 1. World Health Organization and American Diabetes Association criteria for the diagnosis of diabetes mellitus

Criteria for the diagnosis of diabetes mellitus[a]
Symptoms[b] of diabetes mellitus plus casual[c] plasma glucose
    concentrations ≥200 mg/dL (11.1 mM)
    or
FPG ≥126 mg/dL (7.0 mM), where fasting is defined as no caloric
    intake for at least 8 hours
    or
2-hour plasma glucose ≥200 mg/dL (11.1 mM) during an oral
    glucose tolerance test[d]

Criteria for normal FPG and IFG or IGT
FPG
    FPG <110 mg/dL (6.1 mM) = normal fasting glucose
    FPG ≥110 mg/dL (6.1 mM) and <126 mg/dL (7.0 mM) = IFG
    or
Oral glucose tolerance test
    2-hour plasma glucose <140 mg/dL (7.8 mM) = normal
        glucose tolerance
    2-hour plasma glucose ≥140 mg/dL (7.8 mM) and <200 mg/dL
        (11.1 nM) = IGT

---

[a] A confirmatory laboratory test based on measurements of venous plasma glucose must be done on another day in the absence of unequivocal hyperglycemia accompanied by acute metabolic decompensation.
[b] Classic symptoms of diabetes include polyuria, polydipsia, and unexplained weight loss.
[c] Casual is defined as any time of day without regard to time since last meal.
[d] The oral glucose tolerance test should be performed as described by the WHO using a glucose load containing an equivalent of 75 g of anhydrous glucose dissolved in water.
Adapted from Davidson J, Wilkinson AH, Dantal J, et al. New-onset diabetes after transplantation: 2003 international consensus guidelines. Transplantation 2003;7:SS3–24; with permission.

---

mitigate the diabetogenic effect of tacrolimus [6]. It is conceivable that the use of azathioprine or mycophenolate mofetil will allow clinicians to use lower doses of other diabetogenic immunosuppressive medications.

Although early clinical trials suggested that sirolimus was devoid of diabetogenic effect, subsequent studies in animal models and in recipients of renal transplants suggest that sirolimus is associated with reduced insulin sensitivity and a defect in the compensatory β-cell response [10,11]. Studies in diabetic mice transplanted with islet cells suggest that sirolimus is associated with reduced islet engraftment and impaired β-cell function in transplants. In one single-center study, cyclosporine and sirolimus combination therapy was associated with a higher incidence of NODAT when compared with cyclosporine immunosuppression alone [12].

Other potential risk factors for the development of NODAT include the presence of certain HLA antigens such as A30, B27, and B42, increasing HLA mismatches, acute rejection history, cytomegalovirus (CMV) infection, male gender as recipient, and male gender as donor [9]. More recently, polycystic kidney disease has also been suggested to confer an increased risk for diabetes after renal transplantation [13–15]. Suggested risk factors for NODAT are summarized in Fig. 1.

The following sections provide an overview of the literature on post-transplant diabetes mellitus associated with immunosuppressive agents (corticosteroids, cyclosporine, and tacrolimus) and HCV and CMV infection. Suggested potential pathogenic mechanisms associated with individual risk factors are also discussed.

Corticosteroid-associated new onset diabetes

Starlz first described the now well-established contributory role of corticosteroids in NODAT in 1964 in renal transplant recipients [16]. The diabetogenic effect of corticosteroids has been suggested to be dose dependent. In a prospective study of 173 consecutive kidney transplant recipients, overt NODAT and glucose intolerance as assessed by an oral glucose tolerance test developed in 18% and 31%, respectively, at 10 weeks after transplantation. A significant relationship between the prednisolone dose and glucose

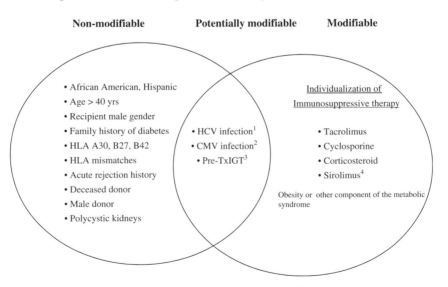

Fig. 1. Risk factors for NODAT. Pre-Tx; pre-transplant, [1]Consider pre-transplant treatment of HCV (see text). [2]Aggressive post-transplant CMV prophylaxis. [3]Counseling on lifestyle modifications (see text). [4]Further studies are needed.

intolerance was demonstrated by univariate and multivariate linear regression analyses. A 0.01 mg/kg/d increase in prednisolone dose was associated with a 5% risk of developing NODAT [17]. Hjelmesaeth and colleagues [18] first demonstrated that a dose reduction in oral prednisolone to 5 mg daily significantly improved glucose tolerance during the first year after transplantation. Multiple linear regression analysis revealed that each 1-mg reduction of the prednisolone dose led to an estimated decline in 2-hour blood glucose of 0.12 mmol/L. In a small study involving 57 stable renal transplant recipients, Midtvedt and colleagues [19] found that a prednisolone dose reduction from a mean of 16 mg daily (range, 10 to 30 mg) to 9 mg (range, 5 to 12.5 mg) resulted in an average increase in the insulin sensitivity index of 24%. Complete withdrawal of 5 mg/d of prednisolone did not influence insulin sensitivity significantly. Whether complete withdrawal of chronic low-dose corticosteroid therapy (prednisolone, 5 mg daily) improves glucose metabolism remains to be studied. The dose-dependent diabetogenic effect of corticosteroid was also observed in recipients of nonrenal organ transplants. In a retrospective review involving 88 heart transplant recipients, Depczynski and colleagues [20] found that patients in whom NODAT developed received higher mean doses of prednisolone at 3 months when compared with those who remained free of diabetes at a mean follow-up of 27 months (0.21 +/− 0.03 mg/kg/d versus 0.19 +/− 0.03 mg/kg/d, $P<.01$).

Experimental animal models have shown that corticosteroids affect glucose metabolism by increasing hepatic glucose production and reducing peripheral insulin sensitivity [21]. Both insulin resistance and relative insulin deficiency have been suggested to have a role in the development of steroid-induced NODAT. Steroid sparing or steroid withdrawal protocols in the early post-transplant period have been shown to reduce insulin resistance and improve glucose metabolism in renal transplant recipients [22]. The precise mechanisms of steroid-induced insulin resistance are not well understood and may be multifactorial. Decreased insulin receptor number and affinity, impaired glucose uptake in skeletal muscles, impaired suppression of endogeneous insulin production, activation of the glucose-free fatty acid cycle, and reduced glycogen synthesis have all been implicated [16,23].

Calcineurin inhibitor–associated new onset diabetes: cyclosporine versus tacrolimus

Although clinical trials comparing the incidence of NODAT in patients treated with cyclosporine versus tacrolimus have yielded mixed results, tacrolimus has more consistently been shown to have a greater diabetogenic effect. Data obtained from the United States Renal Data System revealed that by 2 years post transplant, the incidence of NODAT was approximately 70% greater among patients treated with tacrolimus versus cyclosporine (30% versus 18%, respectively) [24]. The incremental increase in the incidence of

NODAT at 1 year was 15.4% for tacrolimus-treated patients and 9.4% for cyclosporine-treated patients. The corresponding incremental increases in the incidence of NODAT at 2 years were 17.7% and 8.4%, respectively.

The incidence of NODAT after liver transplantation has also been found to be higher in tacrolimus-treated versus cyclosporine-treated patients at 1 year post transplant. In a large randomized trial involving more than 500 liver transplant recipients, NODAT occurred in 26.6% versus 16.1% of patients receiving tacrolimus and cyclosporine immunosuppressive therapy, respectively [25].

Currently, there are limited data on the incidence of NODAT after heart transplants. In small single-center studies, a trend toward a higher incidence of NODAT has been observed in recipients of heart transplants receiving tacrolimus versus cyclosporine-based immunosuppression [26]. In a study involving 85 heart transplant patients, NODAT was observed in 14% and 12% of tacrolimus- and cyclosporine-treated patients, respectively [26]. In a meta-analysis to evaluate the reported incidence of NODAT after solid organ transplantation, Heisel and colleagues [27] found a higher incidence of insulin-dependent diabetes mellitus (IDDM) in tacrolimus versus cyclosporine-treated patients across renal and nonrenal transplant groups including liver, heart, and lung transplants. In renal transplant recipients, IDDM occurred in 9.8% of tacrolimus versus 2.7% of cyclosporine-treated patients ($P<.00001$). Similar trends were observed among recipients of nonrenal organ transplants (11.1% versus 6.2%, respectively [$P<.003$]).

Nonetheless, not all studies show that tacrolimus is more diabetogenic than cyclosporine [28]. It has been suggested that the inconsistent results obtained among studies are due, in part, to the difference in the definitions of NODAT and the difference in calcineurin inhibitor dose and drug levels [28,29]. In a single-center study consisting of 139 patients without known pre-transplant glucose abnormalities, Maes and colleagues [29] showed that a high tacrolimus trough level, particularly a level of greater than 15 ng/mL in the first month after transplant, was a significant risk factor for persistent IFG or diabetes mellitus beyond the first year after transplantation. In a single-center study consisting of 45 orthotopic liver transplant recipients treated with either cyclosporine (n = 9) or high- (n = 15) versus low-dose tacrolimus (n = 13), the incidence of NODAT was 11%, 40%, and 23%, respectively [30]. Of interest, a potential interaction between HCV status and the use of tacrolimus immunosuppression has been suggested. In a retrospective study of more than 400 kidney transplant recipients with no known pre-transplant diabetes, Bloom and colleagues [31] showed that among the HCV-positive cohort, NODAT occurred more often in the tacrolimus versus the cyclosporine-treated groups (57.8% versus 7.7%, $P<.0001$). In contrast, among the HCV-negative cohort, the rate of NODAT was similar between the two calcineurin inhibitor groups (10% for tacrolimus versus 9.4% for cyclosporine, respectively, $P = .521$).

Impaired insulin secretion has been suggested to contribute to the development of calcineurin inhibitor–associated NODAT [21]. Experimental studies have shown that calcineurin inhibitors impair the function of cultured β cells by impairing insulin gene expression [21,32]. In recipients of pancreas transplants, the calcineurin inhibitors cyclosporine and tacrolimus have been shown to cause reversible toxicity to islet cells. In a study of 26 pancreas allograft biopsies from 20 simultaneous kidney-pancreas transplant recipients, a significant correlation was seen between the presence of islet cell damage and serum levels of tacrolimus and cyclosporine, as well as with the tacrolimus peak level [33]. Cytoplasmic swelling and vacuolization and a marked decrease or absence of dense core secretory granules in β cells were demonstrated on electron microscopy. The islet cell damage was more frequent and severe in the tacrolimus group (10 of 13) when compared with the cyclosporine group (5 of 13). Serial biopsies from two patients with hyperglycemia and evidence of islet cell damage receiving tacrolimus immunosuppression demonstrated reversibility of the damage on discontinuation of tacrolimus.

Hepatitis C virus–associated new onset diabetes

The association between HCV infection and IFG or the development of frank type 2 diabetes mellitus in the non-transplant population has long been suggested. Potential mechanisms of the diabetogenic effect of HCV infection include insulin resistance, decreased hepatic glucose uptake and glycogenesis, and a direct cytopathic effect of the virus on pancreatic β cells [34]. Over the last decade, the link between HCV and the development of NODAT has also been increasingly recognized in solid organ transplant recipients. Nevertheless, the pathogenesis of HCV-associated NODAT remains poorly understood. Clinical studies in recipients of orthotopic liver transplants have implicated insulin resistance associated with active HCV infection as a predominant pathogenic mechanism. Independent investigators have shown a temporal relationship between recurrent allograft hepatitis and increasing viral loads and the development of NODAT [3,35]. Furthermore, patients who responded to antiviral therapy were observed to have improvement in glycemic control [3,35,36]. In a small cohort of 17 non-diabetic HCV-positive and 33 non-diabetic HCV-negative orthotopic liver transplant recipients, Baid and colleagues [3] showed that the presence of HCV infection was independently associated with a 62% increase in insulin resistance ($P = .0005$). It was suggested that the virus had a direct effect on insulin resistance, because no difference in β-cell function or hepatic insulin extraction between the HCV-positive and HCV-negative groups was observed.

In a small study consisting of 16 renal transplant candidates with a sustained virologic response to interferon treatment given in the pre-transplant period, none developed NODAT at a mean follow-up of 22.5 months (range, 2 to 88 months) [37]. It is conceivable that successful pre-transplant treatment of hepatitis C could potentially reduce the incidence of NODAT after kidney transplantation.

Cytomegalovirus-associated new onset diabetes

The link between CMV infection and the development of NODAT was first reported in 1985 in a renal transplant recipient [38]. Limited studies suggest that both asymptomatic CMV infection and CMV disease are independent risk factors for the development of NODAT [39]. In a study consisting of 160 consecutive non-diabetic renal transplant recipients who were prospectively monitored for CMV infection during the first 3 months after transplantation, Hjelmesaeth and colleagues [39] found that asymptomatic CMV infection was associated with a fourfold increased risk of new onset diabetes (adjusted relative risk, 4.00; $P = .025$). Patients with active CMV infection had a significantly lower median insulin release when compared with their CMV-negative counterparts, suggesting that impaired pancreatic β-cell insulin release may be involved in the pathogenic mechanism of CMV-associated NODAT. It is speculated that CMV-induced release of proinflammatory cytokines may lead to apoptosis and functional disturbances of pancreatic β cells [40].

Impact of new onset diabetes mellitus after transplantation on patient and allograft outcomes

Clinical studies evaluating the impact of NODAT on patient and allograft outcomes after solid organ transplantation have yielded variable results. Nonetheless, ample literature suggests that kidney transplant recipients in whom NODAT develops are at a two- to three-fold increased risk of fatal and nonfatal cardiovascular disease events when compared with non-diabetic patients [41,42]. In one single-center study, the 8-year (range, 7–9 years) cumulative incidence of major cardiac events defined as cardiac death or nonfatal acute myocardial infarction was 7% in recipients without diabetes (n = 138) versus 20% in those with NODAT (n = 35) [42]. The development of NODAT has also been shown to be associated with an adverse impact on patient survival and an increased risk of graft rejection and graft loss, as well as an increased incidence of infectious complications. In a study consisting of 173 renal transplant recipients, the 1-year patient survival rates for those with versus without NODAT were 83% and 98%, respectively ($P<.01$) [43]. In a single-center study consisting of 40 renal transplant recipients with NODAT and 30 non-diabetic control patients, the 12-year graft survival rate in diabetic and nondiabetic patients was 48% and 70%, respectively ($P = .04$) [44]. Data from the United Renal Data System consisting of over 11,000 Medicare beneficiaries who received primary kidney transplants between 1996 and 2000 demonstrated that in a comparison of patients with "no diabetes," NODAT was associated with a 63% increased risk of graft failure ($P<.0001$), a 46% increased risk of death-censored graft failure ($P<.0001$), and an 87% increased risk of mortality ($P<.0001$) [6].

Similar to the setting of renal transplantation, the development of NODAT after liver transplantation has been reported to be associated with increased morbidity and mortality. Baid and colleagues [3] showed that the development of NODAT after liver transplantation was an independent risk factor for mortality (hazard ratio, 3.67; $P<.0001$). In a subset of HCV-positive patients, the cumulative mortality in those with NODAT was significantly higher than in those without NODAT (56% in HCV-positive, NODAT-positive versus 14% in HCV-positive, NODAT-negative; $P = .001$). In a retrospective study consisting of 46 orthotopic liver transplant recipients with NODAT and 92 age- and sex-matched case-control orthotopic liver transplant recipients who did not have pre- or post-transplant diabetes mellitus, John and colleagues [45] found that in a comparison with the case-control group, the development of NODAT was associated with significant cardiovascular and infectious complications. The incidences of cardiac and major and minor infections in the NODAT group compared with the case-control group were as follows: cardiac complications, 48% versus 24% ($P = .05$); major infections, 41% versus 25% ($P = .07$); and minor infections, 28% versus 5% ($P = .01$). In addition, acute rejection episodes were seen more commonly in the NODAT group (50% versus 30%, $P = .03$).

Currently, there is a paucity of data on the impact of NODAT on post-transplant outcomes after heart transplantation. Experimental animal models and small single-center studies suggest that NODAT may have a pivotal role in the development of cardiac allograft vasculopathy in heart transplant patients, limiting long-term survival in this population [46]. In a study of 66 heart transplant recipients without overt diabetes, hyperglycemia defined as a glucose level greater than 8.9 mmol/L 2 hours after a 75-g oral glucose challenge significantly predicted the development of coronary artery stenosis and death during the subsequent 5 years of follow-up. The probability of freedom from coronary artery disease 5 years after transplantation in patients with hyperglycemia versus those without hyperglycemia was 70 ± 10% and 91 ± 11%, respectively ($P \leq .01$). The corresponding probability of freedom from coronary artery disease death or retransplantation at 5 years was 90 ± 7% versus 100% [47]. It is conceivable that the presence of NODAT confers an increased risk of cardiovascular disease and overall morbidity and mortality across all type of solid organ transplantation.

Detection and management of diabetes mellitus in recipients of solid organ transplants

Early detection and management of cardiovascular disease risk factors in general and of diabetes mellitus in particular should be an integral part of the management of transplant recipients. The following discussion focuses on the diagnosis and management of diabetes mellitus in the pre- and post-transplant period.

Pre-transplant baseline evaluation

The 2004 updated International Consensus Guidelines on New-onset Diabetes after Transplantation suggest that a pre-transplant baseline evaluation should include a complete medical and family history, including documentation of glucose history [7]. FPG should be tested at regular intervals, and a 2-hour oral glucose tolerance test should be performed in those with normal FPG. The use of an oral glucose tolerance test is recommended for screening purposes because it is more predictive of increased cardiovascular disease risk and mortality than FPG testing, particularly in individuals with IGT. Furthermore, it has been suggested that oral glucose tolerance test diagnostic criteria may be more sensitive in identifying patients with IGT than those set for FPG [1]. Patients with evidence of IGT or an abnormal oral glucose tolerance test before transplantation should be counseled on lifestyle modifications including weight control, diet, and exercise. Pre-transplant treatment of HCV-infected renal transplant candidates should be considered. Selection of an immunosuppressive regimen should be tailored to each individual patient, weighing the risk of diabetes after transplantation against the risk of acute rejection. A suggested pre-transplant baseline evaluation of potential transplant candidates is shown in Fig. 2.

Management of established new onset diabetes mellitus after transplantation

The management of NODAT should follow the conventional approach for patients with type 2 diabetes mellitus as recommended by many clinical guidelines established by well-recognized organizations including the ADA. A global guideline for the management of type 2 diabetes mellitus is available through the International Federation Global Guideline Web site at http://www.d4pro.com/diabetesguidelines/index.htm. Further intervention may include an adjustment or modification in immunosuppressive medications and pharmacologic therapy to achieve a target hemoglobin A_{1C} level of less than 6.5%. Corticosteroid dose reduction has been shown to significantly improve glucose tolerance during the first year after transplantation [6]; however, any dose reduction should be weighed against the risk of acute rejection. A steroid sparing regimen or steroid avoidance protocol should be tailored to each individual patient. Tacrolimus to cyclosporine conversion therapy in patients who fail to achieve target glycemic control or in those with difficult to control diabetes has yielded variable results.

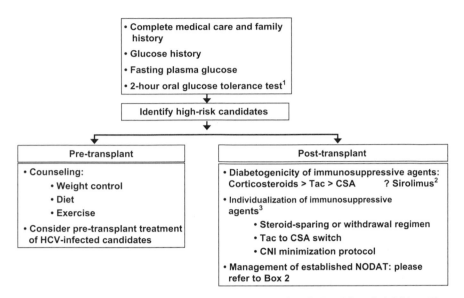

Fig. 2. Pre-transplant baseline evaluation. CSA, cyclosporine; CNI, calcineurin inhibitor; Tac, tacrolimus. [1]Please see text. [2]Further studies are needed. [3]Modification of immunosuppressive regimen should be done at the discretion of the transplant physician.

When lifestyle modification fails to achieve adequate glycemic control, medical intervention is recommended. Orally administered agents can be used alone or in combination with other oral agents or insulin. Although oral hypoglycemic agents may be effective in many patients with corticosteroid or cyclosporine or tacrolimus-induced NODAT, insulin therapy may be necessary in as many as 40% of patients [48], particularly in the early post-transplant period.

The choice of pharmacologic therapy is based on the potential advantages and disadvantages associated with the different classes of oral agents. Although metformin (a biguanide derivative) is the preferred agent for overweight patients, its use should be avoided in patients with impaired allograft function owing to the possibility of lactic acidosis. Care should also be taken when the sulfonylurea derivatives are prescribed to patients with impaired allograft function or to elderly patients due to the increased risk of hypoglycemia. In general, it is best to start with a low dose and to titrate upward every 1 to 2 weeks. The "non-sulfonylureas" meglitinides are insulin secretagogues with a mechanism of action similar to that of the sulfonylureas. Nonetheless, they have a more rapid onset and shorter duration of action and seemingly lower risks of hypoglycemia and weight gain [48,49]. These agents are best suited for patients whose food intake is erratic, for elderly patients, and for patients with impaired graft function. They are best taken before meals; the dose may be omitted if a meal is skipped.

The thiazolidinedione derivatives are insulin sensitizers that may allow for a reduction in insulin requirement. Potential adverse effects of these agents include weight gain, peripheral edema, anemia, pulmonary edema, and congestive heart failure. The incidence of peripheral edema is increased when thiazolidinedione derivatives are used in combination with insulin [49]. More recently, during the A Diabetic Outcome Progression Trial (ADOPT) conducted to compare glycemic control in patients on rosiglitazone, metformin, or glyburide, a higher incidence of fractures in the upper arm, hand, and foot was noted among female patients treated with rosiglitazone [50,51]. Subsequently, pioglitazone was also recognized to be associated with a similar increased risk of fracture in women but not in men, although further studies are needed [51]. The risk of fractures associated with use of the thiazolidinedione derivatives in the transplant setting is currently not known. Nonetheless, thiazolidinedione derivatives should be used with caution, particularly in female transplant recipients who are also receiving steroid immunosuppressive therapy.

Drug-to-drug interactions should also be carefully considered. The meglitinide derivatives repaglinide and, to a lesser extent, nateglinide are metabolized through the cytochrome P-450 isozyme CYP 3A4; therefore, glucose levels should be monitored closely when the patient also receives a strong inhibitor (eg, cyclosporine, gemfibrozil, or the azole antifungal) or inducer (eg, rifampin, carbamazepine, phenytoin, or St. John's wort) of the CYP 3A4 system [48]. The use of gemfibrozil, a CYP 3A4 inhibitor, and repaglinide combination therapy has been shown to dramatically increase the action of the latter, resulting in prolonged hypoglycemia. Coadministration of cyclosporine and repaglinide has also been shown to enhance the blood glucose lowering effect of repaglinide and increase the risk of hypoglycemia [52]. In contrast, rifampin, a strong inducer of CYP 3A4, considerably decreases the plasma concentration of repaglinide and also reduces its effects [53]. Although tacrolimus is also metabolized via the CYP 3A4 system and should be susceptible to many drug interactions similar to those of cyclosporine, these interactions are not as well documented.

Monitoring of patients with post-transplant diabetes mellitus should include measuring the hemoglobin A_{1C} level every 3 months and screening for diabetic complications, including tests for microalbuminuria, regular ophthalmologic examinations, and regular foot care. The hemoglobin A_{1C} level cannot be accurately interpreted within the first 3 months post transplantation due to various factors, including a history of blood transfusion in the early post-transplant period and the presence of anemia or impaired allograft function. The former may render the test invalid until new hemoglobin is formed and the latter (anemia and kidney impairment) can directly interfere with the A_{1C} assay. More recently, an artifactual reduction in the A_{1C} level has been reported in islet cell transplant recipients taking dapsone for *Pneumocystis carinii* (*P jiroveci*) prophylaxis. The cause is not yet known, but a reduction in red blood cell lifespan with or without hemolysis has been implicated [54].

Box 2. Management of new onset diabetes mellitus after transplantation

Dietary modification
Dietitian referral
For diabetic dyslipidemia: a diet low in saturated fats
  and cholesterol and high in complex carbohydrates and fiber
  is recommended

Lifestyle modifications
Exercise
Weight reduction or avoidance of excessive weight gain
Smoking cessation

Adjustment or modification in immunosuppressive medications[a]
Rapid steroid taper, steroid sparing or steroid avoidance
  protocols
Tacrolimus to cyclosporine conversion therapy

Pharmacologic therapy
Acute marked hyperglycemia (may require inpatient
  management): intensive insulin therapy (consider insulin drip
  when glucose $\geq$400 mg/dL)
Chronic hyperglycemia (treat to target HbA_{1C} < 6.5%): oral
  glucose lowering agent monotherapy or combination therapy[b]
  with or without insulin therapy; consider diabetologist referral
  if HbA_{1C} remains $\geq$9.0%

Monitoring of patients with NODAT
Hemoglobin A_{1C} every 3 months
Screening for microalbuminuria
Regular ophthalmologic examination
Regular foot care
Annual fasting lipid profile
Aggressive treatment of dyslipidemia and
  hypertension

---

[a] Clinicians must be familiar with the patient's immune history before manipulating their immunosuppressive therapy (see text).
[b] The choice of a particular agent should be based on the characteristics of each individual patient (see text).
Adapted from Pham PT, Pham PC, Danovitch GM. Cardiovascular disease posttransplant. Seminars Nephrol 2007;27(4):430–44; with permission.

The fasting lipid profile should be measured annually. In transplant recipients with multiple risk factors for cardiovascular disease, more frequent monitoring of the lipid profile should be performed at the discretion of the clinician. Statins or the HMG-CoA reductase inhibitors are the most widely used lipid lowering agents in the non-transplant and transplant settings. Box 2 summarizes the suggested guidelines for the management of NODAT [55]. Suggested guidelines for pharmacologic treatment of post-transplant dyslipidemia are summarized in Fig. 3 [55].

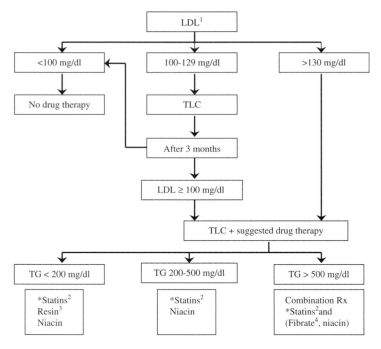

*If LDL targets not achieved with statin monotherapy consider
statins + cholesterol absorption inhibitors[5] combination

Fig. 3. Suggested guidelines for the treatment of post-transplant dyslipidemia. All transplant recipients should be regarded as corornay heart disease. risk equivalent. Goals: low-density lipoprotein (LDL) <100 mg/dL (optional <70 mg/dL), triglyceride (TG) <200 mg/dL, HDL >45 mg/dL. TLC, therapeutic lifestyle change. [1]LDL <70 mg/dL has been suggested for very high-risk patients (NCEP, ATP III guidelines). [2]Statins are the most effective drugs and should be the agents of first choice. Start at low dose in patients on cyclosporine and tacrolimus. Monitor for myositis and transaminitis, particularly in those receiving combination therapy. [3]Bile acid sequestrans should probably not be taken at the same time as cyclosporine. [4]Extreme caution should be used with statin and fibrate combination therapy. [5]Consider cholesterol absorption inhibitors in patients intolerant to statins. (*Adapted from* Pham PT, Danovitch GM, Pham PC. The medical management of the renal transplant recipient. In: Johnson RJ, Feehally J, editors. Comprehensive clincial nephrology. 3rd edition. Philadelphia: Mosby; 2007. p. 1848–53; with permission.)

Summary

NODAT is a serious complication that can adversely impact patient and allograft outcomes. Identification of the high-risk patient and implementation of measures to reduce the incidence of IGT or overt diabetes should be an integral part of the pre- as well as post-transplant management of transplant recipients. The pre-transplant screening process should include obtaining an FPG at regular intervals, and a 2-hour oral glucose tolerance test should be performed in those with normal FPG. Emphasis should be placed on dietary modification, regular aerobic exercise, weight reduction, and tobacco avoidance. Selection of an immunosuppressive regimen should be individualized, and the risk of developing diabetes after transplantation should be weighed against the risk of rejection. In patients with established NODAT, management should include lifestyle changes and pharmacologic therapy to achieve a target hemoglobin A_{1C} level of less than 6.5%. Adjustment or modification in immunosuppressive medications should be performed at the discretion of the transplant physician. Similar to the non-transplant setting, the management of diabetes mellitus after transplantation requires a multidisciplinary approach in which every potential complicating factor must be closely monitored and treated.

References

[1] Davidson J, Wilkinson AH, Dantal J, et al. New-onset diabetes after transplantation: 2003 International Consensus Guidelines. Transplantation 2003;7:SS3–24.

[2] Montori VM, Velosa JA, Basu, et al. Post-transplantation diabetes: a systematic review of the literature. Diabetes Care 2002;25:583–92.

[3] Baid S, Cosimi AB, Farrell ML, et al. Post-transplant diabetes mellitus in liver transplant recipients: risk factors, temporal relationship with hepatitis C virus allograft hepatitis, and impact on mortality. Transplantation 2001;72:1066–72.

[4] Knobler H, Stagnaro-Green A, Wallenstein S, et al. Higher incidence of diabetes in liver transplant recipients with hepatitis C. J Clin Gastroenterol 1998;26:30–3.

[5] Bigam D, Pennington J, Carpentier A, et al. Hepatitis-C related cirrhosis: a predictor of diabetes after orthotopic liver transplantation. Gastroenterology 2000;32:87–90.

[6] Kasiske BL, Snyder JJ, Gilbertson D, et al. Diabetes mellitus after kidney transplantation in the United States. Am J Transplant 2003;3(2):178–85.

[7] Wilkinson AH, Davidson J, Dotta F, et al. Guidelines for the treatment and management of new-onset diabetes after transplantation. Clin Transplant 2005;19:291–8.

[8] The Expert Committee on the Diagnosis and Classification of Diabetes Mellitus. Report of the Expert Committee on the Diagnosis and Classification of Diabetes Mellitus. Diabetes Care 2002;25:S5.

[9] Pham PT, Danovitch GM, Pham PC. The medical management of the renal transplant recipient. In: Johnson RJ, Feehally J, editors. Comprehensive clinical nephrology. 3rd edition. Philadelphia: Mosby; 2007. p. 1085–101.

[10] Teutonico A, Schena PF, Di Paolo S. Glucose metabolism in renal transplant recipients: effect of calcineurin inhibitor withdrawal and conversion to sirolimus. J Am Soc Nephrol 2005;16:3128–35.

[11] Zhang N, Su D, Qu S, et al. Sirolimus is associated with reduced islet engraftment and impaired beta-cell function in transplants. Diabetes 2006;55:2429–36.

[12] Romagnoli J, Citterio F, Nanni E, et al. Incidence of posttransplant diabetes mellitus in kidney transplant recipients immunosuppressed with sirolimus in combination with cyclosporine. Transplant Proc 2006;38:1034–6.

[13] Hamer RA, Chow CL, Ong ACM, et al. Polycystic kidney disease is a risk factor for new-onset diabetes after transplantation. Transplantation 2007;83(1):36–40.

[14] Ducloux D, Motte G, Vautrin P, et al. Polycystic kidney disease as a risk factor for post transplant diabetes mellitus. Nephrol Dial Transplant 1999;14:244–6.

[15] de Mattos AM, Olyaei AJ, Prather JC, et al. Autosomal dominant polycystic kidney disease as a risk factor for post-transplant diabetes mellitus following renal transplantation. Kidney Int 2005;67:714–20.

[16] Jindal RM, Revanur VK, Jardine AG. Immunosuppression and diabetogenicity. In: Hakim N, Stratta R, Gray D, editors. Pancreas and islet transplantation. 1st edition. New York: Oxford University Press; 2002. p. 247–75.

[17] Hjelmesaeth J, Hartmann A, Kofstad J, et al. Tapering off prednisolone and cyclosporine the first year after renal transplantation: the effect on glucose tolerance. Nephrol Dial Transplant 2001;16:829–35.

[18] Hjelmesaeth J, Hartmann A, Kofstad J, et al. Glucose intolerance after renal transplantation depends upon prednisolone dose and recipient age. Transplantation 1997;64(7): 979–83.

[19] Midtvedt K, Hjemesaeth J, Hartmann A, et al. Insulin resistance after renal transplantation: the effect of steroid dose reduction and withdrawal. J Am Soc Nephrol 2004;15(12): 3233–9.

[20] Depcynski B, Daly B, Campbell LV, et al. Predicting occurrence of diabetes mellitus in recipients of heart transplants. Diabet Med 2000;17:15–9.

[21] Crutchlow MF, Bloom RD. Transplant-associated hyperglycemia: a new look at an old problem. Clin J Am Soc Nephrol 2007;2:343–55.

[22] Van Hooff JP, Christiaans MHL, van Duijhoven EM. Evaluating mechanisms of post-transplant diabetes mellitus. Nephrol Dial Transplant 2004;19(Suppl 6):vi8–12.

[23] Venkatesan N, Davidson MB, Huchinson A. Possible role of the glucose-fatty acid cycle in dexamethasone-induced insulin antagonism in rats. Metabolism 1987;36:883–91.

[24] Woodward RS, Schnitzler MA, Baty J, et al. Incidence and cost of new onset diabetes mellitus among US wait-listed and transplanted renal allograft recipients. Am J Transplant 2003;3(5):590–8.

[25] European FK 506 Multicentre Study Group. Randomised trial comparing tacrolimus to cyclosporine in prevention of liver allograft rejection. Lancet 1994;344:423–8.

[26] Taylor DO, Barr ML, Radovancevic B, et al. A randomized, multicenter comparison of tacrolimus and cyclosporine immunosuppressive regimens in cardiac transplantation: decreased hyperlipidemia and hypertension with tacrolimus. J Heart Lung Transplant 1999;18:336–45.

[27] Heisel O, Heisel R, Balshaw R, et al. New onset diabetes mellitus in patients receiving calcineurin inhibitors: a systematic review and meta-analysis. Am J Transplant 2004;4(4): 583–95.

[28] Meiser BM, Uberfuhr P, Fuchs A, et al. Single-center randomized trial comparing tacrolimus (FK506) and cyclosporine in the prevention of acute myocardial rejection. J Heart Lung Transplant 1998;17:782–8.

[29] Maes BD, Kuypers D, Messiaen T, et al. Post-transplant diabetes mellitus in FK-506–treated renal transplant recipients: analysis of incidence and risk factors. Transplantation 2001; 72(10):1655–61.

[30] Cai TH, Esterl RM, Nichols F, et al. Improved immunosuppression with combination tacrolimus (FK506) and mycophenolic acid in orthotopic liver transplantation. Transplant Proc 1998;30:1413–4.

[31] Bloom RD, Rao V, Weng F, et al. Association of hepatitis C with post-transplant diabetes in renal transplant patients on tacrolimus. J Am Soc Nephrol 2002;13:1374–80.

[32] Redmon JB, Olson LK, Armstrong MB, et al. Effects of tacrolimus (FK506) on human insulin gene expression, insulin mRNA levels, and insulin secretion in HIT-T15 cells. J Clin Invest 1996;98:2786–93.

[33] Drachenberg CB, Klassen DK, Weir MR, et al. Islet cell damage associated with tacrolimus and cyclosporine: morphological features in pancreas allograft biopsies and clinical correlation. Transplantation 1999;68(3):396–402.

[34] Bloom RD, Lake JR. Emerging issues in hepatitis C virus-positive liver and kidney transplant recipients. Am J Transplant 2006;6:2232–7.

[35] Delgado-Borrego A, Casson D, Schoenfeld D, et al. Hepatitis C virus is independently associated with increased insulin resistance after liver transplantation. Transplantation 2004;77: 703–10.

[36] Simo R, Lecube A, Genesca J, et al. Sustained virological response correlates with reduction in the incidence of glucose abnormalities in patients with chronic hepatitis C virus infection. Diabetes Care 2006;29:2462–6.

[37] Kamar N, Toupance O, Buchler M, et al. Evidence that clearance of hepatitis C virus RNA after α-interferon therapy in dialysis patients is sustained after renal transplantation. J Am Soc Nephrol 2003;14:2092–8.

[38] Lehr H, Jao S, Waltzer WC, et al. Cytomegalovirus-induced diabetes mellitus in a renal transplant recipient. Transplant Proc 1985;17:2152–4.

[39] Hjelmesaeth J, Sagedal S, Hartmannn A, et al. Asymptomatic cytomegalovirus infection is associated with increased risk for new-onset diabetes and impaired insulin release after renal transplantation. Diabetologia 2004;47(9):1550–6.

[40] Hjelmesaeth J, Muller F, Jenssen T, et al. Is there a link between cytomegalovirus infection and new-onset post-transplant diabetes mellitus? Potential mechanisms of virus induced β-cell damage. Nephrol Dial Transplant 2005;20:2311–5.

[41] Ojo AO. Cardiovascular complications after renal transplantation and their prevention. Transplantation 2006;82:603–11.

[42] Hjelmesaeth J, Hartmann A, Leivestad T, et al. The impact of early-diagnosed new-onset post-transplantation diabetes mellitus on survival and major cardiac events. Kidney Int 2006;69(3):588–95.

[43] Boudreaux JP, McHugh L, Canafax DM, et al. The impact of cyclosporine and combination immunosuppression on the incidence of post transplant diabetes in renal allograft recipients. Transplantation 1987;44(3):376–87.

[44] Miles AM, Sumrani N, Horowitz R, et al. Diabetes mellitus after renal transplantation: as deleterious as non-transplant-associated diabetes? Transplantation 1998;65(3):380–4.

[45] John PR, Thuluvath PJ. Outcomes of patients with new-onset diabetes mellitus after liver transplantation compared with those without diabetes mellitus. Liver Transpl 2002;8(8): 708–13.

[46] Marchetti P. New-onset diabetes after transplantation. J Heart Lung Transplant 2004; 23(5S):S194–201.

[47] Valantine H, Rickenbaker P, Kemna M, et al. Metabolic abnormalities characteristic of dysmetabolic syndrome predict the development of transplant coronary artery disease. Circulation 2001;103:2144–52.

[48] Jindal RM, Hjelmesaeth J. Impact and management of post-transplant diabetes mellitus. Transplantation 2000;70(Suppl 11):SS58–63.

[49] Cheng AYY, Fantus IG. Oral antihyperglycemic therapy for type 2 diabetes mellitus. CMAJ 2005;172(2):213–26.

[50] Kahn SE, Haffner SM, Heise MA. Glycemic durability of rosiglitazone, metformin or glyburide monotherapy for the ADOPT study. N Engl J Med 2006;355:2427–43.

[51] Hampton T. Diabetes drugs tied to fractures in women. JAMA 2007;297:1645–7.

[52] Hatorp V, Hansen KT, Thomsen MS. Influence of drugs interacting with CYP3A4 on the pharmacokinetics, pharmacodynamics and safety of the prandial glucose regulator repaglinide. J Clin Pharmacol 2003;43(6):649–60.

[53] Niemi M, Backman JT, Neuvonen PJ, et al. Rifampin decreases the plasma concentrations and effects of repaglinide. Clin Pharmacol Ther 2000;68(5):495–500.

[54] Tartiana F, Faradji RN, Monroy K, et al. Dapsone-induced artifactual A1C reduction in islet transplant recipients. Transplantation 2007;83(6):824.

[55] Pham PT, Pham PC, Danovitch GM. Post-transplant cardiovascular disease. Seminars in Nephrol 2007;27(4):430–44.

ELSEVIER
SAUNDERS

Endocrinol Metab Clin N Am
36 (2007) 891–905

ENDOCRINOLOGY
AND METABOLISM
CLINICS
OF NORTH AMERICA

Immunosuppressive Agents: Effects on Glucose and Lipid Metabolism

Savitha Subramanian, MD[a],
Dace L. Trence, MD[a,b],*

[a]Division of Metabolism, Endocrinology and Nutrition, University of Washington,
Box 356426, 1959 NE Pacific Street, Seattle, WA 98195, USA
[b]Diabetes Care Center, University of Washington Medical Center,
4225 Roosevelt Way NE, Seattle, WA 98105, USA

Since the first successful kidney transplant in 1959, transplantation medicine has evolved into mainstream medical therapy. Such solid organ transplantation, however, would not have been possible without the development of compounds that can suppress the immune system safely. Agents commonly employed for immunosuppression include glucocorticoids, calcineurin inhibitors, such as cyclosporine and tacrolimus (FK506), and azathioprine. The recent availability of potent immunosuppressive drugs such as mycophenolate mofetil (MMF) and mammalian target of rapamycin (mTOR) inhibitors such as sirolimus (rapamycin) has allowed protocols to be designed to minimize use of calcineurin inhibitors or steroids. Despite their desired action on the immune system, however, immunosuppressive therapies are associated with adverse effects that have deleterious effects on recipient quality of life and survival. Glucocorticoids, cyclosporine, and tacrolimus have been the major offending players affecting glucose homeostasis after solid organ transplantation. Post-transplant diabetes mellitus has been documented in up to 40% of renal and liver transplant recipients [1]. Glucocorticoids, cyclosporine, and sirolimus commonly are associated with hyperlipidemia. Hyperlipidemia is associated not only with an increased risk of cardiovascular disease in renal transplant recipients, but also correlates with allograft survival [2]. Thus, dysregulated glucose and lipid metabolism are well-recognized complications of organ transplantation and immunosuppression. This article focuses on the effects

* Corresponding author. Division of Metabolism, Endocrinology and Nutrition, University of Washington, Box 356426, 1959 NE Pacific Street, Seattle, WA 98195.
E-mail address: dtrence@u.washington.edu (D.L. Trence).

0889-8529/07/$ - see front matter © 2007 Elsevier Inc. All rights reserved.
doi:10.1016/j.ecl.2007.07.003

of immunosuppressive therapies on glucose and lipid metabolism. Adrenal effects of these drugs, where known, also are discussed.

Drugs used for immunosuppression in solid organ transplantation

Glucocorticoids

Effects of glucocorticoids on glucose metabolism

The first description of hyperglycemia associated with glucocorticoid use has been attributed to Ingle in 1941 [3]. The immunosuppressive benefits of glucocorticoid therapy, however, have continued to support its use in maintenance immunosuppressive medication regimens, despite the increased risk of new-onset diabetes mellitus, hyperlipidemia, and other pleiotropic effects of exogenous glucocorticoid use. A review of over 12,000 Medicare beneficiary records of patients receiving kidney transplants between 1996 and 2000 found that glucocorticoids were used as part of the immune regimen in over 97% of individuals [4]. The incidence of post-transplant diabetes mellitus (PTDM) was 9% at 3 months, 16% at 12 months, and 24% at 36 months after transplant. Contributing factors to the development of PTDM with glucocorticoid use are increasing dose used (irrespective of adjustment for weight), older age [2], positive family history of diabetes mellitus, and ethnicity [4,5]. A protective factor is early steroid withdrawal, but this does not affect all ethnicities equally [6].

The mechanisms through which glucocorticoids can induce hyperglycemia are many. Glucocorticoids promote hepatic gluconeogenesis, degradation of proteins to free amino acids in muscle, and lipolysis [7]. In addition, they decrease peripheral insulin sensitivity and inhibit pancreatic insulin production and secretion [8,9]. Glucocorticoids decrease insulin-mediated glucose uptake by mechanisms that are not understood clearly. Although glucocorticoids are the most common cause of drug-induced diabetes mellitus [10], patients who have decreased insulin secretory reserve are much more likely to develop diabetes [11]. Less consistent associations for risk for development of PTDM are human leukocyte antigen types A30, B27, and Bw42, and transplantation using deceased donor kidneys [12].

Effects of glucocorticoids on lipid metabolism

Hyperlipidemia incidence is variable postsolid organ transplant, with overall rates for kidney transplant reported between 16% and 60%, postcardiac transplant between 60% and 80%, and postliver transplant 45%, in settings of immunosuppressive regimens that included glucocorticoid use [13]. Several studies have shown in renal transplant patients that immunosuppressive regimens excluding prednisone, using alternate day, or using lower doses of prednisone are associated with lower cholesterol levels [14–16]. In liver transplant recipients, higher glucocorticoid dose has been associated with hyperlipidemia [17], while in heart transplant recipients, those able to discontinue glucocorticoid from their immunosuppressive regimen had up to 26% lower fasting cholesterol levels than those continuing on glucocorticoid [18].

Glucocorticoids can alter activity of several key enzymes. These include increased activity of acyl coenzyme A carboxylase, fatty acid synthase and HMG CoA reductase, and decreased activity of lipoprotein lipase (LPL). Increased hepatic very low density lipoprotein (VLDL) synthesis and down-regulation of low density lipoprotein (LDL) receptor activity result in increased VLDL, cholesterol, and triglyceride levels and decreased high density lipoprotein (HDL) levels [13,19]. These effects can contribute to risk of cardiovascular disease in post-transplant recipients, and regimens minimizing glucocorticoid dose have engendered increased interest. In a randomized, double-blind study of renal transplant recipients, the effects and feasibility of lower, tapering doses versus regular continued doses of prednisone were studied [20]. All transplant recipients received MMF and cyclosporine also. At baseline, the control group, who were treated with higher prednisone doses ranging from 15 mg to 30 mg daily, had lower cholesterol levels than the intervention group, who received the lower prednisone dosing. At 6 months and 12 months, however, cholesterol and triglyceride levels were significantly higher in the control group, who received higher doses of prednisone, compared to the intervention group, who received low-dose prednisone. Unfortunately, the organ rejection rate for the lower or no prednisone group was 23%, compared with 14% for the control group, suggesting a higher rejection rate, and supported by other steroid withdrawal trials in renal transplantation [21].

Adrenal effects of glucocorticoids

Suppression of the pituitary–adrenal axis occurs rapidly with exogenous glucocorticoid therapy. Fifty milligrams of prednisone daily for 5 days has been associated with decreased responsiveness to insulin-induced hypoglycemia and corticotropin (ACTH) stimulation [22]. Shorter-acting steroids such as prednisone, cortisol, or prednisolone suppress the pituitary axis less than dexamethasone [23], although all have been used either in immunosuppressive maintenance or rescue protocols. Protocols for steroid taper typically should entail small, graduated dose decreases over increments of 1 to 2 weeks for those on long-term glucocorticoid therapy, primarily to prevent precipitating an exacerbation of the immune responses being treated by the glucocorticoid. If steroid withdrawal is considered, assessment of adrenal reserve should be considered when a dose of 5 mg of prednisone or its equivalent is reached. Sequential (monthly) basal morning cortisols have been reported as helpful in guiding rate discontinuation of glucocorticoid therapy [24]. More often, rapid ACTH testing (250 µg of synthetic ACTH given by intravenous bolus followed by a cortisol level drawn 30 to 60 minutes later should yield a cortisol value greater than 20 µg/dL) is a useful test of the pituitary–adrenal axis performed easily in an outpatient setting [25].

Calcineurin inhibitors

Calcineurin inhibitors have played a major role in immunosuppressive regimens since their introduction in 1980. Cyclosporine and tacrolimus, the two drugs under this class, are used in most transplant patients. These agents act against the T cell activator protein, calcineurin, inhibiting T cell activation and cytokine gene expression. Both drugs also inhibit the actions of prolactin, an immune activator, thereby providing a synergistic effect on immunomodulation [26]. Both agents commonly are associated with hyperglycemia and hyperlipidemia as adverse effects. The individual effects of these agents in clinical studies are difficult to interpret, because concomitant administration of steroids almost always occurs as a confounding factor. Although the two drugs in this class are believed to act similarly, cyclosporine does not cause impaired glucose metabolism to the same extent as tacrolimus. In some patients, hyperlipidemia occurs secondary to an underlying genetic predisposition and/or environmental factors [27].

Cyclosporine

Effects of cyclosporine on glucose metabolism. Cyclosporine (Sandimmune, Neoral) is associated with impaired glucose metabolism and post-transplant diabetes mellitus in 5% to 35% of renal transplant recipients. While glucocorticoids increase insulin resistance, cyclosporine appears to decrease insulin secretion.

Studies in animals receiving cyclosporine have demonstrated functional and morphological abnormalities in pancreatic islet cells. Specifically, reduction in insulin secretion, diminished β cell density, and decreased insulin synthesis have been reported. Several in vitro studies have shown that cyclosporine has a direct inhibitory effect on insulin release from human pancreatic islet cells [28]. Alterations in islet cell morphology, including cytoplasmic swelling and vacuolization, and immunohistochemical and ultrastructural loss of secretory granules have been noted in pancreatic islet transplants on biopsy [29]. A recent report suggests altered mitochondrial function of islet β cells exposed to cyclosporine [30]. Some early rat studies also have suggested worsened peripheral insulin resistance, although this has not been demonstrated in human studies.

Some investigators have reported the lack of effects of cyclosporine on glucose in the absence of concomitant administration of steroids [31]. Cyclosporine is believed to decrease metabolism of prednisolone by interfering with the cytochrome P-450 system in renal transplant recipients, thereby worsening potential for hyperglycemia [32]. Hyperglycemic clamp studies in nontransplanted hemodialysis subjects after treatment with cyclosporine have shown a decrease in insulin and C peptide secretion [33]. These subjects showed a decrease in second-phase insulin secretion but no change in first-phase secretion. No differences in insulin sensitivity or glucose clearance were shown. However, the exact mechanism by which cyclosporine causes a reduction in islet insulin secretion is understood poorly. No significant relationship between cyclosporine dosing or cyclosporine blood trough concentration and impaired insulin secretion has been documented. Robertson and colleagues [34] found no abnormalities in pancreatic β cell function as assessed by intravenous glucose tolerance testing before and during a 2-year course of cyclosporine therapy in a small group of patients who had multiple sclerosis.

Effects of cyclosporine on lipid metabolism. After glucocorticoids, cyclosporine is a common offending agent causing post-transplant hyperlipidemia. The exact mechanisms underlying cyclosporine-induced hyperlipidemia have not been elucidated completely, but they appear to be dose- and duration-related. Studies in nontransplant subjects who received cyclosporine show increases in plasma cholesterol with elevation of LDL levels [35]. It has been suggested that cyclosporine inhibits steroid 26-hydroxylase, an important mitochondrial enzyme that enables bile acid synthesis from cholesterol [19]. Inhibition of bile acid synthesis, elevated hepatic cholesterol, and down-regulation of the LDL receptor then results in hypercholesterolemia. Cyclosporine is carried by LDL particles and can bind to the LDL receptor [36]. LDL receptor blockade by cyclosporine can lead to elevated LDL levels and cause hyperlipidemia. Low cholesterol levels therefore can increase toxicity by increasing drug delivery to target tissues. Cyclosporine increases hepatic lipase activity and decreases LPL activity, resulting in impaired VLDL and LDL clearance [37]. Cyclosporine can inhibit prednisone metabolism and thereby worsen lipid abnormalities induced by glucocorticoids. Increased susceptibility of LDL to oxidation has been suggested in a study of renal transplant recipients treated with cyclosporine [38]. The pro-oxidant effect of cyclosporine could increase cardiovascular risk, and could, in part, explain accelerated atherosclerosis seen in transplant recipients. Inhibition of calcineurin by cyclosporine can increase vascular tone and systemic vascular resistance, leading to hypertension. Cyclosporine also elevates lipoprotein (a) levels in renal transplant recipients [39]. Discontinuation of cyclosporine is associated with improvement in hyperlipidemia; this effect could be related to improvement in kidney function and concomitant reduction of steroid doses.

Tacrolimus

The other important calcineurin inhibitor, tacrolimus (Prograf), is a macrolide antibiotic with more potent immunosuppressant activity than cyclosporine. It appears to have significant effects on glucose metabolism and less deleterious effects on lipids.

Effects of tacrolimus on glucose metabolism. Tacrolimus appears to cause significant alterations in blood glucose compared with cyclosporine. In vitro studies have demonstrated that tacrolimus can decrease insulin secretion from islet cells, similar to the effects of cyclosporine. In a human islet cell line, tacrolimus has been shown to decrease insulin mRNA, insulin synthesis, and insulin secretion in a dose-dependent manner [40]. In rats, vacuolation of islet cells and reduction in insulin content and secretion that reverse within 2 weeks of discontinuation of the drug have been demonstrated [41,42]. Consistent with these in vitro and animal data, similar reversible histopathologic changes, including cytoplasmic swelling and vacuolation, apoptosis and loss of secretory granules, have been noted in patients receiving simultaneous kidney–pancreas transplants on tacrolimus regimens [29].

In a cohort of 18 individuals, glucose metabolism was assessed by intravenous glucose tolerance testing before and after renal transplantation. The transplanted patients received only tacrolimus for immunosuppression, but no steroids. After receiving tacrolimus, a significant increase in plasma glucose and decrease in the insulin sensitivity index were found compared with pretransplant measurements [43]. This decrease was noted to be caused by decreased insulin secretion as opposed to worsening insulin resistance, and was worsened when the trough levels of tacrolimus were the highest. In a prospective randomized longitudinal study in renal allograft recipients, tacrolimus caused a reduction in C peptide and insulin secretion 3 weeks after transplantation [44]. At the end of the study in 3 years, however, there were no differences in any parameters of glucose metabolism studied in the groups receiving tacrolimus or cyclosporine. This suggests that there is no chronic cumulative toxicity on the pancreatic beta cell caused by tacrolimus. Similarly, no differences were found in glucose metabolism or pancreatic secretory capacity in islet transplant patients receiving tacrolimus at 3 months or 3 years compared with patients on cyclosporine [45].

A retrospective analysis suggested that conversion of renal transplant recipients from tacrolimus to cyclosporine resulted in significant lowering of blood glucose, reduction in HbA1c, reduction in insulin dosage, or reversal of diabetes without altering graft function [46]. Although some reports have shown that tacrolimus and cyclosporine induced a similar glucose intolerance and hyperinsulinemia after successful allogeneic liver transplantation, other studies show a higher incidence of hyperglycemia or diabetes in tacrolimus-treated patients. In contrast, two studies in patients who received liver transplants did not show any significant diabetogenic adverse effect or dose dependency of tacrolimus treatment [47].

Thus the effect of tacrolimus on glucose metabolism appears to be a reversible, dose-dependent cytotoxicity to the beta cell in animal models and in human clinical studies. Administration of pulse steroids potentially could worsen tacrolimus-induced hyperglycemia.

Effects of tacrolimus on lipid metabolism. Tacrolimus appears to have less adverse effects on lipids than cyclosporine, not explained by concomitant steroid administration [48,49]. In the absence of lipid-lowering therapy, tacrolimus has been associated with lower LDL cholesterol, apolipoprotein B, and triglyceride levels with no differences in HDL cholesterol [50,51]. Combination therapy with glucocorticoids results in increased cholesterol and triglyceride levels in plasma. Cross-over studies in renal and liver transplant patients have shown improvement in lipid profiles after switching to tacrolimus from cyclosporine [52,53]. A retrospective analysis of 150 pancreas–kidney transplantation recipients showed no differences in plasma cholesterol or triglyceride levels 5 years after transplant in patients receiving tacrolimus versus those who did not [54].

Azathioprine

Azathioprine (Imuran) served as a mainstay of immunosuppression along with glucocorticoids until the advent of the calcineurin inhibitors. Azathioprine inhibits purine synthesis and DNA replication. There are no data to suggest that azathioprine disrupts glucose or lipid metabolism.

Mycophenolate mofetil

Mycophenolate (MMF, Cellcept) has found an important role in immunosuppressant therapies, enabling the use of steroid-sparing or low-dose calcineurin inhibitor regimens. The immunosuppressive activity of MMF is thought to derive mainly from inhibition of de novo purine synthesis in T and B lymphocytes and therefore cell proliferation [55].

Effects of mycophenolate on glucose metabolism

In vitro studies in rat islets have shown MMF to inhibit insulin secretion, predominantly through effects on voltage-dependent calcium channels [56] and through induction of beta cell apoptosis [57]. One in vitro study in human islets showed that MMF had no deleterious effects on human islet insulin secretion or insulin gene expression [58]. No effects on glucose metabolism have been noted in clinical trials, although studies are scarce. In liver transplant recipients, addition of MMF to tacrolimus did not decrease the occurrence of glucose intolerance or post-transplant hyperglycemia compared with patients treated with tacrolimus alone [59]. Some studies have shown lower incidence of post-transplant diabetes in patients receiving MMF as part of their immunosuppression, although studies using intravenous glucose tolerance tests and glucose clamp studies are lacking.

Effects of mycophenolate on lipid metabolism

There is an association between hyperlipidemia and mycophenolate mofetil, although, once again, the data are limited. There is no direct evidence that MMF affects lipoprotein metabolism or causes hyperlipidemia. No evidence of significant differences in serum cholesterol or triglycerides have been noted in rabbits fed high-cholesterol diets without or with MMF, but evidence of reduced atherosclerosis has been noted in the latter group [60]. In renal transplant recipients, MMF did not worsen lipid profiles of patients treated with cyclosporine and glucocorticoids [61]. The product information for Cellcept (http://www.rocheusa.com/products/cellcept/pi.pdf), however, states that hypercholesterolemia was noted in 41% of cardiac transplant recipients receiving 3 g/d of MMF. Treatment with other immunosuppressive medications and other risk factors are unknown for this group of patients. An interesting aspect of this drug is that MMF is being studied in animal models as an immune modulator of inflammatory activation in atherosclerosis.

Therefore, in contrast to other available immunosuppressants, MMF appears to lack cardiovascular toxicity or diabetogenic potential, thus making it an excellent candidate for combination regimens.

Mammalian target of rapamycin inhibitors

Sirolimus

Sirolimus or rapamycin (Rapamune) is a macrolide that prevents T cell activation through inhibitory effects on the protein kinase, mTOR. mTOR plays an important role in cell growth and proliferation and has been termed a nutrient sensor regulated by insulin, glucagon, and certain amino acids. Inhibition of mTOR by sirolimus could result in various effects on intermediary metabolism.

Effects of sirolimus on glucose metabolism. The effects of sirolimus on insulin action and secretion are being debated, and data are conflicting. In skeletal muscle cells, long-term exposure to rapamycin has been shown to decrease insulin-dependent glucose uptake and glycogen synthesis and increase fatty acid oxidation [62]. Rapamycin has been shown to modulate glucose transport in 3T3-L1 adipocyte cells, preventing long-term insulin-induced increases in glucose transporter 1 (GLUT 1) protein synthesis and to decrease insulin-mediated glucose uptake and insulin signaling in adipocytes [63,64]. There are also studies showing rapamycin to decrease insulin resistance and partially improve insulin-dependent glucose transport [65].

In vitro effects of sirolimus on islet cells are also conflicting. Some studies have shown deleterious effects of rapamycin on rodent [66] and human islets [67], resulting in reduced insulin secretion and impaired beta cell function at doses higher than used in clinical settings. There is also evidence that sirolimus has no deleterious effects on human islet insulin secretion at levels used for immunosuppression in people. In vivo rodent studies have suggested that sirolimus causes insulin resistance [68]. Studies in mini-pigs treated with sirolimus demonstrated improved basal and glucose-stimulated insulin levels and decreased apoptosis [69]. Therefore, the effects of sirolimus on islets and insulin secretion seem to depend upon the cell lines or animal models used and plasma drug concentrations. In a small cohort of renal transplant recipients, sirolimus caused worsening of glucose intolerance and insulin resistance and insulin secretion even after discontinuation of tacrolimus [70].

Therefore, based on existing evidence, effects of sirolimus on glucose metabolism appear to be cell-, species- and dose-dependent. Overall, it appears to have beneficial effects on islet cells, which could explain its successful use in islet cell transplantation partially. Sirolimus potentially can worsen insulin resistance, but more studies are required, because data are conflicting.

Effects of sirolimus on lipid metabolism. Hyperlipidemia is a well-known consequence of sirolimus therapy in kidney, liver, and pancreas transplant recipients [71,72]. Hyperlipidemia is a serious adverse effect, because it may exacerbate the lipid disturbances associated with cyclosporine, glucocorticoids, and renal disease [73]. The incidence of sirolimus-associated dyslipidemia is as high as 49% in liver transplantation [74,75] and 40% in renal transplantation. In a study in guinea pigs treated with rapamycin, animals that received the drug had higher triglyceride levels, increased VLDL and small dense LDL, and higher glucose and circulating free fatty acid levels [76].

Reversible hypertriglyceridemia that improved after dose reduction or resolved 1 to 2 months after discontinuation of the drug has been noted in patients who received renal transplants in several studies [77,78] . Increased free fatty acid pool has been noted in patients who had sirolimus-related hypertriglyceridemia, possibly due to increased hormone sensitive lipase and decreased lipoprotein lipase activity secondary to elevated apolipoprotein C-III levels. Increased hepatic synthesis and delayed clearance of triglyceride-rich lipoproteins have been implicated as potential mechanisms of sirolimus-induced hypertriglyceridemia [71].

In a cohort of patients with renal allografts who were taking cyclosporine and glucocorticoids, the addition of sirolimus increased the mean fasting serum cholesterol and triglyceride levels as compared with placebo [79]. These levels were significantly higher in patients receiving higher doses, suggesting a dose relationship. These effects however, were reversible with discontinuation of sirolimus. In a retrospective analysis of 55 stable liver transplant recipients who received sirolimus along with tacrolimus and/or MMF, hypercholesterolemia was noted in 15% and hypertriglyceridemia in 10% of patients who received sirolimus. This was not significantly different from the control group of patients who received tacrolimus with MMF. No differences in LDL or HDL were noted [80]. Trotter and colleagues [81] studied a cohort of 57 liver transplant subjects and found worsened hypercholesterolemia and hypertriglyceridemia in subjects treated with the combination of cyclosporine and sirolimus as opposed to tacrolimus and sirolimus.

Overall, the benefits of sirolimus supersede its dyslipidemic effects, because it leads to use of calcineurin inhibitor-sparing regimens, and therefore a lower incidence of nephrotoxicity. It is also interesting to note that sirolimus inhibits smooth muscle cell proliferation and migration and decreases the vascular response to injury in rats. These beneficial effects have led to the development of sirolimus-coated coronary stents used for percutaneous coronary intervention, in an effort to prevent stent restenosis [82].

Everolimus

Everolimus is a semisynthetic derivative of sirolimus that acts by inhibition of mTOR. Safety and efficacy have been established in a few trials involving liver and kidney transplantation. Everolimus also is plagued by dyslipidemic adverse effects, including elevations in cholesterol and triglycerides. Early in vitro data in macrophages suggest disruption of cellular lipid homeostasis, increased cholesterol efflux, and decreased triglyceride synthesis [83]. Everolimus has shown beneficial effects in patients who receive cardiac transplant, however, by reducing allograft vasculopathy [84].

Newer agents

Polyclonal antibodies such as antithymocyte globulin and antilymphocyte globulin are used as part of induction therapy and/or acute rejection treatments. Monoclonal antibodies such as basiliximab, daclizumab, and muromonab (OKT3) are use as antirejection therapies or in treatment of steroid-resistant acute rejection. No known adverse effects on glucose or lipid metabolism are known for any of these preparations.

Summary

Immunosuppression medications contribute to the morbidity of organ transplantation. Adverse effects including dyslipidemia and glucose intolerance are extremely common after transplantation and contribute significantly to cardiovascular morbidity and mortality. Tables 1 and 2 summarize the effects of various immunosuppressants on blood glucose

Table 1
Effects of immunosuppressive drugs on glucose

Drug	Effect on glucose
Glucocorticoids	↑↑↑
Calcineurin inhibitors:	
Cyclosporine	↔ or ↑
Tacrolimus (FK506)	↑↑
Azathioprine	↔
mTOR inhibitors:	
Sirolimus	↔ or ↑
Everolimus	? ↔
Mycophenolate mofetil	↔

Abbreviations: ↑, increased; ↓, decreased; ↔, unchanged.

Table 2
Effects of immunosuppressants on lipids

Drug	Effect on lipids
Glucocorticoids	↑ TG, ↑ cholesterol, ↓ HDL
Calcineurin inhibitors:	
Cyclosporine	↑ TG, ↑ cholesterol, ↑ Apo B
Tacrolimus (FK506)	↓ cholesterol, ↓ TG, ↔ HDL
Azathioprine	↔
mTOR inhibitors:	
Sirolimus	↑ ↑ TG, ↑ cholesterol
Everolimus	↑ TG, ↑ cholesterol
Mycophenolate mofetil	? ↑ cholesterol

Abbreviations: Apo B, apolipoprotein B; HDL, high-density lipoprotein; TG, triglycerides; ↑, increased; ↓, decreased; ↔, unchanged.

and lipids. Immunosuppressive regimens should be chosen carefully to minimize these risks. Until the ideal immunosuppression regimen is developed, individualization of immunosuppression for each patient is necessary. Metabolic alterations induced by glucocorticoids should be identified and treated. Calcineurin inhibitors at lower doses, in conjunction with the newer immunosuppressive agents such as mycophenolate mofetil, appear to have less detrimental effects on glucose metabolism. Dyslipidemia itself should not be a deterrent to use of any of the agents, because therapies for effective lipid lowering are available.

References

[1] Dmitrewski J, Krentz AJ, Mayer AD, et al. Metabolic and hormonal effects of tacrolimus (FK506) or cyclosporin immunosuppression following renal transplantation. Diabetes Obes Metab 2001;3(4):287–92.
[2] Hjelmesaeth J, Hartmann A, Kofstad J, et al. Glucose intolerance after renal transplantation depends upon prednisolone dose and recipient age. Transplantation 1997;64(7):979–83.
[3] Ingle D. The production of glycosuria in the normal rat by means of 17-hydroxy-11-dehydrocorticosterone. Endocrinology 1941;29:649–52.
[4] Kasiske BL, Snyder JJ, Gilbertson D, et al. Diabetes mellitus after kidney transplantation in the United States. Am J Transplant 2003;3(2):178–85.
[5] Davidson J, Wilkinson A, Dantal J, et al. New-onset diabetes after transplantation: 2003 International consensus guidelines. Proceedings of an international expert panel meeting. Barcelona, Spain, 19 February 2003. Transplantation 2003;75(Suppl 10):SS3–24.
[6] Walczak DA, Calvert D, Jarzembowski TM, et al. Increased risk of post-transplant diabetes mellitus despite early steroid discontinuation in Hispanic kidney transplant recipients. Clin Transplant 2005;19(4):527–31.
[7] Rhen T, Cidlowski JA. Anti-inflammatory action of glucocorticoids—new mechanisms for old drugs. N Engl J Med 2005;353(16):1711–23.
[8] Pagano G, Cavallo-Perin P, Cassader M, et al. An in vivo and in vitro study of the mechanism of prednisone-induced insulin resistance in healthy subjects. J Clin Invest 1983;72(5):1814–20.
[9] Rizza RA, Mandarino LJ, Gerich JE. Cortisol-induced insulin resistance in man: impaired suppression of glucose production and stimulation of glucose utilization due to a postreceptor detect of insulin action. J Clin Endocrinol Metab 1982;54(1):131–8.

[10] Bressler P, DeFronzo RA. Drugs and diabetes. Diabetes Rev 1994;(2):53–84.

[11] Mokshagundam SP, Peirs AN. Drug-induced disorders of glucose metabolism. In: Leahy JL, Clark NG, Cefalu WT, et al, editors. Medical management of diabetes mellitus. New York: Marcel Decker; 2000. p. 301–15.

[12] Vesco L, Busson M, Bedrossian J, et al. Diabetes mellitus after renal transplantation: characteristics, outcome, and risk factors. Transplantation 1996;61(10):1475–8.

[13] Miller LW. Cardiovascular toxicities of immunosuppressive agents. Am J Transplant 2002; 2(9):807–18.

[14] Vathsala A, Weinberg RB, Schoenberg L, et al. Lipid abnormalities in cyclosporine–prednisone-treated renal transplant recipients. Transplantation 1989;48(1):37–43.

[15] Turgan C, Russell GI, Baker F, et al. The effect of renal transplantation with a minimal steroid regime on uraemic hypertriglyceridaemia. Q J Med 1984;53(210):271–7.

[16] Hricik DE, Bartucci MR, Mayes JT, et al. The effects of steroid withdrawal on the lipoprotein profiles of cyclosporine-treated kidney and kidney–pancreas transplant recipients. Transplantation 1992;54(5):868–71.

[17] Jindal RM, Sidner RA, Hughes D, et al. Metabolic problems in recipients of liver transplants. Clin Transplant 1996;10(2):213–7.

[18] Renlund DG, Bristow MR, Crandall BG, et al. Hypercholesterolemia after heart transplantation: amelioration by corticosteroid-free maintenance immunosuppression. J Heart Transplant 1989;8(3):214–9 [discussion: 219–20].

[19] Kobashigawa JA, Kasiske BL. Hyperlipidemia in solid organ transplantation. Transplantation 1997;63(3):331–8.

[20] Vanrenterghem Y, Lebranchu Y, Hene R, et al. Double-blind comparison of two corticosteroid regimens plus mycophenolate mofetil and cyclosporine for prevention of acute renal allograft rejection. Transplantation 2000;70(9):1352–9.

[21] Kasiske BL, Chakkera HA, Louis TA, et al. A meta-analysis of immunosuppression withdrawal trials in renal transplantation. J Am Soc Nephrol 2000;11(10):1910–7.

[22] Streck WF, Lockwood DH. Pituitary adrenal recovery following short-term suppression with corticosteroids. Am J Med 1979;66(6):910–4.

[23] Byyny RL. Withdrawal from glucocorticoid therapy. N Engl J Med 1976;295(1): 30–2.

[24] Plotz CM, Knowlton AI, Ragan C. The natural history of Cushing's syndrome. Am J Med 1952;13(5):597–614.

[25] Trence DL. Management of patients on chronic glucocorticoid therapy: an endocrine perspective. Prim Care 2003;30(3):593–605.

[26] Wera S, Belayew A, Martial JA. Rapamycin, FK506. and cyclosporin A inhibit human prolactin gene expression. FEBS Lett 1995;358(2):158–60.

[27] Aguilar-Salinas CA, Diaz-Polanco A, Quintana E, et al. Genetic factors play an important role in the pathogenesis of hyperlipidemia post-transplantation. Am J Kidney Dis 2002; 40(1):169–77.

[28] Nielsen JH, Mandrup-Poulsen T, Nerup J. Direct effects of cyclosporin A on human pancreatic beta cells. Diabetes 1986;35(9):1049–52.

[29] Drachenberg CB, Klassen DK, Weir MR, et al. Islet cell damage associated with tacrolimus and cyclosporine: morphological features in pancreas allograft biopsies and clinical correlation. Transplantation 1999;68(3):396–402.

[30] Dufer M, Krippeit-Drews P, Lembert N, et al. Diabetogenic effect of cyclosporin A is mediated by interference with mitochondrial function of pancreatic B cells. Mol Pharmacol 2001; 60(4):873–9.

[31] Cantarovich D, Dantal J, Murat A, et al. Normal glucose metabolism and insulin secretion in CyA-treated nondiabetic renal allograft patients not receiving steroids. Transplant Proc 1990;22(2):643–4.

[32] Ost L. Impairment of prednisolone metabolism by cyclosporine treatment in renal graft recipients. Transplantation 1987;44(4):533–5.

[33] Hjelmesaeth J, Hagen LT, Asberg A, et al. The impact of short-term cyclosporin A treatment on insulin secretion and insulin sensitivity in man. Nephrol Dial Transplant 2007;22(6): 1743–9.

[34] Robertson RP, Franklin G, Nelson L. Glucose homeostasis and insulin secretion during chronic treatment with cyclosporin in nondiabetic humans. Diabetes 1989;38(Suppl 1): 99–100.

[35] Ballantyne CM, Podet EJ, Patsch WP, et al. Effects of cyclosporine therapy on plasma lipoprotein levels. JAMA 1989;262(1):53–6.

[36] de Groen PC. Cyclosporine, low-density lipoprotein, and cholesterol. Mayo Clin Proc 1988; 63(10):1012–21.

[37] Derfler K, Hayde M, Heinz G, et al. Decreased postheparin lipolytic activity in renal transplant recipients with cyclosporin A. Kidney Int 1991;40(4):720–7.

[38] Apanay DC, Neylan JF, Ragab MS, et al. Cyclosporine increases the oxidizability of low-density lipoproteins in renal transplant recipients. Transplantation 1994;58(6):663–9.

[39] Brown JH, Murphy BG, Douglas AF, et al. Influence of immunosuppressive therapy on lipoprotein(a) and other lipoproteins following renal transplantation. Nephron 1997;75(3): 277–82.

[40] Redmon JB, Olson LK, Armstrong MB, et al. Effects of tacrolimus (FK506) on human insulin gene expression, insulin mRNA levels, and insulin secretion in HIT-T15 cells. J Clin Invest 1996;98(12):2786–93.

[41] Hirano Y, Fujihira S, Ohara K, et al. Morphological and functional changes of islets of Langerhans in FK506-treated rats. Transplantation 1992;53(4):889–94.

[42] Hirano Y, Mitamura T, Tamura T, et al. Mechanism of FK506-induced glucose intolerance in rats. J Toxicol Sci 1994;19(2):61–5.

[43] Duijnhoven EM, Boots JM, Christiaans MH, et al. Influence of tacrolimus on glucose metabolism before and after renal transplantation: a prospective study. J Am Soc Nephrol 2001;12(3):583–8.

[44] van Duijnhoven EM, Christiaans MH, Boots JM, et al. Glucose metabolism in the first 3 years after renal transplantation in patients receiving tacrolimus versus cyclosporine-based immunosuppression. J Am Soc Nephrol 2002;13(1):213–20.

[45] Dieterle CD, Schmauss S, Veitenhansl M, et al. Glucose metabolism after pancreas transplantation: cyclosporine versus tacrolimus. Transplantation 2004;77(10):1561–5.

[46] Bouchta NB, Ghisdal L, Abramowicz D, et al. Conversion from tacrolimus to cyclosporin is associated with a significant improvement of glucose metabolism in patients with new-onset diabetes mellitus after renal transplantation. Transplant Proc 2005;37(4):1857–60.

[47] Fernandez LA, Lehmann R, Luzi L, et al. The effects of maintenance doses of FK506 versus cyclosporin A on glucose and lipid metabolism after orthotopic liver transplantation. Transplantation 1999;68(10):1532–41.

[48] Steinmuller TM, Graf KJ, Schleicher J, et al. The effect of FK506 versus cyclosporine on glucose and lipid metabolism—a randomized trial. Transplantation 1994;58(6):669–74.

[49] Pirsch JD, Miller J, Deierhoi MH, et al. A comparison of tacrolimus (FK506) and cyclosporine for immunosuppression after cadaveric renal transplantation. FK506 Kidney Transplant Study Group. Transplantation 1997;63(7):977–83.

[50] Jindal RM, Popescu I, Emre S, et al. Serum lipid changes in liver transplant recipients in a prospective trial of cyclosporine versus FK506. Transplantation 1994;57(9):1395–8.

[51] Maes BD, Vanrenterghem YF. Cyclosporine: advantages versus disadvantages vis a vis tacrolimus. Transplant Proc 2004;36(Suppl 2):40S–9S.

[52] Aguirrezabalaga J, Fernandez-Selles C, Fraguela J, et al. Lipid profiles after liver transplantation in patients receiving tacrolimus or cyclosporin. Transplant Proc 2002;34(5): 1551–2.

[53] Baid-Agrawal S, Delmonico FL, Tolkoff-Rubin NE, et al. Cardiovascular risk profile after conversion from cyclosporine A to tacrolimus in stable renal transplant recipients. Transplantation 2004;77(8):1199–202.

[54] McCauley J, Shapiro R, Jordan ML, et al. Long-term lipid metabolism in combined kidney–pancreas transplant recipients under tacrolimus immunosuppression. Transplant Proc 2001; 33(1–2):1698–9.

[55] Allison AC, Eugui EM. Purine metabolism and immunosuppressive effects of mycophenolate mofetil (MMF). Clin Transplant 1996;10(1 Pt 2):77–84.

[56] Paty BW, Harmon JS, Marsh CL, et al. Inhibitory effects of immunosuppressive drugs on insulin secretion from HIT-T15 cells and Wistar rat islets. Transplantation 2002;73(3): 353–7.

[57] Li G, Segu VB, Rabaglia ME, et al. Prolonged depletion of guanosine triphosphate induces death of insulin-secreting cells by apoptosis. Endocrinology 1998;139(9):3752–62.

[58] Polastri L, Galbiati F, Bertuzzi F, et al. Secretory defects induced by immunosuppressive agents on human pancreatic beta cells. Acta Diabetol 2002;39(4):229–33.

[59] Eckhoff DE, McGuire BM, Frenette LR, et al. Tacrolimus (FK506) and mycophenolate mofetil combination therapy versus tacrolimus in adult liver transplantation. Transplantation 1998;65(2):180–7.

[60] Romero F, Rodriguez-Iturbe B, Pons H, et al. Mycophenolate mofetil treatment reduces cholesterol-induced atherosclerosis in the rabbit. Atherosclerosis 2000;152(1):127–33.

[61] Akman B, Uyar M, Afsar B, et al. Lipid profile during azathioprine or mycophenolate mofetil combinations with cyclosporine and steroids. Transplant Proc 2007;39(1):135–7.

[62] Sipula IJ, Brown NF, Perdomo G. Rapamycin-mediated inhibition of mammalian target of rapamycin in skeletal muscle cells reduces glucose utilization and increases fatty acid oxidation. Metabolism 2006;55(12):1637–44.

[63] Cho HJ, Park J, Lee HW, et al. Regulation of adipocyte differentiation and insulin action with rapamycin. Biochem Biophys Res Commun 2004;321(4):942–8.

[64] Taha C, Liu Z, Jin J, et al. Opposite translational control of GLUT1 and GLUT4 glucose transporter mRNAs in response to insulin. Role of mammalian target of rapamycin, protein kinase b, and phosphatidylinositol 3-kinase in GLUT1 mRNA translation. J Biol Chem 1999;274(46):33085–91.

[65] Berg CE, Lavan BE, Rondinone CM. Rapamycin partially prevents insulin resistance induced by chronic insulin treatment. Biochem Biophys Res Commun 2002;293(3): 1021–7.

[66] Zhang N, Su D, Qu S, et al. Sirolimus is associated with reduced islet engraftment and impaired beta cell function. Diabetes 2006;55(9):2429–36.

[67] Bell E, Cao X, Moibi JA, et al. Rapamycin has a deleterious effect on MIN-6 cells and rat and human islets. Diabetes 2003;52(11):2731–9.

[68] Larsen JL, Bennett RG, Burkman T, et al. Tacrolimus and sirolimus cause insulin resistance in normal sprague dawley rats. Transplantation 2006;82(4):466–70.

[69] Marcelli-Tourvieille S, Hubert T, Moerman E, et al. In vivo and in vitro effect of sirolimus on insulin secretion. Transplantation 2007;83(5):532–8.

[70] Teutonico A, Schena PF, Di Paolo S. Glucose metabolism in renal transplant recipients: effect of calcineurin inhibitor withdrawal and conversion to sirolimus. J Am Soc Nephrol 2005;16(10):3128–35.

[71] Morrisett JD, Abdel-Fattah G, Hoogeveen R, et al. Effects of sirolimus on plasma lipids, lipoprotein levels, and fatty acid metabolism in renal transplant patients. J Lipid Res 2002;43(8):1170–80.

[72] MacDonald AS. Rapamycin in combination with cyclosporine or tacrolimus in liver, pancreas, and kidney transplantation. Transplant Proc 2003;35(Suppl 3):201S–8S.

[73] Kahan BD. Sirolimus-based immunosuppression: present state of the art. J Nephrol 2004; 17(Suppl 8):S32–9.

[74] Mathe D, Adam R, Malmendier C, et al. Prevalence of dyslipidemia in liver transplant recipients. Transplantation 1992;54(1):167–70.

[75] Morard I, Dumortier J, Spahr L, et al. Conversion to sirolimus-based immunosuppression in maintenance liver transplantation patients. Liver Transpl 2007;13(5):658–64.

[76] Aggarwal D, Fernandez ML, Soliman GA. Rapamycin, an mTOR inhibitor, disrupts triglyceride metabolism in guinea pigs. Metabolism 2006;55(6):794–802.
[77] Brattstrom C, Wilczek HE, Tyden G, et al. Hypertriglyceridemia in renal transplant recipients treated with sirolimus. Transplant Proc 1998;30(8):3950–1.
[78] Brattstrom C, Wilczek H, Tyden G, et al. Hyperlipidemia in renal transplant recipients treated with sirolimus (rapamycin). Transplantation 1998;65(9):1272–4.
[79] Ponticelli C, MacDonald AS, Rajagopalan P, et al. Phase III trial of Rapamune versus placebo in primary renal allograft recipients. Transplant Proc 2001;33(3):2271–2.
[80] Kniepeiss D, Iberer F, Schaffellner S, et al. Dyslipidemia during sirolimus therapy in patients after liver transplantation. Clin Transplant 2004;18(6):642–6.
[81] Trotter JF, Wachs ME, Trouillot TE, et al. Dyslipidemia during sirolimus therapy in liver transplant recipients occurs with concomitant cyclosporine but not tacrolimus. Liver Transpl 2001;7(5):401–8.
[82] Ruygrok PN, Muller DW, Serruys PW. Rapamycin in cardiovascular medicine. Intern Med J 2003;33(3):103–9.
[83] Pascual J. Everolimus in clinical practice—renal transplantation. Nephrol Dial Transplant 2006;21(Suppl 3):iii, 18–23.
[84] Patel JK, Kobashigawa JA. Everolimus: an immunosuppressive agent in transplantation. Expert Opin Pharmacother 2006;7(10):1347–55.

ELSEVIER
SAUNDERS

Endocrinol Metab Clin N Am
36 (2007) 907–922

ENDOCRINOLOGY
AND METABOLISM
CLINICS
OF NORTH AMERICA

Comprehensive Management of Post-Transplant Diabetes Mellitus: From Intensive Care to Home Care

Philip A. Goldberg, MD

*Department of Internal Medicine, Section of Endocrinology and Metabolism,
Yale University School of Medicine, 333 Cedar Street, New Haven, CT 06520, USA*

Post-transplant diabetes mellitus (PTDM) is a common complication of solid organ and hematopoietic transplantation [1,2]. Because of substantial heterogeneity in affected patients and their diseases, reported incidence rates for PTDM vary widely; this condition may develop in up to 50% of at-risk patients [3]. Until recently, post-transplant hyperglycemia was largely ignored, in part, due to a longstanding lack of consensus regarding the proper definition of PTDM. In addition, the broad clinical impact of this disease has only recently been fully appreciated.

We now understand that PTDM, like "standard" type 2 diabetes mellitus (T2DM), increases patients' risk for macrovascular disease of the coronary, cerebral, and peripheral arteries [4–7]. Microvascular complications, including neuropathy, nephropathy, and retinopathy, also occur in patients with PTDM, although published data supporting this association are lacking. Beyond vascular disease, PTDM has been clearly associated with an elevated risk for serious infections, acute graft rejection, and even death [8,9]. Because of the enormous clinical impact and health economic consequences of PTDM [10], all patients undergoing solid organ or hematopoietic transplantation should be actively screened for hyperglycemia, and affected patients should be treated aggressively.

In this comprehensive, clinically oriented article, the author briefly reviews the pathophysiology of PTDM to lay the groundwork for a meaningful discussion regarding therapy. The author then discusses the key clinical aspects of PTDM screening, diagnosis, and management during all phases following transplantation from the ICU, to the inpatient ward, to the outpatient arena.

E-mail address: shayala@pol.net

0889-8529/07/$ - see front matter © 2007 Elsevier Inc. All rights reserved.
doi:10.1016/j.ecl.2007.07.011   *endo.theclinics.com*

Pathophysiology of post-transplant diabetes mellitus

Like T2DM, PTDM results from a combination of insulin resistance and impaired insulin secretion [11]. The predominant mechanism remains a subject of academic debate. In 1998, Midtvedt and colleagues [12] studied 46 renal transplant patients with oral glucose tolerance tests (oGTT) and euglycemic clamps. When compared with non-diabetic controls, patients with PTDM exhibited reduced glucose disposal rates (3.4 ± 1.3 versus 7.1 ± 2.4 mg/kg/min, $P < .05$) and reduced insulin responses (170 ± 128 versus 448 ± 310 pmol/L, $P < .05$). Nam and colleagues [13] then studied 114 patients with normal glucose tolerance before solid organ transplantation. Impaired glucose tolerance (IGT) developed in 51 patients (46%) and PTDM in 27 patients (24%). In this study, patients with PTDM had similar insulin sensitivity to non-diabetic controls; however, insulin responses were 18% lower in PTDM patients ($P < .05$), suggesting a primary role for pancreatic β-cell dysfunction. In 2003, Hagen and colleagues [14] observed 63 patients for 6 years following renal transplantation. In this cohort, impaired insulin secretion accounted for the majority of PTDM cases; however, normalization of IGT was mediated by improved insulin sensitivity without changes in insulin secretory capacity.

Immunosuppressive therapy, not the transplant itself, appears to account for most cases of PTDM [15]. In 2002, Montori and colleagues [16] systematically reviewed 19 clinical studies containing 3611 patients with PTDM. Multiple linear regression analysis estimated that the patients' immunosuppressive regimen (ie, corticosteroids with or without calcineurin inhibitors [CNIs]) accounted for 74% of PTDM cases. Corticosteroids have long been known to induce tissue insulin resistance through several mechanisms, including stimulation of gluconeogenesis, impairment of peripheral glucose utilization and inhibition of tissue lipogenesis [7]. In humans, corticosteroids increase basal insulin levels and first-phase insulin release in an attempt to overcome insulin resistance [12,17]. The diabetogenic effects of corticosteroids are clearly related to the dose and the duration of therapy. Following solid organ transplantation, steroid doses are independently associated with new-onset IGT and PTDM [18].

CNIs, including cyclosporine and tacrolimus, are also involved in the generation of hyperglycemia, predominantly by impairing β-cell insulin release [19]. In vitro and animal studies suggest multiple potential actions on the β cell, including impaired nucleic acid synthesis, islet cell vacuolization, and the promotion of apoptosis [15]. The risk for post-transplant hyperglycemia seems to depend on the specific CNI employed. In early renal transplant studies, patients receiving tacrolimus were five times more likely to develop PTDM than patients receiving cyclosporine [20]. A 2004 meta-analysis of 16 prospective kidney, liver, and heart transplant studies confirmed this observation [21]; among these patients, PTDM developed in 16.6% of those receiving tacrolimus versus 9.8% of those receiving cyclosporine. Rates of insulin-dependent PTDM were also higher in tacro-limus-treated patients (10.4% versus 4.5%, $P < .001$) independent of the organ transplanted or the corticosteroid dose employed. Although prospective head-to-head trials have not been performed, tacrolimus appears to be more diabetogenic than cyclosporine.

Inpatient management

In the hospital, hyperglycemia occurs commonly following transplantation, even in patients without a prior history of diabetes. For decades, retrospective studies have revealed an association between high blood glucose levels and adverse clinical outcomes in hospitalized patients, including those recovering from major surgery. For example, in diabetic patients undergoing open heart procedures, high postoperative blood glucose levels have been associated with an increased risk for deep sternal wound infections [22]. In general surgical patients with diabetes, early postoperative glycemic control predicts nosocomial infection rates [23]. These types of published observations have not been limited to patients with pre-existing diabetes. In a general community hospital, hyperglycemia was a strong independent marker of in-hospital mortality in previously non-diabetic patients [24].

Recent clinical trials have supported intensive glycemic control in critically ill patients, including those recovering from major surgery. In a large series of diabetic patients undergoing open heart surgery, strict glycemic control lowered deep sternal wound infection rates [25] and reduced overall mortality [26]. In a subsequent randomized controlled trial of 1548 intubated patients in a surgical ICU (13% of whom had previous diabetes), aggressive glycemic control with intravenous insulin reduced overall mortality by 42% and also lowered the incidence of septicemia, acute renal failure, severe anemia requiring blood transfusion, and critical illness polyneuropathy [27]. Although some more recent studies from medical and cardiac ICUs have challenged the importance of strict glycemic control in all hospitalized patients [28,29], the benefits of strict glycemic control exceed its risks, particularly in patients recovering from major surgery [30].

Based on these and other key clinical studies, several professional medical organizations have recently addressed target blood glucose levels for hospitalized patients. The American Diabetes Association (ADA) advocates goal blood glucose levels of 80 to 110 mg/dL in the ICU, with intravenous insulin recommended perioperatively; target blood glucose levels outside of the ICU should be less than 110 mg/dL before meals and less than 180 mg/dL at all times [31]. Recent management guidelines from the American College of Endocrinology endorse similarly strict glycemic targets [32]. Inpatient management of PTDM should be broken down as follows:

ICU management
    Intravenous IIP (for critically ill patients)
    Transition protocol: transitioning to subcutaneous insulin

Ward management
Subcutaneous insulin regimens—basal, bolus, correction insulin
Oral agents—sulfonylureas, meglitinides, other oral agents

In critically ill patients, particularly those at increased risk for infection (eg, patients undergoing solid organ or hematopoietic transplantation), intravenous insulin should be administered perioperatively using a standardized insulin infusion protocol (IIP).

Many such protocols have been developed for clinical practice [33–38]. Although the specific details vary, all successful IIPs incorporate three critical factors into a nurse-implemented clinical algorithm: (1) the current blood glucose level, (2) the previous blood glucose level (accounting for the "velocity" of blood glucose change), and (3) the current insulin infusion rate. Among published IIPs, glycemic targets vary slightly. In essence, blood glucose levels should be rendered as normal as possible without undue risk for severe hypoglycemia. For mostly practical reasons, individual IIPs appeal to different clinicians and nurses within a variety of hospital settings. In my view, the successful implementation of a standardized IIP is far more important than the specific protocol selected [36].

In the ICU, once a patient's clinical status improves, and once he or she is eating decent meals, intravenous insulin can usually be transitioned to subcutaneous insulin injections, preferably using a standardized transition protocol. Bode and colleagues [39] extrapolate the last 6 to 8 hours of intravenous insulin to calculate 24-hour insulin requirements. Conservatively, 80% of this figure is then used as the "total daily dose," half of which is given as basal insulin and the other half at mealtimes. Another strategy employs the final intravenous insulin infusion rate (in U/h). Eight times this rate is given as NPH insulin twice daily, and four times this rate is given as regular insulin three times daily with meals [40]. At the author's institution, we extrapolate 24-hour intravenous insulin requirements from the last 8 hours of therapy; clinicians may then reduce this total daily dose by a "safety factor" (up to 25%) in patients at risk for hypoglycemia. This total daily insulin dose is then provided as approximately 50% basal insulin (glargine, Levemir, or neutral protamine Hagedorn [NPH]) and approximately 50% bolus insulin. The latter is preferably a rapid-acting insulin analogue given immediately before meals.

Upon transfer to a general medical or surgical ward, hyperglycemic patients should be managed using a physiologic insulin strategy, employing basal, bolus, and correction (formerly known as "sliding scale") insulin orders [41]. Available basal insulins include NPH, glargine, and detemir [42]. For many patients, the latter two agents offer smoother, more predictable pharmacodynamics with fewer "peaks and valleys" of insulin action. For patients with PTDM, NPH insulin (with onset at 2–4 hours and peak activity from 4–10 hours) can be useful to match the "steroid effect," during which once-daily (morning) steroid doses generate late-day hyperglycemia.

In my clinical experience, combining two basal insulins may provide optimal results. Bedtime glargine or detemir insulin (instead of NPH) reduces the incidence of overnight hypoglycemia, whereas a morning dose of NPH insulin best counteracts the steroid effect. In the hospital, either regular insulin or rapid-acting insulin analogues (lispro, aspart, or glulisine) may be administered with meals. For most patients, rapid-acting agents offer the distinct advantage of reduced between-meal hypoglycemia. Regular insulin may be preferred if more prolonged insulin action is desired, for example, during periods of prolonged steroid-induced hyperglycemia. Despite extensive clinical experience with a variety of insulins, no prospective studies have addressed the relative efficacy of specific insulin regimens for treating PTDM.

The use of oral agents for PTDM is reviewed more extensively in the section on outpatient diabetes management. In the hospital setting, insulin therapy is generally preferred because of its superior predictability and rapid titratability [41]. In well-selected patients (eg, medically stable, eating well, no anticipated radiologic studies), oral agents can safely be employed in the hospital setting. Sulfonylureas are most often used in this capacity; of course, their benefits must be weighed against an increased risk of hypoglycemia, particularly in patients with renal insufficiency. Shorter-acting meglitinides such as repaglinide and nateglinide provide a reasonable inpatient alternative. In general, metformin is best avoided in the hospital owing to its long list of contraindications (including renal or hepatic impairment, heart failure, and pending radiology studies involving intravenous contrast). Thiazolidinediones (TZDs), although generally safe for inpatient use, have a delayed onset of action (days to weeks), limiting their clinical utility.

During hospital-wide implementation of any glycemic strategy, many hospital barriers (highlighted by indifference and a fear of hypoglycemia) must be overcome to safely and effectively administer intensive insulin therapy [36]. In addition, hospital-wide systems issues must be prospectively addressed, preferably by early involvement of clinicians, nurses, pharmacy, and nutrition staff to achieve common goals. As a concrete example, for hospitalized patients eating meals, fingerstick blood glucose levels should always be obtained before meals to facilitate prandial insulin dosing. Ideally, rapid-acting insulin analogues (lispro, aspart, glulisine) should be given only after patients have direct access to their meal. When bedtime fingersticks are obtained, these readings should be used mainly for adjusting basal insulin therapy; bedtime correction insulin orders should be conservative, if employed at all.

Outpatient management

Although the body of literature regarding PTDM is growing, there are few long-term studies on which to base practical guidelines for long-term management. In the general diabetes population, there is strong evidence that strict glycemic control prevents vascular complications [43–45]. As stated previously, transplant patients are at similarly high risk for diabetic complications, and there is no reason to believe that transplant recipients should tolerate hyperglycemia better than others [46]. As a result, PTDM should be managed with similar aggression to T2DM to lower patients' risks for vascular complications, serious infections, graft failure, and even death (Box 1). The 2003 International Consensus Guidelines [47] endorse this aggressive screening and management philosophy, discussed in the following sections.

Box 1. Outpatient management of post-transplant diabetes mellitus

Therapeutic lifestyle modifications
    Diet—limited intake of calories, carbohydrates, and saturated
        fats
    Exercise—aerobic activity, resistance training
    Weight loss and maintenance of ideal body weight
Consider modification of immunosuppressive regimen
    Reduction and/or split dosing of corticosteroid doses
    Reduction and/or alteration of CNI therapy
    "Steroid-sparing" immunosuppressive regimens
Non-insulin pharmacologic therapy
    Sulfonylureas
    Metformin
    Thiazolidinediones
    Meglitinides
    Alpha-glucosidase inhibitors
    Exenitide, DPP-IV inhibitors
Insulin therapy
    Basal insulins—NPH, glargine, detemir
    Bolus insulins—regular, lispro, aspart, glulisine
Management of cardiovascular risk factors
    Hypertension
    Dyslipidemia
    Aspirin therapy
    Smoking cessation
Screening for PTDM complications
    Retinopathy screening—dilated retinal examinations
    Nephropathy screening—creatinine (for glomerular filtration
        rate), urine microalbumin
    Neuropathy screening—tuning fork, monofilament
    Podiatry screening—pulses, skin integrity
    Macrovascular screening (controversial)

Outpatient screening for post-transplant diabetes mellitus

Despite growing clinical attention to PTDM, an alarming number of at-risk patients are still not appropriately screened for hyperglycemia [47]. Simply convincing transplant clinicians to screen for PTDM is an important step. Historically, the lack of an accepted definition for PTDM has hampered efforts to diagnose and treat this condition. Previous clinicians (and researchers) have employed a wide range of definitions based on either arbitrary blood glucose cutoffs or even more arbitrary "requirements" for insulin therapy. To date, no prospective studies have examined the impact of specific blood glucose levels on clinical outcomes in PTDM patients. Nevertheless, because evidence from the general diabetes population is strong and consistent, the 2003 International Consensus Guidelines formally adopted the general diagnostic criteria of the ADA's Expert Committee [47]. Specifically, reproducible fasting plasma glucose levels greater than 126 mg/dL, 2-hour post-challenge plasma glucose levels greater than 200 mg/dL, or casual plasma glucose levels greater than 200 mg/dL with symptoms of diabetes should be used to establish the diagnosis of PTDM [48,49].

When should clinicians screen for PTDM? Hyperglycemia develops most commonly during the early weeks after transplantation; however, PTDM has been reported up to 4 years following solid organ transplantation. A reasonable program should screen early and often, and then periodically thereafter. The 2003 International Consensus Guidelines recommend screening with fasting plasma glucose levels on a weekly basis for 4 weeks following transplant, at 3 and 6 months post transplant, and then annually. Nevertheless, because PTDM occurs in patients with normal fasting plasma glucose levels (eg, postprandial hyperglycemia), fasting plasma glucose levels may lack sufficient sensitivity. In 2005, Shah and colleagues [50] studied this question in 89 consecutive non-diabetic renal transplant recipients. Of these 89 patients, just 5 (5%) met criteria for PTDM based on fasting plasma glucose levels greater than 126 mg/dL. Another 29 (32%) had elevated fasting plasma glucose levels between 111 and 125 mg/dL. These 29 patients were taught to use a home glucose meter and were instructed to check their glucose levels before meals and at bedtime for 3 days. Remarkably, 19 (66%) of these 29 patients were subsequently diagnosed with PTDM. Self-monitoring of glucose levels greatly improved the sensitivity of PTDM screening. As another option, a 75-g, 2-hour oGTT would likely improve the sensitivity of PTDM screening; however, the predictive value and cost-effectiveness of this more cumbersome strategy remain unclear.

Based on the available (and admittedly limited) evidence, I recommend routine screening for PTDM in all post-transplant patients starting with four weekly fasting plasma glucose levels. Fasting plasma glucose levels should then be repeated every 3 months for the first post-transplant year. Transplant patients with impaired fasting glucose levels (100–125 mg/dL) should be further evaluated for PTDM with either a formal oGTT or home glucose monitoring. In addition, patients with risk factors for PTDM, including advanced age (>40 years), high-risk ethnicity (African American, Hispanic, Native American, Pacific Islander), obesity (body mass index >30 kg/m^2), a family history of diabetes (first-degree relative), or hepatitis C positivity, should be considered for more aggressive screening. Hemoglobin A$_{1c}$ levels, although advocated by some authors [51], are not recommended for diagnosis owing to problems with low test sensitivity and confounding variables such as severe anemia, blood transfusions, and abnormal hemoglobins. Of course, hemoglobin A$_{1c}$ levels are valuable to confirm the diagnosis, to assess the extent of disease, and (most importantly) to guide therapeutic lifestyle changes and pharmacologic interventions.

Therapeutic lifestyle changes

As a first step, medical nutrition therapy should be recommended for all patients with PTDM [52]. Patients should be taught to monitor their total caloric and carbohydrate intake and should limit their intake of saturated fat to less than 7% of total calories. If medically feasible, more than 150 minutes per week of moderate intensity physical activity (generating 50%–70% of maximal heart rate) should be recommended, ideally distributed over 3 or more days per week. When possible, regular muscle resistance training is also recommended. For overweight or obese patients, weight loss should be encouraged, with a long-term goal of approaching or maintaining ideal body weight.

Oral agents: metformin, sulfonylureas, and thiazolidinediones

For patients with non–transplant related T2DM, both metformin and the sulfonylurea drugs have a long established safety record for lowering blood glucose levels and for reducing microvascular complications of diabetes [44,45]. Because PTDM is associated with insulin resistance, metformin (which improves insulin sensitivity, most notably in the liver) would seem a logical candidate for therapy; however, metformin has several characteristics that limit its utility (and safety) in PTDM patients. Metformin is contraindicated in patients with renal or hepatic insufficiency or with active alcohol use [53]. This drug is also best avoided during medical procedures, surgeries, and radiologic contrast studies. Given metformin's risk for inducing lactic acidosis under these conditions, it is uncommonly used to treat patients with PTDM, at least during the early stages of the disease. On the other hand, using metformin to treat stable chronic PTDM in patients without active contraindications seems a sensible strategy.

Because PTDM has also been associated with impaired insulin secretion, sulfonylurea drugs would seem another logical choice for therapy. Glyburide, glipizide, and glimepiride are most commonly employed in the United States for this purpose. Despite a lack of published data, there is ample clinical experience using these inexpensive oral agents to treat PTDM; however, sulfonylurea monotherapy is often inadequate to achieve glycemic control in transplant patients [54,55]. In addition, these drugs are associated with an increased risk for hypoglycemia, especially in patients with renal or hepatic insufficiency. Glipizide, with a shorter half-life than other sulfonylureas, may be preferred in this setting [56], although good comparative data are lacking.

In recent years because of the limitations associated with other oral agents, TZDs (which primarily address insulin resistance at the level of skeletal muscle) have been evaluated as a potential therapy for PTDM. Early studies examined the efficacy of troglitazone (an early TZD, no longer marketed) in patients receiving corticosteroid therapy. In 2002, Willi and colleagues [57] examined the metabolic effects of dexamethasone (4 mg/d) in 10 non-diabetic human subjects and then reassessed these effects after subjects completed 4 to 6 weeks of oral troglitazone therapy (400 mg/d). Without troglitazone, 4 days of dexamethasone induced profound insulin resistance, with 2.3-fold and 4.4-fold increases in baseline and 2-hour insulin values, respectively ($P < .001$), as well a 34% reduction in maximal glucose disposal rate. Remarkably, pretreatment with troglitazone completely reversed these metabolic effects. These researchers [58] then evaluated the effectiveness of troglitazone therapy (400 mg/d) in seven actual patients with steroid-induced diabetes. Following 5 to 8 weeks of treatment, hemoglobin A_{1c} levels were reduced from 7.8% to 7.2% ($P < .01$). Troglitazone therapy also led to increased insulin secretion and decreased post-challenge blood glucose levels during oGTTs. Fubiyashi and colleagues [59] reported similar success treating steroid-induced diabetes with troglitazone. These investigators also reported reduced serum leptin concentrations, suggesting that TZDs have beneficial effects on adipocyte metabolism.

Several more recent studies have specifically evaluated rosiglitazone for the treatment of PTDM. As opposed to pioglitazone, rosiglitazone is generally preferred in this setting because it is not metabolized by the CYP3A4 system, lowering the risk for dangerous interactions with CNIs. In 2005, Pietruck and colleagues [60] reported their experience with 22 PTDM patients, 16 of whom were treated successfully with rosiglitazone. In these 16 patients, fasting plasma glucose levels dropped from 182 to 127 mg/dL while hemoglobin A_{1c} levels fell from 7.2% to 6.2%. Five of the six patients poorly controlled with rosiglitazone monotherapy subsequently responded to combination therapy with either glyburide or insulin; in the sixth patient, rosiglitazone was stopped owing to edema. In 2005, Voytovich and colleagues [61] studied 10 patients with PTDM following renal transplantation. In these patients, 4 weeks of rosiglitazone therapy (8 mg/d) improved insulin sensitivity and reduced both fasting and 2-hour plasma glucose levels (from 6.4 to 5.8 mmol/L and 14.2 to 10.6 mmol/L, respectively, both $P \leq .03$).

Baldwin and Duffin [54] recently reported their experience with 18 post-transplant patients treated with rosiglitazone, which was added to insulin or sulfonylurea therapy. Eleven of these 18 patients had diabetes before their organ transplantation. In this study, hemoglobin A_{1c} levels dropped from 8.1% to 6.9% (P = .01). Notably, all seven patients with new-onset PTDM were successfully managed (mean hemoglobin A_{1c}, 6.7%) without insulin therapy. In 2005, Villaneuva and colleagues [55] reported their experience treating 40 consecutive PTDM patients with rosiglitazone. Most of these patients had initially required insulin therapy. Following 3 to 4 months of rosiglitazone therapy, insulin was discontinued in 91% of treated patients, two-thirds of whom also required treatment with sulfonylureas to maintain glycemic target goals. During this study, clinically significant edema developed in 13% of patients. Weight gains were minimal during this brief clinical trial.

Rosiglitazone appears to be a safe and effective treatment for PTDM; however, because corticosteroids are associated with weight gain, special attention must be paid to body weight in patients receiving both drugs. Also, careful monitoring for edema and fluid overload is warranted in all patients treated with TZDs.

Oral agents: other considerations

Repaglinide and nateglinide, which also act on the sulfonylurea receptor, are associated with reduced rates of hypoglycemia when compared with standard sulfonylureas [62]. These agents should be considered for patients experiencing frequent hypoglycemia, especially if renal insufficiency is present. Alpha-glucosidase inhibitors such as acarbose and miglitol might also prove useful in select situations but are limited by common gastrointestinal side effects and limited hemoglobin A_{1c} reductions. Theoretically, GLP-1 agonists such as exenatide and liraglutide would also be sensible therapy; however, the chief side effects of these medications (nausea, diarrhea, dizziness, and headache) may limit their utility in treating PTDM. Oral DPP-IV inhibitors such as sitagliptin and vildagliptin might also prove useful given their placebo-like side effect profile and their utility (dose adjusted) in patients with renal insufficiency; however, none of these newer agents have been studied for use in PTDM.

Insulin therapy

Ultimately, insulin therapy is required for many outpatients with PTDM. Indications for insulin therapy in such patients include extreme hyperglycemia, failure of oral hypoglycemic agents, and intolerance of (or contraindications to) other available therapies. Traditional basal-bolus insulin regimens, such as glargine or detemir insulin combined with rapid-acting analogues [42], may be successful in treating PTDM patients. For patients taking daily steroid therapy, NPH insulin is often useful because its delayed peak action closely mirrors the delayed hyperglycemic effect of once-daily steroid therapy [63]. For patients with evening hyperglycemia induced by morning corticosteroid doses, I find bedtime glargine or detemir plus morning NPH to be an effective, if slightly unorthodox, basal insulin combination. In general, because PTDM patients can be difficult to manage, creative insulin management strategies are often required to optimize glycemic control. For difficult and poorly controlled patients, an experienced endocrinologist should be consulted to assist with patient management.

Tailoring immunosuppression

In patients with poorly controlled PTDM despite therapeutic lifestyle changes and pharmacologic interventions, the components (and doses) of the immunosuppressive regimen should be re-evaluated. In patients with PTDM, blood glucose elevations are correlated with corticosteroid doses [19] and with the choice and dose of CNI [22]. In renal transplant patients, reducing corticosteroid doses (prednisolone ≤ 5 mg/d) improves insulin sensitivity and lowers fasting plasma glucose levels [64–66]. This strategy, while effective for managing PTDM, must obviously be weighed against an increased risk for transplant rejection. In my experience, twice-daily dosing of steroids can also help to smooth out the peaks and valleys of steroid-induced hyperglycemia.

In patients with poorly controlled PTDM, reducing the CNI dose should also be considered. Success with this clinical approach has been reported in small patient series [67]. In renal transplant recipients, reducing tacrolimus doses improves β-cell secretion capacity [65]. In a recent clinical study [20], reducing tacrolimus doses by 30% (within the therapeutic window) increased patients' insulin and C-peptide responses by 24% and 36%, respectively.

Although no prospective trials have addressed this issue, some researchers have suggested that switching from tacrolimus to cyclosporine therapy may be an effective maneuver for treating PTDM. In 1996, Kanzler and colleagues [68] reported the findings in a 41-year-old liver transplant recipient (treated with tacrolimus) who experienced severe hyperglycemia refractory to high-dose intravenous insulin therapy. Following a switch to cyclosporine, this patient no longer required insulin; in fact, the patient had normal oGTT results. In 1998, Lagget and colleagues [69] contributed two additional cases of "disappearing" PTDM following a conversion from tacrolimus to cyclosporine. In 2000, Emre and colleagues [70] retrospectively reviewed the charts of 70 liver transplant patients requiring conversion (for various reasons, most commonly neurotoxicity and PTDM) of tacrolimus to cyclosporine. In this series, blood glucose levels responded dramatically; 15 patients with new-onset PTDM became nondiabetic following conversion of tacrolimus to cyclosporine therapy.

Although the clinical evidence is largely anecdotal, tailoring of immunosuppression should be considered in patients with poorly controlled PTDM. Therapeutic options include dose reductions of corticosteroids, CNIs, or both. In patients receiving tacrolimus, conversion to cyclosporine may also be considered. Ongoing trails of steroid-sparing regimens (eg, adjunctive antibody treatments) may provide additional therapeutic options in the near future.

Cardiovascular risk factor modification

Patients with PTDM, like patients with T2DM, are at increased risk for macrovascular and (probably) microvascular complications. In affected patients, glycemic control reduces the incidence of these complications [44,45]. Patients with PTDM are also at risk for obesity, hypertension, high triglyceride levels, and reduced high-density lipoprotein (HDL) cholesterol levels, that is, the metabolic syndrome, conveying further increased risk for cardiovascular disease [71]. As a result, cardiovascular risk factors should be managed aggressively in PTDM patients.

In patients with PTDM, blood pressure should ideally be lowered to less than 130/80 mm Hg [48,72,73] Low-density lipoprotein (LDL) cholesterol levels should be lowered to less than 100 mg/dL, with an optional goal of less than 70 mg/dL in high-risk patients. Triglyceride and HDL levels should be managed as secondary lipid targets, often with combination therapy [48,72,74]. Aspirin therapy (81–162 mg daily) should be considered for primary prevention in patients with an increased cardiovascular risk and is indicated for secondary prevention in patients with known cardiovascular disease. Smoking cessation should be advised for all patients with PTDM.

Screening for vascular complications

Like patients with T2DM, patients with PTDM should be screened for microvascular complications starting within 3 to 5 years of diagnosis [48,49,51]. Nephropathy screening should consist of a serum creatinine level (to estimate the glomerular filtration rate) and a spot urine microalbumin collection. Comprehensive ophthalmologic examinations, including dilated retinal examinations, should be performed annually. Detailed foot evaluations should include a visual examination, palpation of skin temperature and pedal pulses, and the use of a standard monofilament or tuning fork to detect sensory neuropathy. All PTDM patients with advanced neuropathy, foot deformities, or impaired skin integrity should be referred for podiatric care.

Screening regimens for macrovascular disease in diabetic patients are far more controversial. Cardiac stress testing (or stress echocardiography) should be performed in patients with cardiac symptoms or an abnormal EKG and should be considered for all high-risk patients. Carotid artery ultrasonography should be performed in patients with carotid bruits or a history of focal neurologic symptoms. Pulse volume recordings or lower extremity Doppler examinations may be considered in patients with claudication or diminished pedal pulses. These macrovascular screening recommendations are a matter of academic debate, the scope of which extends well beyond the focus of this article.

Summary

PTDM results from impaired insulin secretion and peripheral insulin resistance, largely generated by chronic immunosuppression. In transplanted patients, hyperglycemia is associated with an increased risk for cardiovascular disease, serious infections, graft rejection, and even death. As a result, meticulous screening programs are indicated, and PTDM should be treated in a comprehensive and aggressive manner. In the beginning, all patients should be screened for T2DM before transplantation and then periodically thereafter via fasting plasma glucose levels, home glucose monitoring, or selective oGTTs. Patients with PTDM should be counseled regarding therapeutic lifestyle modifications focused on proper nutrition, exercise, and maintenance of ideal body weight. When possible, reduction of corticosteroid doses or changes in CNI therapy should be considered. When pharmacologic therapy is indicated, it should be tailored to the patient and the degree (and pattern) of hyperglycemia. Inpatient management should focus on intensive insulin therapy, ranging from intravenous insulin protocols in the ICU to subcutaneous insulin regimens on the ward. First-line regimens for outpatient management of PTDM include the sulfonylureas, TZDs, or subcutaneous insulin therapy. For optimal management of difficult cases, specialty input may be required. Recognizing that PTDM (like T2DM) is associated with cardiovascular complications, careful attention should be paid to managing risk factors including hypertension, dyslipidemia, and prothrombotic states. Careful screening for diabetic complications is also warranted.

References

[1] Viberti G. Diabetes mellitus: a major challenge in transplantation. Transplant Proc 2001; 33(Suppl 5A):3S–7S.

[2] Woo M, Przepiorka D, Ippoliti C, et al. Toxicities of tacrolimus and cyclosporine A after allogeneic blood stem cell transplantation. Bone Marrow Transplant 1997;20:1095–8.

[3] Reisaeter AV, Hartmann A. Risk factors and incidence of posttransplant diabetes mellitus. Transplant Proc 2001;33(Suppl 5A):8S–18S.

[4] Jindal RM, Hjelmesaeth J. Impact and management of posttransplant diabetes mellitus. Transplantation 2000;70(Suppl):SS58–63.

[5] Kasiske BL, Guijarro C, Massy ZA, et al. Cardiovascular disease after renal transplantation. J Am Soc Nephrol 1996;7:158–65.

[6] Lindholm A, Albrechtsen D, Frodin L, et al. Ischemic heart disease—major cause of death and graft loss after renal transplantation in Scandinavia. Transplantation 1995;60:451–7.

[7] Ojo AO, Hanson JA, Wolfe RA, et al. Long-term survival in renal transplant recipients with graft function. Kidney Int 2000;57:307–13.

[8] Markovitz LJ, Wiechmann RJ, Harris N, et al. Description and evaluation of a glycemic management protocol for patients with diabetes undergoing heart surgery. Endocr Pract 2002;8:10–8.

[9] Miles AMV, Nabil S, Horowitz R, et al. Diabetes mellitus after renal transplantation: as deleterious as non-transplant-associated diabetes? Transplantation 1998;65:380–4.

[10] Chilcott JB, Whitby SM, Moore R. Clinical impact and health economic consequences of posttransplant type 2 diabetes mellitus. Transplant Proc 2001;33(Suppl 5A):32S–9S.

[11] Ekstrand AV, Eriksson JG, Gronhagen-Riska C, et al. Insulin resistance and insulin deficiency in the pathogenesis of posttransplant diabetes in man. Transplantation 1992;53: 563–9.

[12] Midtvedt K, Hartmann A, Hjelmesaeth J, et al. Insulin resistance is a common denominator of post-transplant diabetes mellitus and impaired glucose tolerance in renal transplant recipients. Nephrol Dial Transplant 1998;13:427–31.

[13] Nam JH, Mun JI, Kim SI, et al. B-cell dysfunction rather than insulin resistance is the main contributing factor for the development of postrenal transplantation diabetes mellitus. Transplantation 2001;71:1417–23.

[14] Hagen M, Hjelmesaeth J, Jenssen T, et al. A 6-year prospective study on new onset diabetes mellitus, insulin release and insulin sensitivity in renal transplant recipients. Nephrol Dial Transplant 2003;18:2154–9.

[15] Weir M. Impact of immunosuppressive regimens on posttransplant diabetes mellitus. Transplant Proc 2001;33(Suppl 5A):23S–6S.

[16] Montori VM, Basu A, Erwin PJ, et al. Posttransplantation diabetes: a systematic review of the literature. Diabetes Care 2002;25:583–92.

[17] Meachem LR, Abdul-Latif H, Sullivan K, et al. Predictors of change in insulin sensitivity during glucocorticoid treatment. Horm Metab Res 1997;29:172–5.

[18] Hjelmesaeth J, Hartmann A, Kofstad J, et al. Glucose intolerance after renal transplantation depends on prednisolone dose and recipient age. Transplantation 1997;64:979–83.

[19] Van Hooff JP, Christians MHL, van Duijnhoven EM. Evaluating mechanisms of post-transplant diabetes mellitus. Nephrol Dial Transplant 2004;19(Suppl 6):vi8–12.

[20] Knoll GA, Bell RC. Tacrolimus versus cyclosporine for immunosuppression in renal transplantation: meta-analysis of randomized trials. BMJ 1999;318:1104–7.

[21] Heisel O, Heisel R, Balshaw R, et al. New-onset diabetes mellitus in patients receiving calcineurin inhibitors: a systematic review and meta-analysis. Am J Transplant 2004;4:583–95.

[22] Zerr KJ, Furnary AP, Grunkemeier GL, et al. Glucose control lowers the risk of wound infection in diabetics after open heart operations. Ann Thorac Surg 1997;63:356–61.

[23] Pomposelli JJ, Baxter JK III, Babineau TJ, et al. Early postoperative glucose control predicts nosocomial infection rate in diabetic patients. J Parenter Enteral Nutr 1998;22:77–81.

[24] Umpierrez GE, Isaacs SD, Bazargan N, et al. Hyperglycemia: an independent marker of in-hospital mortality in patients with undiagnosed diabetes. J Clin Endocrinol Metab 2002;87: 978–82.

[25] Furnary AP, Zerr KJ, Grunkmeier GL, et al. Continuous intravenous insulin infusion reduces the incidence of deep sternal wound infection in diabetic patients after cardiac surgical procedures. Ann Thorac Surg 1999;67:352–62.

[26] Furnary AP, Gao G, Grunkemeier GL, et al. Continuous insulin infusion reduces mortality in patients undergoing coronary artery bypass grafting. J Thorac Cardiovasc Surg 2003;125: 1007–21.

[27] Van den Berghe G, Wouters P, Weekers F, et al. Intensive insulin therapy in critically ill patients. N Engl J Med 2001;345:1359–67.

[28] Cheung NW, Wong VW, McLean M. The Hyperglycemia: Intensive Insulin Infusion in Infarction (HI-5) study: a randomized controlled trial of insulin infusion therapy for myocardial infarction. Diabetes Care 2006;29:765–70.

[29] Van den Berghe G, Wilmer A, Hermans G, et al. Intensive insulin therapy in the medical ICU. N Engl J Med 2006;354:449–61.

[30] Van den Berghe G, Wilmer A, Milants I, et al. Intensive insulin therapy in mixed medical/surgical intensive care units: benefit versus harm. Diabetes 2006;55:3151–9.

[31] Clement S, Braithwaite SS, Magee MF, et al. On behalf of the Diabetes in Hospitals Writing Committee. Diabetes Care 2004;27:553–91.

[32] American College of Endocrinology Task Force on Inpatient Diabetes and Metabolic Control. American College of Endocrinology position statement on inpatient diabetes and metabolic control. Endocr Pract 2004;10:77–82.

[33] DeSantis AJ, Schmeltz LR, Schmidt K, et al. Inpatient management of hyperglycemia: the Northwestern experience. Endocr Pract 2006;12:491–505.

[34] Goldberg PA, Siegel MD, Sherwin RS, et al. Implementation of a safe and effective insulin infusion protocol in a medical intensive care unit. Diabetes Care 2004;27:461–7.

[35] Goldberg PA, Roussel MG, Inzucchi SE. Clinical results of an updated insulin infusion protocol in critically ill patients. Diabetes Spectrum 2005;18:188–91.

[36] Goldberg PA, Inzucchi SE. Selling root canals: lessons learned from implementing a hospital insulin infusion protocol. Diabetes Spectrum 2005;18:28–33.

[37] Markell M. Clinical impact of posttransplant diabetes mellitus. Transplant Proc 2001; 33(Suppl 5A):19S–22S.

[38] Trence DL, Kelly JL, Hirsch IB. The rationale and management of hyperglycemia for inpatients with cardiovascular disease: time for change. J Clin Endocrinol Metab 2003;88: 2430–7.

[39] Bode BW, Braithwaite SS, Steed RD, et al. Intravenous insulin therapy: indications, methods, and transition to subcutaneous insulin therapy. Endocr Pract 2004;10(Suppl 2): 71–80.

[40] Abern M, Boland E, Rothenberg DM, et al. Intensive insulin therapy (IIT) after coronary artery bypass graft (CABG) surgery: from latest IV infusion rate, provide 8 times rate as NPH insulin plus 4 times rate as regular insulin [abstract]. Diabetes 2004;53(suppl 2):A116.

[41] Inzucchi SE. Clinical practice: management of hyperglycemia in the hospital setting. N Engl J Med 2006;355:1903–11.

[42] Hirsch IB. Drug therapy: insulin analogues. N Engl J Med 2005;352:174–83.

[43] Diabetes Control and Complications Trial Research Group. The effect of intensive treatment of diabetes on the development and progression of long-term complications in insulin-dependent diabetes mellitus. N Engl J Med 1993;329:977–86.

[44] United Kingdom Prospective Diabetes Group. Intensive blood-glucose control with sulfonylureas or insulin compared with conventional treatment and risk of complications in patients with type 2 diabetes (UKPDS 33). Lancet 1998;352:837–53.

[45] United Kingdom Prospective Diabetes Group. Tight blood pressure control and risk of macrovascular complications in type 2 diabetes (UKPDS 38). BMJ 1998;317:703–13.

[46] Hjelmesaeth J, Jenssen T, Hartmann A. Diagnosing PTDM [letter]. Transplantation 2003; 75:1761.

[47] Davidson J, Wilkinson A, Dantal J, et al. New-onset diabetes after transplantation: 2003 international consensus guidelines. Transplantation 2003;75(suppl):SS3–24.

[48] American Diabetes Association. Standards of medical care in diabetes—2007. Diabetes Care 2007;30(Suppl 1):S4–41.

[49] American Diabetes Association. Diagnosis and classification of diabetes mellitus. Diabetes Care 2007;30(Suppl 1):S42–7.

[50] Shah A, Kendall G, Demme RA, et al. Home glucometer monitoring markedly improves diagnosis of post renal transplant diabetes mellitus in renal transplant recipients. Transplantation 2005;80:775–81.

[51] Hoban R, Gielda B, Temkit M, et al. Utility of HbA1c in the detection of subclinical post renal transplant diabetes. Transplantation 2006;81:379–83.

[52] Sherwin RS. Diabetes mellitus. In: Arend WP, Armitage JO, Drzaen JM, editors. Cecil textbook of medicine. 22nd edition. Philadelphia: W.B. Saunders; 2004.

[53] Kirpichnikov D, MacFarlane SI, Sowers JR. Metformin: an update. Ann Intern Med 2002; 137:25–33.

[54] Baldwin D Jr, Duffin KE. Rosiglitazone treatment of diabetes mellitus after solid organ transplantation. Transplantation 2004;77:1009–14.

[55] Villaneuva G, Baldwin D. Rosiglitazone therapy of posttransplant diabetes mellitus. Transplantation 2005;80:1402–5.

[56] Del Prato S, Aragona M, Copelli A. Sulfonylureas and hypoglycaemia. Diabetes Nutr Metab 2002;15:444–50.

[57] Willi SM, Kennedy A, Wallace P, et al. Troglitazone antagonizes metabolic effects of glucocorticoids in humans. Diabetes 2002;51:2895–902.

[58] Willi SM, Kennedy A, Brant BP, et al. Effective use of thiazolidinediones for the treatment of glucocorticoid-induced diabetes. Diabetes Res Clin Pract 2002;58:87–96.

[59] Fujibayashi K, Nagasaka S, Itabashi N, et al. Troglitazone efficacy in a subject with gluco-corticoid-induced diabetes. Diabetes Care 1999;22:2088–9.

[60] Pietruck F, Kribben A, Van TN, et al. Rosiglitazone is a safe and effective treatment option of new-onset diabetes mellitus after renal transplantation. Transpl Int 2005;18:483–6.

[61] Voytovich MH, Simonsen C, Jenssen T, et al. Short-term treatment with rosiglitazone improves glucose tolerance, insulin sensitivity and endothelial function in renal transplant recipients. Nephrol Dial Transplant 2005;20:413–8.

[62] Blickle JF. Meglitinide analogues: a review of clinical data focused on recent trials. Diabetes Metab 2006;32:113–20.

[63] Pasternak JJ, McGregor DG, Lanier WL. Effect of single-dose dexamethasone on blood glucose concentration in patients undergoing craniotomy. J Neurosurg Anesthesiol 2004; 16:122–5.

[64] Boots JMM, Van Duijnhoven EM, Christiaans MHL, et al. Glucose metabolism in renal transplant recipients on tacrolimus: the effect of steroid withdrawal and tacrolimus trough level reduction. J Am Soc Nephrol 2002;13:221–7.

[65] Hjelmesaeth J, Hartmann A, Kofstad J, et al. Tapering off prednisolone and cyclosporine the first year after renal transplantation: the effect on glucose tolerance. Nephrol Dial Transplant 2001;16:829–35.

[66] Midtvedt K, Hjelmesaeth J, Hartmann A, et al. Insulin resistance after renal transplantation: the effect of steroid dose reduction and withdrawal. J Am Soc Nephrol 2004;15:3233–9.

[67] Scantlebury V, Shapiro R, Fung J, et al. Transplant Proc 1991;23:3169–70.

[68] Kanzler S, Lohse AW, Schirmacher P, et al. Complete reversal of FK 506 induced diabetes in a liver transplant recipient by change of immunosuppression to cyclosporine A. Z Gastroenterol 1996;34:128–31.

[69] Lagget M, Marzano A, Actis GC, et al. Disappearance of diabetes mellitus after conversion from FK 506 to Neoral in two liver transplant patients. Transplant Proc 1998;30: 1863–5.

[70] Emre S, Genyk Y, Schluger LK, et al. Treatment of tacrolimus-related adverse events by conversion to cyclosporine in liver transplant recipients. Transpl Int 2000;13:73–8.

[71] Hjelmesaeth J, Hartmann A, Midtvedt K, et al. Metabolic syndrome after renal transplantation. Nephrol Dial Transplant 2001;16:1047–52.

[72] Expert Panel on Detection, Evaluation, and Treatment of High Blood Cholesterol in Adults. Executive summary of the third report of the National Cholesterol Education Program (NCEP) expert panel on detection, evaluation, and treatment of high blood cholesterol in adults (Adult Treatment Panel III). JAMA 2001;285:2486–97.

[73] Chobanian AV, Bakris GL, Black HR, et al. the National High Blood Pressure Education Program Writing Program Coordinating Committee. The seventh report of the Joint National Committee on Prevention, Detection, Evaluation, and Treatment of High Blood Pressure: the JNC 7 report. JAMA 2003;289:2560–72.

[74] Grundy SM, Cleeman JI, Merz CNB, et al. for the Coordinating Committee of the National Cholesterol Education Program. Implications of recent clinical trials for the National Cholesterol Education Program Adult Treatment Panel III guidelines. Circulation 2004; 110:227–39.

ELSEVIER
SAUNDERS

Endocrinol Metab Clin N Am
36 (2007) 923–935

ENDOCRINOLOGY
AND METABOLISM
CLINICS
OF NORTH AMERICA

Calcium and Bone Metabolism Pre- and Post-Kidney Transplantation

Neveen A.T. Hamdy, MD

Department of Endocrinology and Metabolic Diseases,
Leiden University Medical Center, Albinusdreef 2, 2333 ZA Leiden, the Netherlands

Chronic kidney disease (CKD) is associated with significant disturbances in bone and mineral metabolism representing a major cause of skeletal and cardiovascular morbidity, particularly in end-stage CKD. Successful kidney transplantation corrects many of these disturbances, but the degree of improvement is often incomplete, and disorders of bone remodeling may persist or worsen after transplantation. Because the function of a renal graft deteriorates with time, disturbances are likely to reappear within the 10- to 12-year life span of a kidney transplant.

The aim of this article is to review the scope of disturbances in bone and mineral metabolism observed in the patient with end-stage CKD before and after kidney transplantation.

Disturbances in mineral metabolism before kidney transplantation

The pathogenesis of disturbances in bone and mineral metabolism encountered in CKD is complex and multifactorial [1]. Central to the evolution of these disturbances is the mobilization of homeostatic mechanisms to maintain serum calcium and phosphate concentrations within a physiologic range at the expense of an ever-increasing parathyroid hormone (PTH) secretion, PTH synthesis, and parathyroid hyperplasia [2–5].

Hyperphosphatemia

In progressive CKD, a decreasing glomerular filtration rate (GFR) results in a decreased ability of the failing kidney to excrete phosphate. The resulting hyperphosphatemia stimulates constitutive FGF-23 secretion, the

---

E-mail address: n.a.t.hamdy@lumc.nl

phosphaturic effect of which maintains normal phosphate levels until the late stages of CKD at the expense of an increasing concentration of FGF-23 [6,7]. An additional effect of the high levels of FGF-23 is to suppress the activity of the 1α-hydroxylase enzyme, contributing to decreased calcitriol synthesis [8,9]. Phosphate retention also contributes to hyperparathyroidism by directly stimulating pre-pro-PTH mRNA transcription [1]. Although controlling hyperphosphatemia is one of the main goals of the management of bone and mineral metabolism before transplantation, this is often difficult to achieve, and a significant number of patients have increased serum phosphate levels at the time of transplantation.

Calcitriol deficiency

The kidney is the major site of synthesis of the active metabolite of vitamin D, calcitriol, the genomic action of which is mediated by a receptor of the steroid-nuclear receptor superfamily—the vitamin D receptor (VDR). In CKD, the decrease in renal mass results in a progressive decrease in the availability of the 1α-hydroxylase enzyme leading to a decreased synthesis of calcitriol when creatinine clearance falls below 50 to 60 mL/min. Low levels of 25-hydroxyvitamin D, the substrate for calcitriol, are often observed in patients with CKD and contribute to the low calcitriol levels [10]. Hyperphosphatemia and high FGF-23 levels also inhibit the 1α-hydroxylase enzyme, further contributing to the decreased synthesis of calcitriol. Calcitriol deficiency impairs intestinal absorption of calcium, leading to hypocalcemia. Acting through the calcium-sensing receptor (CaSR) on the parathyroids, a decrease in ionized calcium concentration is the most potent stimulus for PTH secretion, synthesis, and, eventually, parathyroid cell proliferation. Independently of prevailing serum calcium concentrations, calcitriol deficiency can also directly stimulate pre-pro-PTH gene transcription. Deficiency of calcitriol also increases the skeletal resistance to the calcemic effect of PTH. These direct and indirect effects of calcitriol deficiency result in continuous stimulation of the parathyroid cells eventually leading to parathyroid cell proliferation and hyperplasia [1–5,11]. In the late stages of CKD, diffuse hyperplasia of the parathyroid glands is associated with a downregulation of both CaSR and VDR, rendering the parathyroids more resistant to the action of calcium and calcitriol. With the further evolution of CKD, monoclonal changes take place leading to nodular hyperplasia of the parathyroid glands with further reduction in the expression of CaSR and VDR [12,13]. The nonsuppressible component of PTH release becomes greater as parathyroid gland mass increases, and autonomous hyperparathyroidism develops, often associated with hypercalcemia. High serum calcium concentrations may also occur as a result of vitamin D intoxication or spontaneously in the absence of increased PTH levels in patients with low turnover or adynamic bone disease. Other causes of hypercalcemia should be excluded.

Disturbances in skeletal metabolism before kidney transplantation

In CKD, the various homeostatic mechanisms set into motion to control mineral metabolism result in a broad spectrum of disturbances in skeletal metabolism collectively termed *renal osteodystrophy*. These disturbances include high or low bone turnover lesions, osteomalacia, and osteoporosis, and any of these bone lesions may be associated with an increased risk for fractures [2–4]. Disturbances in bone metabolism start early in the course of progressive CKD, and histologic abnormalities can be found in 75% of patients with a creatinine clearance of less than 50 mL/min [14]. The pattern of renal osteodystrophy has changed over the years, probably because of the modulating effect of therapeutic interventions. Although hyperparathyroid bone disease remains prominent, there has been a virtual disappearance of aluminum bone disease and a higher prevalence of adynamic bone lesions [15–17]. Over the last decade, there has also been growing awareness about the potential relationship between disturbances in bone and mineral metabolism and cardiovascular morbidity and mortality [18–20].

In hyperparathyroid bone disease, high circulating concentrations of PTH increase the number and activity of osteoclasts and osteoblasts, and most trabecular bone surfaces become occupied by active resorption and formation. The rapid rate of bone turnover results in the haphazard deposition of woven rather than lamellar bone matrix. In severe cases, variable fibrosis in bone marrow cavities results in the histologic pattern of osteitis fibrosa cystica, and fibrous tissue infiltration may lead to bone marrow suppression, contributing to chronic anemia and potential resistance to treatment with erythropoietin. High bone turnover lesions are characteristically associated with increased serum alkaline phosphatase activity and high PTH levels. Hyperphosphatemia is often observed, and hypercalcemia develops when the parathyroids become autonomous. The combination of both mineral abnormalities leads to a high Ca × P product, heightening the risk of extraskeletal and vascular calcifications [18–20].

High bone turnover also has significant effects on the net flux of calcium from bone, with the finite deficit occurring proportional to the rate of bone turnover and leading to a decrease in bone mass and osteoporosis [21]. Bone mass has been shown to progressively decrease in CKD, particularly at cortical sites, proportional to decreases in the GFR [22]. Bone loss is also exacerbated in patients treated with corticosteroids for intrinsic renal disease. Osteomalacia is characterized by an increase in the amount of unmineralized bone matrix. It is most commonly associated with hyperparathyroid bone disease, when it is termed *mixed osteodystrophy*. Severe 25-hydroxyvitamin D deficiency has superseded aluminum intoxication as the main cause of isolated osteomalacia.

At the other end of the spectrum of renal osteodystrophy is the histologic pattern of the adynamic bone lesion, histologically characterized by a paucity of active osteoblasts and osteoclasts, a normal or decreased osteoid seam, and a marked decrease in bone formation with an overall low bone turnover. This lesion is biochemically associated with low serum alkaline phosphatase activity and normal or low PTH levels. Patients tend to develop hypercalcemia spontaneously or following the use of vitamin D metabolites, probably because of failure of calcium accretion into bone by dysfunctional osteoblasts. Pathogenetically, the adynamic bone lesion was originally associated with aluminum bone disease, but this histologic pattern has been increasingly reported in non-users of aluminum-containing phosphate binders. The patients most at risk for an adynamic bone lesion are the elderly, those with iron overload or diabetes mellitus, those treated with calcium salts or continuous ambulatory peritoneal dialysis, those with a history of total parathyroidectomy, and those in whom PTH levels are inappropriately suppressed [17,23,24]. The low bone turnover resulting from cellular insufficiency may potentially increase the risk of microfractures and overt fractures, and adynamic bone disease has also been associated with an increased risk for extraskeletal and vascular calcifications [19,20].

A definition of osteoporosis based strictly on bone mineral density (BMD) is not applicable to CKD patients, because bone quality is altered and fracture risk increased across the spectrum of osteodystrophy [20]. The correlation of BMD with biochemical markers or histologic features is poor, and the risk of fracture cannot be confidently predicted by BMD measurements alone [25]. In end-stage CKD, the prevalence of vertebral fractures is reported to be as high as 21%, and the relative risk for hip fracture is increased by 2- to 14-fold [25–28]. Axial fractures are more frequently seen in patients with low turnover bone disease and appendicular fractures in those with high turnover disease. Other contributory factors to the increased fracture risk include advanced age, menopausal status, glucocorticoid use, nutritional status, and a sedentary lifestyle [29]. A new histologic classification based on bone turnover, mineralization, and volume has recently been proposed for the uniform evaluation of renal osteodystrophy in CKD patients [30].

Management of disturbances in calcium and bone metabolism pre-kidney transplantation

The ultimate goal of treatment of disturbances of bone and mineral metabolism before kidney transplantation remains the prevention of chronic exposure of the skeleton to persistently elevated PTH levels without swaying the pendulum too far by over-suppressing PTH secretion. Achieving the right balance should prevent bone loss and decrease the risk of fragility fractures as well as prevent the development of vascular and visceral calcifications, thereby significantly reducing morbidity. Control of hyperphosphatemia and correction of calcitriol deficiency are of prime importance, and treatment should be started early if parathyroid hyperplasia is to be prevented or reversed [14]. The Kidney Disease Outcomes Quality Initiative (NKF-KDOQI) clinical practice guidelines for bone metabolism and disease in chronic kidney disease were proposed to achieve these goals by carefully balancing the use of phosphate binders and vitamin D and its analogues [31]. Nevertheless, several publications appearing since the publication of these guidelines have highlighted the difficulties encountered in achieving these goals, and it is rare to encounter an end-stage CKD patient awaiting a transplant who has no underlying disturbance in bone and mineral metabolism.

Disturbances in mineral metabolism after kidney transplantation

The disturbances in bone and mineral metabolism observed after kidney transplantation are largely determined by pre-existing disturbances at the time of transplantation and by factors inherent to the transplant status, such as kidney graft function and the use of immunosuppressive agents [32].

Persistent hyperparathyroidism

Hyperparathyroidism is nearly universal in patients with end-stage CKD. Persistently increased PTH concentrations may be found in as many as 75% of patients a year after transplantation [32–34], largely due to failure of the enlarged parathyroid glands to involute [34–36]. Although PTH concentrations decrease significantly within the first 3 months after transplantation, they are nevertheless found to be normal in only about 50% of patients a year after transplantation [36–39]. A main determinant of persistent hyperparathyroidism after transplantation is the severity of hyperparathyroidism at the time of transplantation, corresponding to pre-transplantation PTH levels. The presence of pre-transplantation hypercalcemia also reflects autonomy of the parathyroid glands, most likely owing to the development of nodular or monoclonal hyperplasia. Other determinants of persistent hyperparathyroidism after transplantation are the number of years on dialysis therapy and failure of establishment of adequate graft function or its subsequent deterioration [38–40]. The role of the commonly observed low levels of 25-hydroxyvitamin D, independent of those of calcitriol, in the pathogenesis of hyperparathyroidism and bone loss after kidney transplantation has also been recently highlighted [31,41–43]. More than 85% of transplant recipients studied cross-sectionally had levels of 25-hydroxyvitamin D below 30 ng/mL [41], and in a study from Spain, hardly lacking in sunshine, only 11.5% of patients had levels of 25-hydroxyvitamin D above 30 ng/mL [43]. Despite the prevalence of persistent autonomous hyperparathyroidism, only about 5% of patients require a parathyroidectomy after kidney transplantation, the indications for which are persistent severe hypercalcemia, which may jeopardize graft function, calciphylaxis, or progressive bone loss associated with fractures [34,44,45].

Post-transplantation hypercalcemia

Persistent post-transplantation hyperparathyroidism is characterized by an autonomous pattern of PTH secretion often associated with overt hypercalcemia and hypophosphatemia [34,36,46]. Hypercalcemia generally develops some weeks after transplantation, possibly related to the removal of the suppressing effect of high doses of corticosteroids used in the immediate postoperative period on bone turnover. It is widely regarded as benign and transient but may be prolonged in as many as 50% of patients. Parameters of bone turnover are often increased in these patients, in which case bisphosphonates, by normalizing bone turnover, may have a calcium-lowering effect, although normocalcemia is rarely achieved owing to the unopposed effect of high PTH levels on renal tubular reabsorption of calcium [47]. A further potential mechanism for transient post-transplant hypercalcemia is the resolution of extraskeletal calcifications [34,48]. Malignant disease must be excluded.

Post-transplantation hypophosphatemia

Hypophosphatemia is reported in as many as 93% of patients in the first few months after kidney transplantation. It is usually transient and asymptomatic, disappearing almost completely a year after transplantation [49,50], although it may persist for up to 10 years [51]. Hyperparathyroidism is an aggravating factor, but low phosphate levels may persist after normalization of PTH levels [50,52–54]. A characteristic feature of post-transplant hypophosphatemia is the association of renal phosphate wasting with inappropriately low calcitriol levels despite the establishment of good renal function [37,39,55]. This association is analogous to that observed in disorders of FGF-23 excess in which high levels of FGF-23 induce phosphaturia while inhibiting the renal 1α-hydroxylase enzyme [56]. It has been postulated that the persistent hypophosphatemia observed after successful kidney transplantation may be due primarily to persistence of high levels of FGF-23 after establishment of good renal function rather than to persistently elevated PTH levels. Although serum FGF-23 levels were shown to decrease by 50%, 4 to 5 days after transplantation, they remained 10-fold increased, and an inverse correlation was observed between serum FGF-23 and phosphorus levels [57]. There was also a strong correlation between persistently elevated FGF-23 levels and persistently suppressed calcitriol levels [58]. Renal phosphate wasting may also persist long after normalization of serum phosphate [59]. Other pathogenetic factors for post-transplant hypophosphatemia include the impact of immunosuppressive agents. High-dose glucocorticoids and tacrolimus have both been linked to renal phosphate wasting after kidney transplantation although not after other solid organ transplants in which these agents are used at even higher doses [60]. The importance of persistent post-transplant hypophosphatemia lies in its potential to induce mineralization defects, a characteristic feature of bone disease after kidney transplantation, which may occur despite normal concentrations of 25-hydroxyvitamin D [61,62]. Persistent hypophosphatemia is also associated with cardiovascular morbidity in the form of cardiac arrhythmias and can lead to impaired muscle contractility, respiratory failure, and neurologic complications [63].

Although treatment with phosphorus has been recommended in the management of persistent hypophosphatemia after kidney transplantation [31], caution should be advocated with its use because it may increase PTH concentrations and inhibit calcitriol production, as well as further stimulate FGF-23 secretion, potentially worsening renal phosphate wasting rather than improving it. Phosphorus administration should only be considered in severe persistent hypophosphatemia, when it should be used in conjunction with active metabolites of vitamin D [64].

Bone disease after kidney transplantation

Over the last 2 decades, post-transplantation bone disease has emerged as a common and challenging complication of the transplantation process [31,32,65–67]. As outlined previously, the kidney transplant recipient comes to transplantation with the unique disadvantage among other solid organ recipients of having a form of pre-existing renal osteodystrophy, which is difficult to predict from routine laboratory or radiologic investigations and which may persist, improve, or worsen after transplantation. The most important features of bone disease after kidney transplantation include the development or worsening of pre-existing osteoporosis and an increased risk for fractures, which may or may not be related to bone loss. Since the widespread use of newer immunosuppressants, there has been a clear decrease in the risk of osteonecrosis, although the morbidity associated with this skeletal pathology when it develops remains appreciable [68].

Prevalence of osteoporosis and fractures after kidney transplantation

The early post-transplantation period is characterized by dramatic bone loss, reported to range between 4% and 9% at the lumbar spine and 5% and 8% at the hip, predominantly attributed to glucocorticoid use [69–75]. Glucocorticoids have been the cornerstone of induction and maintenance of immunosuppression after solid organ transplantation and are still routinely used in most immunosuppression protocols after kidney transplantation. These agents result in profound suppression of bone formation, rapid bone loss, and an increased fracture rate [76,77]. Glucocorticoids also have direct effects on calcium metabolism, decreasing intestinal absorption of calcium and increasing its renal excretion, leading to a negative calcium balance [78].

The calcineurin inhibitors cyclosporine and tacrolimus (FK506) have also been implicated in the bone loss observed after kidney transplantation [79].

Cyclosporine is associated with high turnover bone loss in rat models, but an effect on bone resorption remains controversial in humans [80–82]. Tacrolimus may cause less bone loss than cyclosporine in humans [74,83]. Sirolimus (rapamycin), mycophenolate mofetil, and azathioprine appear to have little effect on bone mass [74,84]. Data from in vitro studies on animal and human cells and in vivo experiments in rodents suggest that the new immunosuppressant everolimus may suppress cathepsin K expression by osteoclasts and may have the potential of inhibiting bone resorption and preventing bone loss [85].

The later transplant phase is characterized by slower bone loss or even recovery of bone mass in the 6 to 18 months after tapering or discontinuing glucocorticoids. Nevertheless, most studies show decreased BMD as long as 20 years after kidney transplantation [73,86]. Other factors contributing to bone loss include age-related factors, menopausal status, hypogonadism, immobilization, and the use of bone-modulating medications such as diuretics [29,31]. The prevalence of osteoporosis is variably reported to be 17% to 49% at the lumbar spine, 11% to 56% at the femoral neck, and 22% to 52% at the distal radius after kidney transplantation. The reported incidence of fractures varies from 5% to 44%, with a fourfold increase when compared with pre-transplantation fracture rates [65–67,87,88]. The fracture rate increases with time after transplantation [65], and fracture is more common in the appendicular than in the axial skeleton [88]. Patients with diabetes have the highest incidence of fractures, reported to be as high as 40% to 49% after transplantation [89].

Histologic patterns of osteodystrophy after kidney transplantation

A double-tetracycline labeled bone biopsy remains the gold standard for the accurate diagnosis of the type of post-transplantation osteodystrophy, but available data are scarce. Underlying bone disease is heterogeneous at the time of transplantation and remains so thereafter [15,16,89–91]. Except for bone alkaline phosphatase, none of the biochemical markers, including PTH concentrations, are useful in predicting histologic findings after kidney transplantation, the same applying for BMD measurements [92,93]. Identifying the nature of the underlying bone disease is of paramount importance because it would provide a better rationale for devising therapies directed at preventing or reversing the bone loss nearly universally observed in long-term survivors of kidney transplantation [17].

Management of disturbed bone and mineral metabolism post-kidney transplantation

The KDOQI [31] and equivalent European guidelines [94] recommend a systematic evaluation of skeletal status, close monitoring of serum calcium, phosphate, and PTH concentrations, yearly BMD measurements, and adjustment of immunosuppressive regimens to the lowest effective dose of glucocorticoids to avoid bone loss, the risk of fractures, and osteonecrosis after kidney transplantation. Nevertheless, a thorough review of all available literature revealed a remarkable scarcity of data-based evidence on which to recommend further management of bone disease after kidney transplantation. Correcting vitamin D deficiency is strongly advised, but it is also suggested that treatment with nitrogen-containing bisphosphonates be considered based on the severity of osteoporosis or rate of bone loss [31,94]. A later systematic review of randomized controlled trials for preventing bone disease in kidney transplant recipients revealed that, although treatment with bisphosphonates, vitamin D analogues, or calcitonin had a favorable effect on BMD when administered at any time after renal transplantation, there were no available data on anti-fracture efficacy for any of the agents or regimens used [94]. Kidney transplant recipients have a different pattern of fracture when compared with postmenopausal women with osteoporosis. Potential concerns with the use of bisphosphonates after kidney transplantation include not only the expected increase in total body retention due to suboptimal renal function but also the presence of a difficult to predict complex underlying skeletal pathology, including low bone turnover or adynamic bone disease in kidney transplant recipients [17]. In this setting, the therapeutic implications of using bisphosphonates should include the possibility that further suppression of bone remodeling, even if resulting in increases in bone mass, may potentially not be associated with an improvement in bone quality or with a reduction in fracture risk. For all of these reasons, and although it is seemingly reasonable and desirable to treat kidney transplant patients at high risk for fractures with bisphosphonates, caution should be advocated with the use of these agents until firm evidence is obtained from large randomized controlled trials on their long-term efficacy and safety after kidney transplantation [95,96]. More specific aspects of the management of post-transplant osteoporosis are detailed elsewhere in this issue.

References

[1] Slatopolsky E, Delmez JA. Pathogenesis of secondary hyperparathyroidism. Am J Kidney Dis 1994;23:229–36.
[2] Elder G. Pathophysiology and recent advances in the management of renal osteodystrophy. J Bone Miner Res 2002;17:2094–105.
[3] Hruska KA, Teitelbaum SL. Renal osteodystrophy. N Engl J Med 1995;333:166–74.
[4] Kanis JA, Cundy T, Hamdy NAT. Renal osteodystrophy. In: Martin TJ, editor. Metabolic bone disease. Baillieres Clin Endocrinol Metab 1998;2:193–241.
[5] Goodman WG, Quarles LD. Development and progression of secondary hyperparathyroidism in chronic kidney disease: lessons from molecular genetics. Kidney Int 2007;1–13 [online publication].
[6] Larsson T, Nisbeth U, Ljunggreen O, et al. Circulating concentration of FGF-23 increases as renal function declines in patients with chronic kidney disease, but does not change in response to phosphate intake in healthy volunteers. Kidney Int 2003;64:2272–9.

[7] Imanishi Y, Inaba M, Nakatsuka K, et al. FGF-23 in patients with end-stage renal disease on hemodialysis. Kidney Int 2004;65:1943–6.

[8] Gutierrez O, Isakova T, Rhee E, et al. Fibroblast growth factor-23 mitigates hyperphosphatemia but accentuates calcitriol deficiency in chronic kidney diseases. J Am Soc Nephrol 2005;16:2205–15.

[9] Shigematsu T, Kazama JJ, Yamashita T, et al. Possible involvement of circulating fibroblast growth factor 23 in the development of secondary hyperparathyroidism associated with renal insufficiency. Am J Kidney Dis 2004;44:250–6.

[10] LaClair RE, Hellman RN, Karp SL, et al. Prevalence of calcidiol deficiency in CKD: a cross-sectional study across latitudes in the United States. Am J Kidney Dis 2005;45:1026–33.

[11] Parfitt AM. The hyperparathyroidism of chronic renal failure: a disorder of growth. Kidney Int 1997;52:3–9.

[12] Kifor O, Moore FD Jr, Wang P, et al. Reduced immunostaining for the extracellular Ca2+-sensing receptor in primary, uremic hyperparathyroidism. J Clin Endocrinol Metab 1996;81: 1598–606.

[13] Tokumoto M, Tsuruya K, Fukuda K, et al. Reduced p21, p27 and vitamin D receptor in the nodular hyperplasia in patients with advanced secondary hyperparathyroidism. Kidney Int 2002;62:1196–207.

[14] Hamdy NAT, Kanis JA, Beneton MNC, et al. Effect of alfacalcidol on natural course of renal bone disease in mild to moderate renal failure. Br Med J 1995;310:358–63.

[15] Hamdy NAT. The spectrum of renal bone disease. Nephrol Dial Transplant 1995;10(Suppl 4):14–8.

[16] Sherrard DJ, Hercz G, Pei Y, et al. The spectrum of bone disease in end-stage renal failure: an evolving disorder. Kidney Int 1993;43:436–42.

[17] Goodman WG. Perspectives on renal bone disease. Kidney Int 2006;70:S59–63.

[18] Block GA. Prevalence and clinical consequences of elevated Ca × P product in hemodialysis patients. Clin Nephrol 2000;54:318–24.

[19] Goldsmith D, Ritz E, Covic A. Vascular calcification: a stiff challenge for the nephrologist. Does preventing bone disease cause arterial disease? Kidney Int 2004;66:1315–33.

[20] Ketteler M, Gross ML, Ritz E. Calcification and cardiovascular problems in renal failure. Kidney Int 2005;94(Suppl):S120–7.

[21] Cunningham J, Sprague SM. Osteoporosis Work Group: osteoporosis in chronic kidney disease. Am J Kidney Dis 2004;43:566–71.

[22] Rix M, Andreassen H, Eskildsen P, et al. Bone mineral density and biochemical markers of bone turnover in patients with predialysis chronic renal failure. Kidney Int 1999;56:1084–93.

[23] Hercz G, Pei Y, Greenwood C, et al. Aplastic osteodystrophy without aluminum: the role of "suppressed" parathyroid function. Kidney Int 1993;44:860–6.

[24] Sherrard DJ, Hercz G, Pei Y, et al. The aplastic form of renal osteodystrophy. Nephrol Dial Transplant 1996;11(Suppl 3):29–31.

[25] Atsumi K, Kushida K, Yamazaki K, et al. Risk factors for vertebral fractures in renal osteodystrophy. Am J Kidney Dis 1999;33:287–93.

[26] Alem AM, Sherrard DJ, Gillen DL, et al. Increased risk of hip fracture among patients with end-stage renal disease. Kidney Int 2000;58:396–9.

[27] Coco M, Rush H. Increased incidence of hip fractures in dialysis patients with low serum parathyroid hormone. Am J Kidney Dis 2000;36:1115–21.

[28] Stehman-Breen CO, Sherrard DJ, Alem AM, et al. Risk factors for hip fracture among patients with end-stage renal failure. Kidney Int 2000;58:2200–5.

[29] NIH Consensus Development Panel on Osteoporosis Prevention, Diagnosis and Therapy. Osteoporosis prevention, diagnosis, and therapy. JAMA 2001;285:785–95.

[30] Moe S, Drueke T, Cunningham J, et al. Definition, evaluation and classification of renal osteodystrophy: a position statement from Kidney Disease: Improving Global Outcomes (KDIGO). Kidney Int 2006;69:1945–53.

[31] National Kidney Foundation. K-DOQI clinical practice guidelines for bone metabolism and disease. Am J Kidney Dis 2003;42(Suppl 3):S1–202.
[32] Torres A, Lorenzo V, Salido E. Calcium metabolism and skeletal problems after transplantation. J Am Soc Nephrol 2002;13:551–8.
[33] Reinhardt W, Bartelworth H, Jockenhovel F, et al. Sequential changes of biochemical parameters after kidney transplantation. Nephrol Dial Transplant 1998;13:436–42.
[34] Parfitt AM. Hypercalcemic hyperparathyroidism following renal transplantation: differential diagnosis, management and implications for cell population control in the parathyroid gland. Miner Electrolyte Metab 1982;8:92–112.
[35] Alsina J, Gonzales MT, Bonnin R, et al. Long-term evolution of renal osteodystrophy after renal transplantation. Transplant Proc 1989;21:2151–8.
[36] Messa P, Sindici C, Canella G, et al. Persistent secondary hyperparathyroidism after renal transplantation. Kidney Int 1998;54:1704–13.
[37] Claesson K, Hellman P, Frodin L, et al. Prospective study of calcium homeostasis after renal transplantation. World J Surg 1998;22:635–41.
[38] Evenepoel P, Claes K, Kuyper D, et al. Natural history of parathyroid function and calcium metabolism after kidney transplantation: a single center study. Nephrol Dial Transplant 2004;19:1281–7.
[39] Saha HH, Salmela KT, Ahonen PJ, et al. Sequential changes in vitamin D and calcium metabolism after successful renal transplantation. Scand J Urol Nephrol 1994;28:21–7.
[40] McCarron DA, Muther RS, Lenfesty B, et al. Parathyroid function in persistent hyperparathyroidism: relationship to gland size. Kidney Int 1982;22:662–70.
[41] Lomonte C, Antonelli M, Vernaglione L, et al. Are low plasma levels of 25-(OH) vitamin D a major risk factor for hyperparathyroidism independent of calcitriol in renal transplant patients? J Nephrol 2005;18:96–101.
[42] De Sevaux RG, Hoitsma AJ, van Hood HJ, et al. Abnormal vitamin D metabolism and loss of bone mass after renal transplantation. Nephron Clin Pract 2003;93:C21–8.
[43] Gomez Alonso G, Naves Diaz M, Rodriguez Garcia M, et al. Review of the concept of vitamin D "sufficiency and insufficiency". Nefrologia 2003;23(Suppl 2):S73–7.
[44] D'Alessandro AM, Melzer JS, Pirsch JD, et al. Tertiary hyperparathyroidism after renal transplantation: operative indications. Surgery 1989;106:1049–55.
[45] Schmid T, Muller P, Spelsberg F. Parathyroidectomy after renal transplantation: a retrospective analysis of long-term outcome. Nephrol Dial Transplant 1997;12:2393–6.
[46] Cundy T, Kanis JA, Heynen G, et al. Calcium metabolism and hyperparathyroidism after renal transplantation. Q J Med 1983;205:67–8.
[47] Hamdy NAT, Gray RES, McCloskey EV, et al. Clodronate in the medical management of hyperparathyroidism. Bone 1987;8:S69–77.
[48] McGregor D, Burn J, Lynn K, et al. Rapid resolution of tumoral calcinosis after renal transplantation. Clin Nephrol 1999;51:54–8.
[49] Ambuhl PM, Meier D, Wolf B, et al. Metabolic aspects of phosphate replacement therapy for hypophosphatemia after renal transplantation: impact on muscular phosphate content, mineral metabolism and acid/base homeostasis. Am J Kidney Dis 1999;34:875–83.
[50] Levi M. Post-transplant hypophosphatemia. Kidney Int 2001;59:2377–87.
[51] Felsenfeld AJ, Gutman RA, Drezner M, et al. Hypophosphatemia in long-term renal transplant recipients: effects on bone histology and 1,25-dihydroxycholecalciferol. Miner Electrolyte Metab 1986;12:333–41.
[52] Parfitt AM, Kleerekoper M, Cruz C. Reduced phosphate reabsorption unrelated to parathyroid hormone after renal transplantation: implications for the pathogenesis of hyperparathyroidism in chronic renal failure. Miner Electrolyte Metab 1986;12:356–62.
[53] Rosenbaum RW, Hruska KA, Korkor A, et al. Decreased phosphate reabsorption after renal transplantation: evidence for a mechanism independent of calcium and parathyroid hormone. Kidney Int 1981;19:568–78.

[54] Green J, Debby H, Lederer E, et al. Evidence for a PTH-independent humoral mechanism in post-transplant hypophosphatemia and phosphaturia. Kidney Int 2001;60:1182–96.

[55] Riancho JA, de Francisco AL, del Arco C, et al. Serum levels of 1,25-dihydroxyvitamin D after renal transplantation. Miner Electrolyte Metab 1988;14:332–7.

[56] Shimada T, Hasegawa H, Yamazaki Y, et al. FGF-23 is a potent regulator of vitamin D metabolism and phosphate homeostasis. J Bone Miner Res 2004;19:429–35.

[57] Pande S, Ritter CS, Rothstein M, et al. FGF-23 and sFRP-4 in chronic kidney disease and post-renal transplantation. Nephron Physiol 2006;104:23–32.

[58] Bahn I, Shah A, Holmes J, et al. Post-transplant hypophosphatemia: tertiary "hyper-phosphatoninism?". Kidney Int 2006;70:1486–94.

[59] Ghanekar H, Welch BJ, Moe OW, et al. Post-renal transplantation hypophosphatemia: a review and novel insights. Curr Opin Nephrol Hypertens 2006;15:97–104.

[60] Falkiewicz K, Nahaczewska W, Boratynska M, et al. Tacrolimus decreases tubular phosphate wasting in renal allograft recipients. Transplant Proc 2003;35:2213–5.

[61] Carlini RG, Rojas E, Weisinger JR, et al. Bone disease in patients with long-term renal transplantation and normal renal function. Am J Kidney Dis 2000;36:160–6.

[62] Monier-Faugere MC, Mawad H, Qi Q, et al. High prevalence of low bone turnover and occurrence of osteomalacia after kidney transplantation. J Am Soc Nephrol 2000;11:1093–9.

[63] Rubin MF, Narins RG. Hypophosphatemia: pathophysiological and practical aspects of its therapy. Semin Nephrol 1990;10:536–45.

[64] Caravaca F, Fernadez MA, Ruiz-Calero R, et al. Effects of oral phosphorus supplementation on mineral metabolism of renal transplant recipients. Nephrol Dial Transplant 1998; 13:2605–11.

[65] Sprague SM, Josephson MA. Bone disease after kidney transplantation. Semin Nephrol 2004;24:82–90.

[66] Cunningham J. Post-transplantation bone disease. Transplantation 2005;79:629–34.

[67] Maalouf NM, Shane E. Osteoporosis after solid organ transplantation. J Clin Endocrinol Metab 2005;90:2456–65.

[68] Hamdy NAT. Osteonecrosis and organ transplantation. In: Compston J, Shane E, editors. Bone disease of organ transplantation. London: Elsevier Academic Press; 2005. p. 353–71.

[69] Julian BA, Laskow DA, Dubovsky J, et al. Rapid loss of vertebral mineral density after renal transplantation. N Engl J Med 1991;325:544–50.

[70] Kwan JT, Almond MK, Evans K, et al. Changes in total body bone mineral content and regional bone mineral density in renal patients following renal transplantation. Miner Electrolyte Metab 1992;18:166–8.

[71] Epstein S, Inzerillo AM, Caminis J, et al. Disorders associated with acute rapid and severe bone loss. J Bone Miner Res 2003;18:2083–94.

[72] Almond MK, Kwan JT, Evans K, et al. Loss of regional bone mineral density in the first 12 months after renal transplantation. Nephron 1994;66:52–7.

[73] Grotz WH, Mundinger FA, Gugel B, et al. BMD after kidney transplantation: a cross-sectional study in 190 graft recipients up to 20 years after transplantation. Transplantation 1995;7:982–6.

[74] Aroldi A, Tarantino A, Montagnino G, et al. Effects of three immunosuppressive regimens on vertebral bone density in renal transplant recipients: a prospective study. Transplantation 1997;63:380–6.

[75] Pichette V, Bonnardeaux A, Prudhomme L, et al. Long-term bone loss in kidney transplant recipients: a cross-sectional and longitudinal study. Am J Kidney Dis 1996;28: 105–14.

[76] Canalis E. Mechanisms of glucocorticoid action in bone: implications to glucocorticoid-induced osteoporosis. J Clin Endocrinol Metab 1996;81:3441–7.

[77] Weinstein RS, Jilka RL, Parfitt AM, et al. Inhibition of osteoblastogenesis and promotion of apoptosis of osteoblasts and osteocytes by glucocorticoids: potential mechanisms of their deleterious effects on bone. J Clin Invest 1998;102:274–82.

[78] Canalis E. Mechanisms of glucocorticoid-induced osteoporosis. Curr Opin Rheumatol 2003; 15:454–7.
[79] Epstein S. Post-transplantation bone disease: the role of immunosuppressive agents and the skeleton. J Bone Miner Res 1995;11:1–7.
[80] Grotz W, Mundinger A, Gugel B, et al. Missing impact of cyclosporine on osteoporosis in renal transplant recipients. Transplant Proc 1994;26:2652–3.
[81] McIntyre HD, Menzies B, Rigby R, et al. Long-term bone loss after renal transplantation: comparison of immunosuppressive regimen. Clin Transplant 1995;9:20–4.
[82] Westeel FP, Mazouz H, Ezaitouni F, et al. Cyclosporine bone remodeling effect prevents steroid osteopenia after kidney transplantation. Kidney Int 2000;58:1788–96.
[83] Goffin E, Devogelaer JP, Depresseux G, et al. Evaluation of bone mineral density after renal transplantation under a tacrolimus-based immunosuppression: a pilot study. Clin Nephrol 2003;59:190–5.
[84] Goodman GR, Dissanayake IR, Sodam BR, et al. Immunosuppressant use without bone loss- implications for bone loss after transplantation. J Bone Miner Res 2001;16:72–8.
[85] Kneissel M, Luong-Nguyen N-H, Baptist M, et al. Everolimus suppresses cancellous bone loss, bone formation, and cathepsin K expression by osteoclasts. Bone 2004;35:1144–56.
[86] Durieux S, Mercadal L, Orcel P, et al. BMD and fracture prevalence in long-term kidney graft recipients. Transplantation 2002;74:496–500.
[87] Grotz WH, Mundiger FA, Gugel B, et al. Bone fracture and osteodensitometry with dual energy X-ray absorptiometry in kidney transplant recipients. Transplantation 1994;58: 912–5.
[88] Ramsey-Goldman R, Dunn JE, Dunlop DD, et al. Increased risk of fracture in patients receiving solid organ transplants. J Bone Miner Res 1999;14:456–63.
[89] Nisbeth U, Lindh E, Junghall S, et al. Increased fracture rate in diabetes mellitus and in females after renal transplantation. Transplantation 1999;67:1218–22.
[90] Bellorin-Font E, Rojas E, Carlini RG, et al. Bone remodeling after renal transplantation. Kidney Int 2003;63:S125–8.
[91] Cueto-Manzano AM, Konel S, Hutchinson AJ, et al. Bone loss in long-term renal transplantation: histopathology and densitometry analysis. Kidney Int 1999;55:2021–9.
[92] Cruz EAS, Lugon JR, Jorgetti V, et al. Histologic evolution of bone disease 6 months after successful kidney transplantation. Am J Kidney Dis 2004;44:747–56.
[93] Bravenboer N, Lips P, Holzmann PJ, et al. Bone alkaline phosphatase activity as a predictor of bone histomorphometric parameters of bone turnover a year after successful kidney transplantation. J Bone Miner Res 2003;18(Suppl 2):S394.
[94] European best practice guidelines for renal transplantation. Section IV. Long-term management of the transplant recipient. Nephrol Dial Transplant 2002;17(Suppl 4):43–8.
[95] Palmer S, McGregor DO, Strippoli GF. Interventions for preventing bone disease in kidney transplant recipients. Cochrane Database Syst Rev 2005;18:CD005015.
[96] Weber TJ, Quarles LD. Preventing bone loss after renal transplantation with bisphosphonates: we can but should we? Kidney Int 2000;57:735–7.

ELSEVIER
SAUNDERS

Endocrinol Metab Clin N Am
36 (2007) 937–963

ENDOCRINOLOGY
AND METABOLISM
CLINICS
OF NORTH AMERICA

Post-Transplantation Osteoporosis

Emily Stein, MD[a], Peter Ebeling, MD[b],
Elizabeth Shane, MD[a],*

[a]Division of Endocrinology, Department of Medicine, College of Physicians & Surgeons,
Columbia University, 630 West 168th Street, PH8-864, New York, NY 10032, USA
[b]Department of Medicine, Western Hospital, The University of Melbourne,
Gordon Street, Footscray, Victoria 3011, Australia

Survival after solid-organ and bone marrow transplantation (BMT) has improved markedly during the past 2 decades, mainly because of the addition of calcineurin inhibitors, cyclosporine A (CsA) and tacrolimus, to posttransplantation immunosuppressive regimens. With improved survival has come a greater appreciation of complications such as osteoporosis and vertebral fractures that adversely influence patients' quality of life. Osteoporosis after transplantation is related both to pretransplantation factors and to early, rapid posttransplantation bone loss, probably caused by the concomitant administration of high-dose glucocorticoids (GCs) and calcineurin inhibitors. This article discusses the factors that contribute to low bone mass in candidates for transplantation and transplant recipients and the studies that have assessed various treatment strategies for prevention and treatment of transplantation osteoporosis. The reader also is referred to several recent reviews and articles on this topic [1–5] that contain detailed references.

Bone disease in patients awaiting transplantation

A summary of specific factors contributing to bone disease in candidates awaiting transplantation is presented in Box 1.

Chronic kidney disease

Patients who have end-stage kidney disease generally have some form of renal osteodystrophy, the most complex form of pretransplantation bone disease [6]. For a complete discussion of renal osteodystrophy, the reader is referred to the article by Hamdy in this issue.

---

* Corresponding author.
E-mail address: es54@columbia.edu (E. Shane).

0889-8529/07/$ - see front matter © 2007 Elsevier Inc. All rights reserved.
doi:10.1016/j.ecl.2007.07.008   *endo.theclinics.com*

**Box 1. Specific factors contributing to bone disease
in candidates awaiting transplantation**

Heart failure
Renal insufficiency
Vitamin D deficiency and secondary hyperparathyroidism
Failure to attain peak bone mass (in patients who have congenital
    heart disease)
Exposure to loop diuretics, heparin

End-stage liver disease
Vitamin D deficiency and secondary hyperparathyroidism
Low body weight
Alcohol abuse
Cholestasis
Hypogonadism

End-stage lung disease
Hypercapnia
Tobacco use
Glucocorticoids
Pancreatic insufficiency (in patients who have cystic fibrosis)
Hypogonadism (in patients who have cystic fibrosis)
Inactivity (in patients who have cystic fibrosis)
Failure to attain peak bone mass (in patients who have cystic
    fibrosis)

Bone marrow transplant recipients
Glucocorticoids
Hypogonadism
Growth hormone deficiency (in children)

Congestive heart failure

Approximately 8% to 10% of patients awaiting cardiac transplantation meet World Health Organization criteria for osteoporosis, and 40% to 50% have low bone mass [7]. Mild renal insufficiency, vitamin D deficiency, secondary hyperparathyroidism (SHPT), and biochemical evidence of increased bone resorption are seen frequently in patients who have end-stage congestive heart failure and may contribute to the prevalence of low BMD among these patients.

End-stage liver disease

Patients who have end-stage liver disease have numerous risk factors that predispose them to the development of abnormal mineral metabolism, osteoporosis, and fractures [4,8]. Studies have reported osteoporosis at the spine or hip (T score < -2.5 or Z score < -2) in 11% to 52% of patients awaiting liver transplantation [2,9–12]. In a recent study of 243 candidates for liver transplantation [13], serum concentrations of 25-hydroxyvitamin D (25-OHD), parathyroid hormone (PTH), osteocalcin, and testosterone were significantly lower than in healthy controls [9]. Low bone mineral density (BMD) in this group was associated with older age, lower body weight, and the presence of cholestatic liver disease [9].

Chronic respiratory failure

Hypoxia, hypercapnia, tobacco use, and GCs contribute to the extremely high prevalence of osteoporosis in patients awaiting lung transplantation [14,15]. Osteoporosis, defined either by World Health Organization BMD criteria or as a BMD Z score of -2.0 or lower, has been reported in 29% to 61% of patients who have end-stage pulmonary disease. A recent study found that chronic GC use, low body mass index, and worse pulmonary function were associated with low BMD [16]. In patients who have cystic fibrosis (CF), additional risk factors (pancreatic insufficiency, vitamin D deficiency, calcium malabsorption, hypogonadism, and inactivity) contribute to low bone mass [17–19]. In adult patients who have CF, vertebral and rib fractures are 10- to 100-fold more common than among the general population. Recent studies also have documented high rates of osteopenia and osteoporosis in patients who have primary pulmonary hypertension [20] and diffuse parenchymal lung disease [21].

Candidates for bone marrow transplantation

Bone loss occurs in BMT candidates as a direct result of their underlying disease and of the various treatments they receive, including chemotherapy and irradiation [22]. In patients studied after chemotherapy but before BMT, osteopenia was present in 24% and osteoporosis was present in in 4% [23]. GCs induce bone loss in these patients through decreases in bone formation and serum 1,25-dihydroxyvitamin D (1,25(OH)$_2$D). Hypogonadism commonly occurs, precipitated by many factors including high-dose chemotherapy, total body irradiation, and GCs. The adverse effects of total body irradiation and chemotherapy on gonadal function are seen more frequently in women, the majority of whom develop ovarian insufficiency, although young, premenarchal girls may recover ovarian function. In most men, testosterone levels decline acutely after BMT and subsequently normalize [24,25]. Long-term impairment of spermatogenesis with elevated follicle-stimulating hormone has been reported in 47% of men [26]. Growth hormone deficiency may contribute to low BMD in children following BMT.

Skeletal effects of immunosuppressive drugs

Glucocorticoids

GCs, well-known causes of osteoporosis, are used in most immuno-suppressive regimens after transplantation. Typically, high doses (eg, $\geq$ 50 mg/d of prednisone or prednisolone) are prescribed immediately after transplantation, with subsequent reduction over several weeks. Doses may be increased transiently during rejection episodes. The extent of GC exposure is determined by several factors, including the type of organ transplanted, the frequency and management of rejection episodes, and the specific practices of different transplantation programs. Newer agents, including CsA, tacrolimus, and, more recently, rapamycin and daclizumab, reduce GC requirements and have enabled some programs to adopt steroid-free regimens. Significant exposure to GCs still occurs in many patients, particularly during the first few months after transplantation, and can result in substantial bone loss.

The skeletal effects of GCs are manifold. GCs decrease osteoblast replication, differentiation, and lifespan. Additionally, they inhibit genes for type I collagen, osteocalcin, insulin-like growth factors, bone morphogenetic proteins and other bone matrix proteins, transforming growth factor beta, and the receptor activator for nuclear factor kappa B ligand (RANK-L). These combined actions result in direct and profound reductions in bone formation. In comparison, the direct effects of GCs on bone resorption are less prominent. GCs may increase bone resorption indirectly through inhibition of gonadal steroid synthesis. Through reduction of intestinal and renal calcium absorption, GCs can induce SHPT. Although hyperparathyroidism is thought to be of minor importance in the pathogenesis of steroid-induced bone loss, it may be substantially more important in the setting of organ transplantation. GCs lower BMD at trabecular sites in particular. Treatment with GCs, even in small doses, is associated with a markedly increased risk of fracture [27].

Calcineurin inhibitors: cyclosporine A and tacrolimus

The introduction of CsA, a small fungal cyclic peptide that inhibits the T-cell phosphatase calcineurin, into transplantation regimens has led to a marked reduction in rejection episodes and improved survival. Recent studies have suggested that calcineurin may regulate both osteoblast [28] and osteoclast differentiation [29]. CsA may cause bone loss by direct effects on calcineurin genes expressed in osteoclasts [30] or indirectly through alterations in T-cell function [31]. CsA reduces T-cell function through suppression of regulatory genes for interleukin-2, interleukin receptors, and the proto-oncogenes H-ras and c-myc [32]. As might therefore be expected, in vitro studies have shown that CsA inhibits bone resorption. In contrast, however, in vivo rodent studies suggest that CsA may have independent adverse effects on bone and mineral metabolism that contribute to posttransplantation bone loss [32]. In the rat, CsA administration resulted in significant losses of trabecular bone, marked increases in resorption and formation, and increased levels of osteocalcin and $1,25(OH)_2D$ [32]. CsA-mediated bone loss is independent of renal function [32], is attenuated by parathyroidectomy [33], is associated with testosterone deficiency [34], and is prevented by antiresorptive agents such as estrogen, raloxifene, calcitonin, and alendronate [32]. Although the results of animal studies suggest that CsA may be responsible for the high-turnover aspects of posttransplantation bone disease, studies of the effects of CsA on the human skeleton have found conflicting results. Several studies of kidney transplant recipients who received CsA but otherwise were managed with a GC-free regimen did not report any bone loss [35–37]. In contrast, a small study found similar rates of bone loss among kidney transplant recipients receiving long-term CsA monotherapy and those taking prednisolone and azathioprine [38]. In another recent study, cumulative CsA dose was associated with bone loss during the first 2 years after transplantation, independent of the effects of steroids [39].

Tacrolimus (FK506), another calcineurin inhibitor, inhibits cytokine gene expression and T-cell activation and proliferation but also causes trabecular bone loss in the rat [32]. The skeletal effects of FK506 in humans are not well studied. Rapid bone loss with FK506 has been reported in both cardiac [40] and liver [41] transplant recipients. There also is evidence, however, that FK506 may cause less bone loss in humans than CsA [42,43], probably because its use permits lower doses of GCs. Liver transplant recipients receiving FK506 were exposed to less prednisone and had significantly higher femoral neck (FN) BMD 2 years after transplantation than those taking CsA [43]. Similarly, in a small group of kidney transplant recipients followed for 1 year, those who received FK506 and low-dose steroids had a small net increase in BMD, compared with a loss in those who received CsA and normal-dose steroids [42].

Other immunosuppressive agents

The effects of other immunosuppressive drugs on BMD and bone metabolism have yet to be elucidated clearly. Azathioprine, mycophenolate mofetil, and sirolimus (rapamycin) do not cause bone loss in the rat model. Recent open-label studies demonstrated that markers of bone turnover, osteocalcin and N-telopeptide, were lower in kidney transplant recipients who received sirolimus than in those who received CsA; it is unclear whether the different drugs resulted in differing rates of bone loss, because BMD was not measured [44]. The skeletal effects of newer agents, including daclizumab, have not been studied. These agents may be beneficial to the skeleton by reducing GC requirements.

Clinical features of transplantation osteoporosis

Kidney and kidney-pancreas transplantation

Osteoporosis following kidney transplantation is discussed in the article by Hamdy in this issue.

Cardiac transplantation

Osteoporosis is prevalent in long-term cardiac transplant recipients; densitometric osteoporosis at the lumbar spine (LS) has been reported in approximately 28% and at the FN in approximately 20%. In a cross-sectional study of long-term heart transplant recipients, low bone density (T score < −1.0) was observed in 26% at the LS and in 66% at the FN [45]. Adults who had received cardiac transplants as adolescents had lower BMD at the LS, FN, and distal radius (DR) than age-matched controls, perhaps because of a failure to achieve peak bone mass [46].

The most rapid rate of bone loss occurs during the first year after transplantation [1,2,47]. BMD at the LS decreases by 3% to 10% over the first 6 months and then seems to stabilize. Some studies have observed partial recovery of LS BMD in later years. BMD at the FN decreases 6% to 11% during the first year and subsequently stabilizes. Perhaps reflecting posttransplantation SHPT, BMD at the proximal radius, a primarily cortical site, declines during the second and third years. More extreme bone loss during the first year is associated with vitamin D deficiency, with testosterone deficiency (in men), and with GC dose in some studies. There may, however, be less bone loss in more recent studies than was documented in the late 1980s and early 1990s [48].

Prevalent vertebral fractures have been found in 22% to 35% of long-term cardiac transplant recipients. In one study, the majority of fractures involved the spine and occurred within the first 6 months after transplantation; the incidence of vertebral fracture was 36% during the first year after cardiac transplantation [49]. In a European study of 105 patients, one third had sustained a vertebral fracture by the end of the third year. Patients who had LS T scores below −1.0 had a threefold increased risk of vertebral fracture [50]. In a more recent study, the incidence of vertebral fractures was 14% during the first posttransplantation year [48].

In the initial period after transplantation, there are transient increases in markers of bone resorption and decreases in markers of bone formation (osteocalcin). These indices typically return to the upper end of the normal range by 6 to 12 months after transplantation. In contrast to the low-turnover state and decreased osteocalcin levels found in patients receiving GCs alone, however, some studies have observed a persistent state of high bone turnover. This elevation may be related to CsA-induced renal insufficiency and resultant SHPT documented by some authors.

Liver transplantation

Osteoporosis also is a common finding after liver transplantation, as has been detailed in several recent reviews [8,51,52]. The progression of bone loss is similar to that following liver and cardiac transplantation [50]. In the first 6 to 12 months, the rates of bone loss and fracture are highest. Early studies reported decreases in spine BMD of 2% to 24%. In contrast, one recent study documented preservation of spinal BMD and bone loss of only 2.3% at the FN during the first year after liver transplantation [53], and another found increases in BMD at 1 year [54]. Fracture rates range from 17% to 65% and, as with cardiac transplantation, most commonly affect the ribs and vertebrae. Several studies have suggested potential risk factors for bone loss and fracture following liver transplantation. Female gender and higher GC dose were associated with lower BMD in cross-sectional [55] and retrospective studies [56]. Whether the type of underlying liver disease predicts bone loss and fracture is controversial. Some authors report higher rates of bone loss and fracture in patients who have alcoholic cirrhosis [57], primary biliary cirrhosis, and primary sclerosing cholangitis [12]. In a study of 360 patients after liver transplantation, higher rates of LS bone loss were seen in recipients who had higher baseline BMD, shorter duration of liver disease, ongoing cholestasis, and younger age, and in smokers [12]. In recent prospective studies, the risk of posttransplantation fractures was related to older age [9] and pretransplantation BMD at the LS and FN [9,11]. Pretransplantation vertebral fractures also have been shown to predict posttransplantation vertebral fractures [50,58]. Recovery of BMD at the LS and hip has been documented during the second and third years after transplantation in patients receiving no treatment to prevent bone loss.

In contrast with the decreased bone formation and low turnover observed before liver transplantation, a state of high turnover is seen afterward. The increase in turnover may result from resolution of cholestasis or hypogonadism, increased PTH secretion, or CsA or FK506 administration. Although PTH levels usually are normal after liver transplantation, significant increases in PTH have been observed during the first 3 to 6 months [9,54], possibly related to a decline in renal function caused by CsA or FK506 treatment and resultant SHPT. Significant elevations in osteoprotegerin and RANK-L levels during the first 2 weeks after liver transplantation [59] provide further evidence of high bone turnover.

Lung transplantation

Osteoporosis is extremely prevalent among lung transplant recipients, seen in up to 73%. Rates of bone loss at the LS and FN range from 2% to 5% in the first year after lung transplantation [1,2,60,61]. Fracture rates also are high, ranging from 18% to 37% during the first year, even in patients who receive antiresorptive therapy. In a 10-year follow-up study, of 28 (29%) of lung transplant recipients who had survived, 11% had prevalent vertebral fractures [62]. Some [63], but not all [64], studies have found a correlation between GC dose and bone loss. Markers of bone turnover reveal increased resorption and formation [64]. In a posttransplantation bone biopsy study of patients who had CF, increased osteoclastic and decreased osteoblastic activity were observed [65].

Bone marrow transplantation

Most patients who undergo BMT or stem cell transplantation for hematologic malignancies survive for many years. Bone loss following allogeneic BMT is related both to treatment effects and direct effects on the bone marrow stromal cell compartment [61,66,67]. The early, rapid bone loss that occurs in these patients also is associated with increased bone resorption and decreased bone formation [24,67,68]. The distinctive pattern of bone loss following allogeneic BMT has been described in several longitudinal studies [24,67–69]. Rapid bone loss occurs in the first 6 to 12 months after BMT and then stabilizes with little additional loss. Although the degree of bone loss is variable, most patients lose more bone from the proximal femur than the spine and total body. The dramatic losses from the proximal femur are not regained, according to studies of long-term BMT survivors [70]. Spinal bone mass may partially recover 6 to 12 months after BMT. Low bone mass (T scores < -1.0) has been found in up to 29% of BMT recipients at the LS and in 52% at the FN [71]. Low BMD in patients who are younger than 18 years at the time of BMT may be related to smaller bone size and a failure to acquire adequate bone mass during adolescence [72]. Rates of bone loss are lower after autologous BMT (about 4%) than after allogeneic BMT. In this group, proximal femoral bone loss occurs as early as 3 months and persists at 2 years, although LS BMD returns to baseline [73].

Many factors contribute to the complex pathogenesis of bone loss after BMT [22], including GC exposure, whether administered before BMT or for treatment of graft-versus-host disease (GVHD), CsA exposure [69], and the direct effects of GVHD on bone cells. Bone turnover after BMT also may be affected by abnormal cellular or cytokine-mediated bone marrow function [74]. Early cytokine release is stimulated by both myeloablative treatment and BMT [74]. Bone marrow osteoprogenitors are damaged by BMT; osteocyte viability is decreased [75], and osteocytes are replaced by differentiation of host stromal cells [76]. Osteoblastic differentiation from osteoprogenitor cells is reduced by many factors including high-dose chemotherapy, total body irradiation, GCs, and CsA. A reduction in colony-forming unit fibroblasts (CFU-f) can be seen for up to 12 years after BMT [66,71]. It is probably through this mechanism that high-dose chemotherapy has adverse effects on bone that are independent of effects on gonadal function [66].

Osteomalacia and avascular necrosis also are common among these patients. Abnormalities in bone resorption markers and vitamin D deficiency can be found in allogeneic BMT survivors, even more than 6 years after BMT [77]. In patients who have vitamin D deficiency and intestinal GVHD, vitamin D repletion improves BMD [78,79]. Avascular necrosis develops in 10% to 20% of allogeneic BMT survivors, usually in the setting of GC treatment for chronic GVHD, typically 12 months after transplantation [69,71]. Avascular necrosis is less common after autologous BMT, occurring in 1.9% of patients. In one study men who had avascular necrosis were shown to have greater FN bone loss [69]. The development of avascular necrosis after BMT may be facilitated by a deficit in bone marrow stromal stem cell regeneration and low osteoblast numbers. In vitro, avascular necrosis seems to be related to decreased numbers of bone marrow CFU-f colonies but not to BMD values [80].

Mechanisms of post-transplantation bone loss

The mechanisms of posttransplantation bone loss and fracture differ depending on the amount of time that has elapsed since transplantation. Table 1 outlines the major factors contributing to bone loss and fractures after transplantation. There seem to be two main phases of bone loss that can be differentiated by the presence or absence of high-dose GCs in the immunosuppressive regimen.

The doses of GCs used during the first 6 months after transplantation profoundly suppress bone formation. Serum markers of bone formation, particularly osteocalcin, are almost universally suppressed in the early posttransplantation period. Urinary markers of bone resorption are consistently elevated

Table 1
Factors contributing to post-transplantation bone loss and fractures

Contributing factors	Mechanisms
Aging	Lower pretransplantation BMD
Hypogonadism	
Calcium and vitamin D deficiencies	
Tobacco use	
Alcohol abuse	
Organ failure	
High-dose prednisone	Decreased bone formation through
	Decreased gonadal function
	Reduced calcium transport
	in the gastrointestinal tract,
	kidneys, and parathyroids
Calcineurin inhibitors:	Increased bone resorption through
cyclosporine or FK506	Decreased renal function and 1,25(OH)$_2$D
	Increased parathyroid hormone secretion
	Possible direct effect

during this period. This increase is related to the suppressive effects of GCs on several systems: osteoblast synthesis of osteoprotegerin, calcium transport across the intestinal, renal tubular, and parathyroid cell membranes, and the hypothalamic-pituitary-gonadal axis. CsA and FK506 have nephrotoxic effects and result in measurable declines in renal function and impaired synthesis of $1,25(OH)_2D$, which results in decreased intestinal calcium transport. Through these mechanisms, both calcineurin inhibitors and GCs have the potential to cause secondary increases in PTH secretion and consequently to increase osteoclast-mediated bone resorption. Both CsA and FK506 also may increase bone resorption directly. Therefore, uncoupling of bone resorption and formation occurs with the simultaneous administration of high-dose GCs and CsA (or FK506). Consequently, bone loss is rapid, and fracture rates are high during this early phase of the posttransplantation period.

As GC doses are tapered (ie, to prednisone doses below 5 mg/d), osteoblast function begins to recover, and there is a recovery of bone formation markers. Bone resorption remains elevated, however, in part because of the persistence of adverse effects of CsA and FK506, which include both direct effects on the skeleton and indirect effects mediated by SHPT resulting from the nephrotoxic effects of these drugs. The recovery of bone formation that occurs as GCs are tapered, however, results in "recoupling" of bone turnover. Rates of bone loss decline, and BMD may recover, particularly at the spine. When graft rejection or periods of stress necessitate increased steroid doses, the underlying bone pathophysiology reverts to the first phase.

In addition to the effects of GCs and calcineurin inhibitors, several other factors contribute to low bone mass in these patients. These factors include decreasing kidney function with persistent or recurrent hyperparathyroidism, hypophosphatemia, and calcitriol deficiency. Vitamin D deficiency is prevalent among kidney transplant recipients: more than 95% of patients were found to have low serum 25-OHD concentrations [81]. Whether similar deficiencies occur in other organ transplant recipients and the role of vitamin D deficiency in development of bone disease remains to be elucidated.

Prevention and management of osteoporosis

Before transplantation

The high prevalence of osteoporosis and abnormal bone and mineral metabolism in patients awaiting transplantation as well as the morbidity related to fractures that occur afterward strongly indicate that all candidates for organ transplantation should have an evaluation of bone health. Before transplantation, preferably at the time of acceptance to the waiting list, BMD should be measured, and spine radiographs should be performed to detect prevalent fractures. Low BMD should prompt an evaluation for correctable secondary causes of osteoporosis and specific treatment if appropriate. All transplantation candidates should receive the recommended daily allowance for calcium (1000–1500 mg, depending on age and menopausal status) and vitamin D (400–800 IU), or as necessary to maintain serum 25-OHD levels above 30 ng/mL. Patients who have end-stage kidney disease should be evaluated and treated for renal osteodystrophy (see article elsewhere in this issue).

It is not known whether osteoporosis therapy given before transplantation reduces the risk of fracture after transplantation. Antiresorptive therapy clearly increases BMD and reduces fractures in other populations, including patients who have GC-induced osteoporosis. Because bisphosphonates suppress bone resorption for up to 12 months after discontinuation of therapy, transplantation after administration of bisphosphonates may prevent the increase in resorption that develops immediately after grafting. Individuals awaiting lung, liver, or cardiac transplantation who have osteopenia or osteoporosis should be evaluated and treated. Significant improvements in BMD frequently can be attained during the pretransplantation waiting period, which can be 1 to 2 years or longer.

After organ transplantation

Bone loss is most rapid immediately after transplantation. Fractures affect patients who have both low and normal BMD before transplantation and may occur very early. Therefore, preventive therapy should be instituted immediately after transplantation even in patients who have normal BMD. In addition, it is important to have a high degree of vigilance for the detection and treatment of osteoporosis in long-term transplant recipients.

Table 2 summarizes the major randomized, controlled trials using vitamin D metabolites and bisphosphonates to prevent bone loss in the immediate period after heart, liver, lung, and bone marrow transplants.

Vitamin D and analogues

Vitamin D metabolites influence posttransplantation bone loss through several mechanisms: they reverse GC-induced decreases in intestinal calcium absorption, limit the resultant SHPT, promote differentiation of osteoblast precursors into mature cells, and may potentiate the immunosuppressive activity of CsA [82–84]. Although parent vitamin D, in doses of 400 to 1000 IU, does not significantly prevent posttransplantation bone loss, active forms of vitamin D have been more effective. Calcidiol (25-OHD) prevents bone loss and increases LS BMD in cardiac transplant recipients [3]. Alfacalcidol given immediately after renal transplantation prevents or attenuates LS and FN bone loss [85–87].

Calcitriol (1,25(OH)$_2$D) has been studied in recipients of heart, lung, and liver transplants, with somewhat conflicting results. Beneficial effects have been seen with the use of 0.5 µg/d or more. A randomized study of heart or lung transplant recipients who received placebo or calcitriol (0.5–0.75 µg/d) for either 12 or 24 months after transplantation found that LS bone loss did not differ between groups [88]. Those who had received calcitriol for the

Table 2
Randomized, controlled clinical trials using vitamin D analogues or bisphosphonates for prevention of bone loss immediately following heart, lung, liver, and bone marrow transplantation

First author	Transplant type	Sample size	Duration	Treatment regimen	Control regimen	Findings
Sambrook et al, [88]	Heart and lung	65	24 months	Calcitriol, 0.5–0.75 µg for 12 months or 24 months; Calcium, 600 mg/d	Placebo; Calcium, 600 mg/d	BMD: FN (but not LS) bone loss was attenuated in the calcitriol groups at 12 months (−6.6% in controls versus −3.9% and −1.2% in the treatment groups). LS bone loss was similar among all three groups (−2.7%–5.6%). In those who discontinued calcitriol after 12 months, FN bone loss was similar to control at 24 months. Fracture: 22 new vertebral fractures occurred in four control subjects. One new vertebral fracture occurred in a calcitriol subject. (Not powered to assess difference in fracture rates).

Study	Organ	N	Duration	Treatment	Control	Results
Aris et al, [91]	Lung (CF)	37	24 months	Pamidronate, 30 mg IV q 3 months; Calcium, 1000 mg/d; Vitamin D, 800 IU/d	Calcium, 1000 mg/d; Vitamin D, 800 IU/d	BMD: LS and TH BMD increased significantly more in the pamidronate group (8.8% and 8.2%) versus controls (2.6% and 0.3%). Fracture: No significant difference
Hommann et al, [95]	Liver and multivisceral	36	12 months	Ibandronate, 2 mg IV q 3 months; Calcium, 1000 mg/d; Vitamin D, 1000 IU/d	Calcium, 1000 mg/d; Vitamin D, 1000 IU/d	BMD: LS, FN, and forearm BMD decreased initially in both groups. Reversal of bone loss with ibandronate was seen after 12 months.
Ninkovic et al, [53]	Liver	99	12 months	Pamidronate, 60 mg IV given once before transplantation	No treatment	BMD: Significant, comparable bone loss at FN in pamidronate (5.2%) and control groups (2.3%). No significant LS losses in either group. Fracture: No significant difference.

(continued on next page)

Table 2 (continued)

First author	Transplant type	Sample size	Duration	Treatment regimen	Control regimen	Findings
Tauchmanova et al, [113]	BMT	34	12 months	Risedronate, 5 mg/d; Calcium, 1 g/d; Vitamin, D 800 IU/d	Calcium, 1 g/d;Vitamin D, 800 IU/d	BMD: LS BMD increased significantly in risedronate group at 6 months (4.4%) and at 12 months (5.9%) and decreased in the control group at 6 months (4.3%) and increased slightly at 12 months (1.1%). FN BMD did not change significantly in the risedronate group but decreased significantly in the control group (4.3%) at 6 months only.
Shane et al, [48]	Heart	149[a]	12 months	Alendronate, 10 mg/d, or calcitriol, 0.5 μg/d; Calcium, 945 mg/d; Vitamin D, 1000 IU/d	Nonrandomized reference group	BMD: Similar small losses at LS and TH in both groups. Significantly less bone loss at LS and TH than in reference group. Fracture: Incidence of vertebral fracture was 6.8% in alendronate group, 3.6% in calcitriol group, and 13.6% in reference group. Differences were not statistically significant.

| Kanenen et al, [25] | BMT | 99 | 12 months | Pamidronate, 60 mg IV administered before transplantation and 1, 2, 3, 6, and 9 months after transplantation; Calcium, 1000 mg/d; Vitamin D, 800 IU/d; Estrogen (women); Testosterone (men) | Calcium, 1000 mg/d; Vitamin D, 800 IU/d; Estrogen (women); Testosterone (men) | BMD: At 12 months, difference in bone loss from baseline was less in the pamidronate group (versus no infusion group) by 2.9% at LS and by 2.3% at TH. The difference in bone loss from baseline was not significant at the FN (2.0%). Fracture: Not powered to assess. |
| Crawford et al, [103] | Liver | 62 | 12 months | Zoledronic acid, 4 mg IV administered within 7 days of transplantation and at months 1, 3, 6, and 9 after transplantation; Calcium, 600 mg/d; Vitamin D, 1000 IU/d | Placebo; Calcium, 600 mg/d; Vitamin D, 1000 IU/d | BMD: At 3 months, difference in bone loss from baseline was decreased in zoledronic acid group (versus placebo group) by 4.0% at LS, by 4.7% at FN, and by 3.8% at TH[b]. At 12 months, the difference in percent bone loss between the groups was less: 1.1% at LS, 2.7% at FN, and 2.4% at TH. Fracture: not powered to assess. |

(continued on next page)

Table 2 (continued)

First author	Transplant type	Sample size	Duration	Treatment regimen	Control regimen	Findings
Grigg (2006) [111]	BMT	116	24 months	Pamidronate, 90 mg IV administered before transplantation and every month after transplantation for 12 months; Calcium, 1000 mg/d; Calcitriol, 0.25 μg/d	Calcium, 1000 mg/d; Calcitriol, 0.25 μg/d	BMD: At 12 months, difference in bone loss from baseline was decreased in pamidronate group (versus no infusion group) by 5.6% at LS, by 7.7% at FN, and by 4.9% at TH. At 24 months, the difference in bone loss from baseline was significant only at the TH (3.9%). Fracture: Not powered to assess.

Abbreviations: BMD, bone mineral density; BMT, bone marrow transplantation; CF, cystic fibrosis; FN, femoral neck; IV, intravenously; q, every.

a Number randomized to alendronate or calcitriol; 27 prospectively recruited, nonrandomized patients served as controls.

b Comparison made after adjustment for baseline weight and serum parathyroid level.

entire 24-month had significantly less FN bone loss, however. Fracture rates were lower in the calcitriol-treated subjects, although this study was inadequately powered to be definitive. These results suggest that rapid bone loss resumes after cessation of calcitriol in heart and lung transplant recipients [88]. In regard to long-term transplant recipients, two studies of heart transplant recipients [89,90] found no benefit. Frequent monitoring of urine and serum calcium is required in patients being treated with vitamin D metabolites, because hypercalcemia and hypercalciuria are common side effects and may develop at any point during treatment. In the authors' opinion, their limited effectiveness and narrow therapeutic window indicate that active vitamin D metabolites should not be regarded as first-line treatment.

Bisphosphonates

Several recent studies have shown that intravenous bisphosphonates prevent bone loss after transplantation [91–101]. A reduction in fractures with intravenous bisphosphonates has been reported by some [94], but not all [91], authors. Repeated doses of intravenous pamidronate prevented LS and FN bone loss in heart [92,99], liver [102], and lung [91,98] transplant recipients. When administered 1 to 3 months before liver transplantation in a placebo-controlled trial, a single dose of intravenous pamidronate had no effect on BMD or fracture; FN BMD fell comparably, and LS BMD did not decline significantly in either group during the first year after transplantation [53]. In contrast, when administered to patients who had pre-existing osteopenia or osteoporosis every 3 months for 1 year following liver transplantation, a significant increase in LS BMD was observed, although FN BMD decreased [102].

Ibandronate and zoledronic acid, the more potent intravenous bisphosphonates, also have been shown in randomized trials to have significant protective effects on BMD at 6 and 12 months in liver transplant recipients [95,103]. Repeated doses of zoledronic acid before and at 1, 3, and 6 months following liver transplantation prevented LS, FN, and total hip bone loss compared with placebo [103]. One year after transplantation, the difference in LS BMD was no longer significant, because BMD increased in the placebo group; however, the between-groups difference at the FN and total hip was maintained (Fig. 1).

The efficacy of oral bisphosphonates also has been demonstrated in heart and liver transplant recipients. In long-term cardiac transplant recipients, clodronate has been shown to increase BMD [104]. Alendronate has been studied in both immediate [48,105] and long-term [106–108] transplant recipients. A randomized trial comparing alendronate (10 mg/d) and calcitriol (0.25 μg twice daily) for 1 year in patients directly after cardiac transplantation found that both regimens prevented bone loss at the LS and hip when compared with reference subjects who received only calcium and vitamin D (Fig. 2) [48]. In the second year after cardiac transplantation, BMD

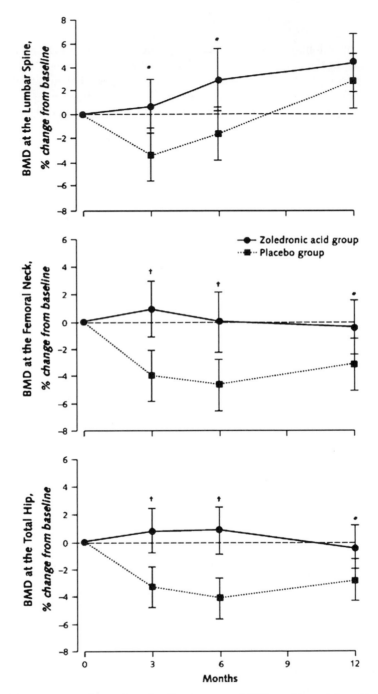

Fig. 1. The percentage change from baseline (means and 95% confidence intervals) in bone mineral density. (*From* Crawford BA, Kam C, Pavlovic J, et al. Zoledronic acid prevents bone loss after liver transplantation: a randomized, double-blind, placebo-controlled trial. Ann Intern Med 2006;144(4):239–48; with permission.)

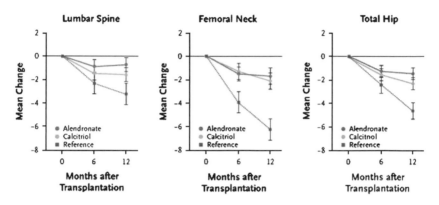

Fig. 2. Intention-to-treat analysis of the mean (± SE) percent change in bone mineral density from base line. (*From* Shane E, Addesso V, Namerow PB, et al. Alendronate versus calcitriol for the prevention of bone loss after cardiac transplantation. N Engl J Med 2004;350(8):767–76; with permission.)

remained stable, although alendronate and calcitriol were discontinued [109]. Alendronate similarly has been shown to prevent bone loss in liver transplant recipients [57,110].

Treatment of bone loss in BMT recipients is particularly complex. Two large, randomized trials of patients who had received allogeneic BMT have found that intravenous pamidronate therapy prevented LS bone loss and reduced proximal femoral bone loss [25,111]. In one of the studies, however, some loss at the proximal femur still occurred, despite doses of 90 mg monthly [111]. The lack of efficacy may result from the failure of pamidronate to inhibit matrix metalloproteinase–mediated bone resorption or to reverse defects in osteoblast function that occur as a result of BMT [112]. Both spinal and proximal femoral bone loss were prevented 12 months after BMT by risedronate [113] and intravenous zoledronate [114]. A small, uncontrolled, prospective study of a single infusion of zoledronate given soon after BMT also reduced spinal and proximal femoral bone loss [115]. The effects of zoledronate may be related to improved osteoblast recovery and increased osteoblast numbers after BMT resulting from increases in ex vivo growth of the bone marrow CFU-f derived from iliac crest biopsies [114].

Although bisphosphonates presently are the most promising agents for the management of transplantation osteoporosis, several issues pertaining to their use have yet to be resolved. These issues include the optimal drug and route of administration, whether continuous or intermittent (cyclical) therapy should be used, and the duration of therapy. Questions related to kidney disease, namely the level of renal impairment at which bisphosphonates are no longer safe and whether they should be used in kidney transplant recipients who have adynamic bone disease, remain unclear. The utility of bisphosphonates in pediatric transplant recipients also is not known. Most importantly, fracture prevention has yet to be demonstrated clearly.

Calcitonin

Calcitonin is relatively ineffective in preventing bone loss after transplantation.

Hormone replacement therapy

Hormone replacement therapy (HRT) has been shown to protect the skeleton in postmenopausal women after lung [98] and liver [116] transplantation and after BMT [117]. In premenopausal women who develop amenorrhea after BMT, a common occurrence, HRT should be administered, provided there are no contraindications. HRT is associated with greater risks than benefits in postmenopausal women, and it should not be used to treat transplant-related bone loss in this population.

Hypogonadism is common in male transplant recipients, related to chronic illness and suppressive effects of CsA and GCs on the hypothalamic-pituitary-gonadal axis. Testosterone levels have been shown to fall immediately after cardiac transplantation and to normalize 6 to 12 months later. In a recent study, hypogonadal men treated with ibandronate had improved BMD at 1 year if also treated with testosterone [118]. Because the potential risks of testosterone therapy, namely prostatic hypertrophy, hyperlipidemia, and abnormal liver enzymes, may have particularly adverse consequences in the transplant population, only men who are truly hypogonadal should receive testosterone.

Other treatment modalities

A few studies have investigated the effects of other treatments on bone loss after transplantation. Resistance exercise significantly improved LS BMD after lung [119] and heart [120] transplantation when used alone and in combination with alendronate. These studies, however, were very small and used lateral BMD measurements, which are highly variable and produce greater percent changes than are typically reported. A recent small study, which was not randomized or controlled, found that liver transplant recipients treated with intravenous prostaglandin E_1 for 12 days after transplantation had less LS and FN BMD loss at 3 and 6 months after transplantation, but no difference was seen at the subsequent 24-month follow-up [121]. The methodological flaws in this study, including using the change in T score as an end point, make the validity of these findings questionable.

Summary

Osteoporosis is prevalent among transplantation candidates. Bone loss in the early posttransplantation period, namely the first 6 months, is associated with a biochemical pattern consistent with uncoupled bone turnover: an increase in markers of bone resorption and a decrease in markers of bone formation. During this period, and through the first year after transplantation, there is clear evidence of rapid bone loss and a high incidence of fragility fractures. In the later posttransplantation period, as GC doses are tapered, bone formation begins to increase, and the underlying pathophysiology reflects high bone turnover osteoporosis. Although rates of bone loss and fracture reported in recent studies are lower than those of a decade ago, they remain unacceptably high. Further, it is not possible to predict fracture risk in an individual patient, because vertebral fractures have been shown to occur even in patients who have normal BMD. Of the presently available treatment modalities, bisphosphonates are the most consistently effective for both prevention and treatment of osteoporosis in transplant recipients. Promising areas of investigation include anabolic agents that stimulate bone formation, namely PTH (1-34) or PTH (1-84), RANKL antagonists, and cathepsin K inhibitors. All patients should be assessed before transplantation and should be treated for prevalent bone disease. Because the greatest amount of bone loss occurs during the first few months after grafting, primary prevention therapy should commence immediately after transplantation. A high degree of vigilance should be maintained for osteoporosis in long-term transplant recipients, as well. There has been tremendous progress in the understanding of the natural history, pathogenesis, and optimal treatment of transplantation osteoporosis. Although many questions remain unanswered, it now is possible and imperative to prevent and treat this debilitating disease.

References

[1] Shane E. Transplantation osteoporosis. In: Orwoll E, Bliziotes M, editors. Osteoporosis: pathophysiology and clinical management. Totowa (NJ): Humana Press; 2003. p. 537–67.
[2] Cohen A, Shane E. Osteoporosis after solid organ and bone marrow transplantation. Osteoporos Int 2003;14(8):617–30.
[3] Cohen A, Sambrook P, Shane E. Management of bone loss after organ transplantation J Bone Miner Res 2004;19(12):1919–32.
[4] Maalouf NM, Shane E. Osteoporosis after solid organ transplantation. J Clin Endocrinol Metab 2005;90(4):2456–65.
[5] Kulak CA, Borba VZ, Kulak J Jr, et al. Transplantation osteoporosis. Arq Bras Endocrinol Metabol 2006;50(4):783–92.
[6] Martin K, Al-Aly Z, Gonzalez E. Renal osteodystrophy. In: Favus M, editor. Primer on the metabolic bone diseases and other disorders of bone and mineral metabolism, vol. 6. Washington DC: American Society for Bone and Mineral Research; 2006. p. 359–66.
[7] Shane E, Mancini D, Aaronson K, et al. Bone mass, vitamin D deficiency and hyperparathyroidism in congestive heart failure. Am J Med 1997;103:197–207.
[8] Hay JE. Osteoporosis in liver diseases and after liver transplantation. J Hepatol 2003;38(6): 856–65.
[9] Monegal A, Navasa M, Guanabens N, et al. Bone disease after liver transplantation: a long-term prospective study of bone mass changes, hormonal status and histomorphometric characteristics. Osteoporos Int 2001;12(6):484–92.
[10] Sokhi RP, Anantharaju A, Kondaveeti R, et al. Bone mineral density among cirrhotic patients awaiting liver transplantation. Liver Transpl 2004;10(5):648–53.

[11] Carey EJ, Balan V, Kremers WK, et al. Osteopenia and osteoporosis in patients with end-stage liver disease caused by hepatitis C and alcoholic liver disease: not just a cholestatic problem. Liver Transpl 2003;9(11):1166–73.

[12] Guichelaar MM, Kendall R, Malinchoc M, et al. Bone mineral density before and after OLT: long-term follow-up and predictive factors. Liver Transpl 2006;12(9):1390–402.

[13] Ninkovic M, Love SA, Tom B, et al. High prevalence of osteoporosis in patients with chronic liver disease prior to liver transplantation. Calcif Tissue Int 2001;69(6):321–6.

[14] Aris R, Neuringer I, Weiner M, et al. Severe osteoporosis before and after lung transplantation. Chest 1996;109:1176–83.

[15] Shane E, Silverberg SJ, Donovan D, et al. Osteoporosis in lung transplantation candidates with end stage pulmonary disease. Am J Med 1996;101:262–9.

[16] Tschopp O, Boehler A, Speich R, et al. Osteoporosis before lung transplantation: association with low body mass index, but not with underlying disease. Am J Transplant 2002;2(2): 167–72.

[17] Aris RM, Renner JB, Winders AD, et al. Increased rate of fractures and severe kyphosis: sequelae of living into adulthood with cystic fibrosis. Ann Intern Med 1998;128: 186–93.

[18] Donovan DS Jr, Papadopoulos A, Staron RB, et al. Bone mass and vitamin D deficiency in adults with advanced cystic fibrosis lung disease. Am J Respir Crit Care Med 1998;157(6 Pt 1):1892–9.

[19] Ott SM, Aitken ML. Osteoporosis in patients with cystic fibrosis. Clin Chest Med 1998; 19(3):555–67.

[20] Tschopp O, Schmid C, Speich R, et al. Pretransplantation bone disease in patients with primary pulmonary hypertension. Chest 2006;129(4):1002–8.

[21] Caplan-Shaw CE, Arcasoy SM, Shane E, et al. Osteoporosis in diffuse parenchymal lung disease. Chest 2006;129(1):140–6.

[22] Ebeling PR. Bone disease after bone marrow transplantation. In: Compston JE, Shane E, editors. Bone disease of organ transplantation. Burlington (MA): Elsevier, Academic Press; 2005. p. 339–52.

[23] Schulte C, Beelen D, Schaefer U, et al. Bone loss in long-term survivors after transplantation of hematopoietic stem cells: a prospective study. Osteoporos Int 2000;11:344–53.

[24] Valimaki M, Kinnunen K, Volin L, et al. A prospective study of bone loss and turnover after allogeneic bone marrow transplantation: effect of calcium supplementation with or without calcitonin. Bone Marrow Transplant 1999;23:355–61.

[25] Kananen K, Volin L, Laitinen K, et al. Prevention of bone loss after allogeneic stem cell transplantation by calcium, vitamin D, and sex hormone replacement with or without pamidronate. J Clin Endocrinol Metab 2005;90(7):3877–85.

[26] Tauchmanova L, Selleri C, Rosa GD, et al. High prevalence of endocrine dysfunction in long-term survivors after allogeneic bone marrow transplantation for hematologic diseases. Cancer 2002;95(5):1076–84.

[27] van Staa TP. The pathogenesis, epidemiology and management of glucocorticoid-induced osteoporosis. Calcif Tissue Int 2006;79(3):129–37.

[28] Sun L, Blair HC, Peng Y, et al. Calcineurin regulates bone formation by the osteoblast. Proc Natl Acad Sci U S A 2005;102(47):17130–5.

[29] Sun L, Peng Y, Zaidi N, et al. Evidence that calcineurin is required for the genesis of bone-resorbing osteoclasts. Am J Physiol Renal Physiol 2007;292(1):F285–91.

[30] Awumey E, Moonga B, Sodam B, et al. Molecular and functional evidence for calcineurin alpha and beta isoforms in the osteoclasts. Novel insights into the mode of action of cyclosporine A. Biochem Biophys Res Commun 1999;254:248–52.

[31] Buchinsky FJ, Ma Y, Mann GN, et al. T lymphocytes play a critical role in the development of cyclosporin A-induced osteopenia. Endocrinology 1996;137(6):2278–85.

[32] Epstein S. Post-transplantation bone disease: the role of immunosuppressive agents on the skeleton. J Bone Miner Res 1996;11:1–7.

[33] Epstein S, Dissanayake A, Goodman GR, et al. Effect of the interaction of parathyroid hormone and cyclosporine A on bone mineral metabolism in the rat. Calcif Tissue Int 2001;68: 240–7.

[34] Bowman AR, Sass DA, Dissanayake IR, et al. The role of testosterone in cyclosporine-induced osteopenia. J Bone Miner Res 1997;12(4):607–15.

[35] Ponticelli C, Aroldi A. Osteoporosis after organ transplantation. Lancet 2001;357(9268): 1623.

[36] Grotz WH, Mundinger A, Gugel B, et al. Bone fracture and osteodensitometry with dual energy X-ray absorptiometry in kidney transplant recipients. Transplantation 1994;58: 912–5.

[37] McIntyre HD, Menzies B, Rigby R, et al. Long-term bone loss after renal transplantation: comparison of immunosuppressive regimens. Clin Transplant 1995;9(1):20–4.

[38] Cueto-Manzano AM, Konel S, Crowley V, et al. Bone histopathology and densitometry comparison between cyclosporine A monotherapy and prednisolone plus azathioprine dual immunosuppression in renal transplant patients. Transplantation 2003;75(12):2053–8.

[39] Josephson MA, Schumm LP, Chiu MY, et al. Calcium and calcitriol prophylaxis attenuates posttransplant bone loss. Transplantation 2004;78(8):1233–6.

[40] Stempfle HU, Werner C, Echtler S, et al. Rapid trabecular bone loss after cardiac transplantation using FK506 (tacrolimus)-based immunosuppression. Transplant Proc 1998;30(4): 1132–3.

[41] Park KM, Hay JE, Lee SG, et al. Bone loss after orthotopic liver transplantation: FK 506 versus cyclosporine. Transplant Proc 1996;28(3):1738–40.

[42] Goffin E, Devogelaer JP, Lalaoui A, et al. Tacrolimus and low-dose steroid immunosuppression preserves bone mass after renal transplantation. Transpl Int 2002;15(2–3):73–80.

[43] Monegal A, Navasa M, Guanabens N, et al. Bone mass and mineral metabolism in liver transplant patients treated with FK506 or cyclosporine A. Calcif Tissue Int 2001;68:83–6.

[44] Campistol JM, Holt DW, Epstein S, et al. Bone metabolism in renal transplant patients treated with cyclosporine or sirolimus. Transpl Int 2005;18(9):1028–35.

[45] Chou NK, Su IC, Kuo HL, et al. Bone mineral density in long-term Chinese heart transplant recipients: a cross-sectional study. Transplant Proc 2006;38(7):2141–4.

[46] Cohen A, Addonizio LJ, Lamour JM, et al. Osteoporosis in adult survivors of adolescent cardiac transplantation may be related to hyperparathyroidism, mild renal insufficiency, and increased bone turnover. J Heart Lung Transplant 2005;24(6):696–702.

[47] Cohen A, Shane E. Bone disease in patients before and after cardiac transplantation. In: Compston JE, Shane E, editors. Bone disease of organ transplantation. Burlington (MA): Elsevier Academic Press; 2005. p. 287–301.

[48] Shane E, Addesso V, Namerow PB, et al. Alendronate versus calcitriol for the prevention of bone loss after cardiac transplantation. N Engl J Med 2004;350(8):767–76.

[49] Shane E, Rivas M, Staron RB, et al. Fracture after cardiac transplantation: a prospective longitudinal study. J Clin Endocrinol Metab 1996;81:1740–6.

[50] Leidig-Bruckner G, Hosch S, Dodidou P, et al. Frequency and predictors of osteoporotic fractures after cardiac or liver transplantation: a follow-up study. Lancet 2001;357:342–7.

[51] Compston JE. Osteoporosis after liver transplantation. Liver Transpl 2003;9(4):321–30.

[52] Maalouf NM, Sakhaee K. Treatment of osteoporosis in patients with chronic liver disease and in liver transplant recipients. Curr Treat Options Gastroenterol 2006;9(6):456–63.

[53] Ninkovic M, Love S, Tom BD, et al. Lack of effect of intravenous pamidronate on fracture incidence and bone mineral density after orthotopic liver transplantation. J Hepatol 2002; 37(1):93–100.

[54] Floreani A, Mega A, Tizian L, et al. Bone metabolism and gonad function in male patients undergoing liver transplantation: a two-year longitudinal study. Osteoporos Int 2001;12(9): 749–54.

[55] Smallwood GA, Burns D, Fasola CG, et al. Relationship between immunosuppression and osteoporosis in an outpatient liver transplant clinic. Transplant Proc 2005;37(4):1910–1.

[56] Shah SH, Johnston TD, Jeon H, et al. Effect of chronic glucocorticoid therapy and the gender difference on bone mineral density in liver transplant patients. J Surg Res 2006;135(2): 238–41.

[57] Millonig G, Graziadei IW, Eichler D, et al. Alendronate in combination with calcium and vitamin D prevents bone loss after orthotopic liver transplantation: a prospective single-center study. Liver Transpl 2005;11(8):960–6.

[58] Ninkovic M, Skingle SJ, Bearcroft PW, et al. Incidence of vertebral fractures in the first three months after orthotopic liver transplantation. Eur J Gastroenterol Hepatol 2000; 12(8):931–5.

[59] Fabrega E, Orive A, Garcia-Unzueta M, et al. Osteoprotegerin and receptor activator of nuclear factor-kappaB ligand system in the early post-operative period of liver transplantation. Clin Transplant 2006;20(3):383–8.

[60] Epstein S, Shane E. In: Marcus R, Feldman D, Kelsey J, editors. Osteoporosis. Transplantation osteoporosis, vol. 2. San Diego (CA): Academic Press; 2001. p. 327–40.

[61] Shane E, Epstein S. Transplantation osteoporosis. Transplant Rev 2001;15(1):11–32.

[62] Rutherford RM, Fisher AJ, Hilton C, et al. Functional status and quality of life in patients surviving 10 years after lung transplantation. Am J Transplant 2005;5(5):1099–104.

[63] Spira A, Gutierrez C, Chaparro C, et al. Osteoporosis and lung transplantation: a prospective study. Chest 2000;117(2):476–81.

[64] Shane E, Papadopoulos A, Staron RB, et al. Bone loss and fracture after lung transplantation. Transplantation 1999;68:220–7.

[65] Haworth CS, Webb AK, Egan JJ, et al. Bone histomorphometry in adult patients with cystic fibrosis. Chest 2000;118(2):434–9.

[66] Banfi A, Podesta M, Fazzuoli L, et al. High-dose chemotherapy shows a dose-dependent toxicity to bone marrow osteoprogenitors: a mechanism for post-bone marrow transplantation osteopenia. Cancer 2001;92(9):2419–28.

[67] Lee WY, Cho SW, Oh ES, et al. The effect of bone marrow transplantation on the osteoblastic differentiation of human bone marrow stromal cells. J Clin Endocrinol Metab 2002;87(1):329–35.

[68] Kang MI, Lee WY, Oh KW, et al. The short-term changes of bone mineral metabolism following bone marrow transplantation. Bone 2000;26(3):275–9.

[69] Ebeling P, Thomas D, Erbas B, et al. Mechanism of bone loss following allogeneic and autologous hematopoietic stem cell transplantation. J Bone Miner Res 1999;14:342–50.

[70] Lee WY, Kang MI, Baek KH, et al. The skeletal site-differential changes in bone mineral density following bone marrow transplantation: 3-year prospective study. J Korean Med Sci 2002;17(6):749–54.

[71] Tauchmanova L, Serio B, Del Puente A, et al. Long-lasting bone damage detected by dual-energy x-ray absorptiometry, phalangeal osteosonogrammetry, and in vitro growth of marrow stromal cells after allogeneic stem cell transplantation. J Clin Endocrinol Metab 2002;87(11):5058–65.

[72] Nysom K, Holm K, Michaelsen KF, et al. Bone mass after allogeneic BMT for childhood leukaemia or lymphoma. Bone Marrow Transplant 2000;25(2):191–6.

[73] Gandhi MK, Lekamwasam S, Inman I, et al. Significant and persistent loss of bone mineral density in the femoral neck after haematopoietic stem cell transplantation: long-term follow-up of a prospective study. Br J Haematol 2003;121(3):462–8.

[74] Lee WY, Kang MI, Oh ES, et al. The role of cytokines in the changes in bone turnover following bone marrow transplantation. Osteoporos Int 2002;13(1):62–8.

[75] Michelson JD, Gornet M, Codd T, et al. Bone morphology after bone marrow transplantation for Hodgkin's and non- Hodgkin's lymphoma. Exp Hematol 1993;21(3): 475–82.

[76] Athanasou NA, Quinn J, Brenner MK, et al. Origin of marrow stromal cells and haemopoietic chimaerism following bone marrow transplantation determined by in situ hybridisation. Br J Cancer 1990;61(3):385–9.

[77] Kananen K, Volin L, Tahtela R, et al. Recovery of bone mass and normalization of bone turnover in long-term survivors of allogeneic bone marrow transplantation. Bone Marrow Transplant 2002;29(1):33–9.

[78] Arekat MR, And G, Lemke S, et al. Dramatic improvement of BMD following vitamin D therapy in a bone marrow transplant recipient. J Clin Densitom 2002;5(3):267–71.

[79] Hattori M, Morita N, Tsujino Y, et al. Vitamins D and K in the treatment of osteoporosis secondary to graft-versus-host disease following bone-marrow transplantation. J Int Med Res 2001;29(4):381–4.

[80] Tauchmanova L, De Rosa G, Serio B, et al. Avascular necrosis in long-term survivors after allogeneic or autologous stem cell transplantation: a single center experience and a review. Cancer 2003;97(10):2453–61.

[81] Shirsat M, Josephson MA, Sprague SM. Vitamin D deficiency following renal transplantation. J Am Soc Nephrol, in press.

[82] Briffa NK, Keogh AM, Sambrook PN, et al. Reduction of immunosuppressant therapy requirement in heart transplantation by calcitriol. Transplantation 2003;75(12):2133–4.

[83] Lemire JM. Immunomodulatory role of 1,25 Dihydroxyvitamin D3. J Cell Biochem 1992; 49:26–31.

[84] Lemire JM, Archer DC, Reddy GS. Dihydroxy-24-oxo-16-ene-vitamin D3, a renal metabolite of the vitamin D analog 1,25-dihydroxy-16ene-vitamin D3, exerts immunosuppressive activity equal to its parent without causing hypercalcemia in vivo. Endocrinology 1994;135: 2818–21.

[85] El-Agroudy AE, El-Husseini AA, El-Sayed M, et al. Preventing bone loss in renal transplant recipients with vitamin D. J Am Soc Nephrol 2003;14(11):2975–9.

[86] De Sevaux RG, Hoitsma AJ, Corstens FH, et al. Treatment with vitamin D and calcium reduces bone loss after renal transplantation: a randomized study. J Am Soc Nephrol 2002;13(6):1608–14.

[87] El-Agroudy AE, El-Husseini AA, El-Sayed M, et al. A prospective randomized study for prevention of postrenal transplantation bone loss. Kidney Int 2005;67(5):2039–45.

[88] Sambrook P, Henderson NK, Keogh A, et al. Effect of calcitriol on bone loss after cardiac or lung transplantation. J Bone Miner Res 2000;15(9):1818–24.

[89] Stempfle HU, Werner C, Echtler S, et al. Prevention of osteoporosis after cardiac transplantation: a prospective, longitudinal, randomized, double-blind trial with calcitriol. Transplantation 1999;68(4):523–30.

[90] Stempfle HU, Werner C, Siebert U, et al. The role of tacrolimus (FK506)-based immunosuppression on bone mineral density and bone turnover after cardiac transplantation: a prospective, longitudinal, randomized, double-blind trial with calcitriol. Transplantation 2002; 73(4):547–52.

[91] Aris RM, Lester GE, Renner JB, et al. Efficacy of pamidronate for osteoporosis in patients with cystic fibrosis following lung transplantation. Am J Respir Crit Care Med 2000;162 (3 Pt 1):941–6.

[92] Bianda T, Linka A, Junga G, et al. Prevention of osteoporosis in heart transplant recipients: a comparison of calcitriol with calcitonin and pamidronate. Calcif Tissue Int 2000;67: 116–21.

[93] Fan S, Almond MK, Ball E, et al. Pamidronate therapy as prevention of bone loss following renal transplantation. Kidney Int 2000;57:684–90.

[94] Shane E, Rodino MA, McMahon DJ, et al. Prevention of bone loss after heart transplantation with antiresorptive therapy: a pilot study. J Heart Lung Transplant 1998;17(11): 1089–96.

[95] Hommann M, Abendroth K, Lehmann G, et al. Effect of transplantation on bone: osteoporosis after liver and multivisceral transplantation. Transplant Proc 2002;34(6): 2296–8.

[96] Grotz W, Nagel C, Poeschel D, et al. Effect of ibandronate on bone loss and renal function after kidney transplantation. J Am Soc Nephrol 2001;12(7):1530–7.

[97] Arlen DJ, Lambert K, Ioannidis G, et al. Treatment of established bone loss after renal transplantation with etidronate. Transplantation 2001;71(5):669–73.

[98] Trombetti A, Gerbase MW, Spiliopoulos A, et al. Bone mineral density in lung-transplant recipients before and after graft: prevention of lumbar spine post-transplantation-accelerated bone loss by pamidronate. J Heart Lung Transplant 2000;19(8):736–43.

[99] Krieg M, Seydoux C, Sandini L, et al. Intravenous pamidronate as a treatment for osteoporosis after heart transplantation: a prospective study. Osteoporos Int 2001;12:112–6.

[100] Haas M, Leko-Mohr Z, Roschger P, et al. Zoledronic acid to prevent bone loss in the first 6 months after renal transplantation. Kidney Int 2003;63(3):1130–6.

[101] Coco M, Glicklich D, Faugere MC, et al. Prevention of bone loss in renal transplant recipients: a prospective, randomized trial of intravenous pamidronate. J Am Soc Nephrol 2003; 14(10):2669–76.

[102] Pennisi P, Trombetti A, Giostra E, et al. Pamidronate and osteoporosis prevention in liver transplant recipients. Rheumatol Int 2007;27(3):251–6.

[103] Crawford BA, Kam C, Pavlovic J, et al. Zoledronic acid prevents bone loss after liver transplantation: a randomized, double-blind, placebo-controlled trial. Ann Intern Med 2006; 144(4):239–48.

[104] Ippoliti G, Pellegrini C, Campana C, et al. Clodronate treatment of established bone loss in cardiac recipients: a randomized study. Transplantation 2003;75(3):330–4.

[105] Kovac D, Lindic J, Kandus A, et al. Prevention of bone loss in kidney graft recipients. Transplant Proc 2001;33(1–2):1144–5.

[106] Giannini S, Dangel A, Carraro G, et al. Alendronate prevents further bone loss in renal transplant recipients. J Bone Miner Res 2001;16(11):2111–7.

[107] Jeffery JR, Leslie WD, Karpinski ME, et al. Prevalence and treatment of decreased bone density in renal transplant recipients: a randomized prospective trial of calcitriol versus alendronate. Transplantation 2003;76(10):1498–502.

[108] Koc M, Tuglular S, Arikan H, et al. Alendronate increases bone mineral density in long-term renal transplant recipients. Transplant Proc 2002;34(6):2111–3.

[109] Cohen A, Addesso V, McMahon DJ, et al. Discontinuing antiresorptive therapy one year after cardiac transplantation: effect on bone density and bone turnover. Transplantation 2006;81(5):686–91.

[110] Atamaz F, Hepguler S, Karasu Z, et al. The prevention of bone fractures after liver transplantation: experience with alendronate treatment. Transplant Proc 2006;38(5): 1448–52.

[111] Grigg AC, Shuttleworth P, Reynolds J, et al. Pamidronate therapy for one year after allogeneic bone marrow transplantation (AlloBMT) reduces bone loss from the lumbar spine, femoral neck and total hip. Blood 2004;104:A2253.

[112] Ebeling PR. Defective osteoblast function may be responsible for bone loss from the proximal femur despite pamidronate therapy. J Clin Endocrinol Metab 2005;90(7):4414–6.

[113] Tauchmanova L, Selleri C, Esposito M, et al. Beneficial treatment with risedronate in long-term survivors after allogeneic stem cell transplantation for hematological malignancies. Osteoporos Int 2003;14(12):1013–9.

[114] Tauchmanova L, Ricci P, Serio B, et al. Short-term zoledronic acid treatment increases bone mineral density and marrow clonogenic fibroblast progenitors after allogeneic stem cell transplantation. J Clin Endocrinol Metab 2005;90(2):627–34.

[115] D'Souza AB, Grigg AP, Szer J, et al. Zoledronic acid prevents bone loss after allogeneic haemopoietic stem cell transplantation. Int Med J 2006;36:600–3.

[116] Isoniemi H, Appelberg J, Nilsson CG, et al. Transdermal oestrogen therapy protects postmenopausal liver transplant women from osteoporosis. A 2-year follow-up study. J Hepatol 2001;34(2):299–305.

[117] Branco CC, Rovira M, Pons F, et al. The effect of hormone replacement therapy on bone mass in patients with ovarian failure due to bone marrow transplantation. Maturitas 1996; 23:307–12.

[118] Fahrleitner A, Prenner G, Tscheliessnigg KH, et al. Testosterone supplementation has additional benefits on bone metabolism in cardiac transplant recipients receiving intravenous bisphosphonate treatment: a prospective study. J Bone Miner Res 2002;17(Suppl 1): S388.

[119] Braith RW, Conner JA, Fulton MN, et al. Comparison of alendronate vs alendronate plus mechanical loading as prophylaxis for osteoporosis in lung transplant recipients: a pilot study. J Heart Lung Transplant 2007;26(2):132–7.

[120] Braith RW, Magyari PM, Fulton MN, et al. Comparison of calcitonin versus calcitonin + resistance exercise as prophylaxis for osteoporosis in heart transplant recipients. Transplantation 2006;81(8):1191–5.

[121] Hommann M, Kammerer D, Lehmann G, et al. Prevention of early loss of bone mineral density after liver transplantation by prostaglandin E1. Transplant Proc 2007;39(2):540–3.

ENDOCRINOLOGY
AND METABOLISM
CLINICS
OF NORTH AMERICA

Endocrinol Metab Clin N Am
36 (2007) 965–981

ELSEVIER
SAUNDERS

Cardiac Allograft Vasculopathy and Insulin Resistance—Hope for New Therapeutic Targets

Luciano Potena, MD, PhD[a],
Hannah A. Valantine, MD, MRCP, FACC[b],*

[a]Institute of Cardiology, Academic Hospital S.Orsola-Malpighi, via Massarenti 9,
Building 21, 40138 Bologna, Italy
[b]Cardiovascular Medicine, Stanford University School of Medicine, 300 Pasteur Drive,
Falk CVRC, Stanford, CA 94305-5406, USA

Cardiac allograft vasculopathy (CAV) is a major cause of death in patients surviving more than 1 year after heart transplantation [1–3]. Although numerous immune-mediated and metabolic risk factors have been implicated in the pathogenesis of CAV [4], to date no effective treatment is available to eliminate CAV and its related adverse outcomes fully. Thus, the main therapeutic strategy against CAV is the prevention and treatment of the factors known to trigger or accelerate the disease. An important cluster of CAV risk factors are those that occur as a consequence of insulin resistance and manifest as part of the metabolic syndrome (Box 1) [5]. Indeed, insulin resistance and its associated hypertension, dyslipidemia, diabetes, and systemic inflammation often affect candidates for heart transplantation and are frequent adverse effects of immunosuppressive therapy. These consequences of insulin resistance, individually and collectively, seem to affect negatively the prognosis of patients undergoing heart transplantation. This article first summarizes the pathologic features of CAV and then reviews the contribution of the major components of insulin resistance in CAV development and progression. It focuses on the few studies that have analyzed the impact of the individual metabolic abnormalities and inflammation and on therapeutic strategies to minimize the clinical manifestation of insulin resistance after heart transplantation. The central

This work has been supported by a grant from the National Institutes of Health (PO1 AI-50153), and by grants from the Luisa Fanti Melloni and Banca del Monte foundations.

* Corresponding author.
E-mail address: hvalantine@stanford.edu (H.A. Valantine).

Box 1. Abnormalities associated with insulin resistance

Some degree of glucose intolerance
    Impaired fasting glucose
    Impaired glucose tolerance
Dyslipidemia
    ↑ Triglycerides
    ↓ High-density lipoprotein cholesterol
    ↓ Low-density lipoprotein particle diameter
    ↑ Postprandial accumulation of triglyceride-rich lipoproteins
Endothelial dysfunction
    ↑ Monocyte cell adhesion
    ↑ Plasma concentration of cellular adhesion molecules
    ↑ Plasma concentration of asymmetric dimethylarginine
    ↓ Endothelial-dependent vasodilatation
Procoagulant factors
    ↑ Plasminogen activator inhibitor-1
    ↑ Fibrinogen
Hemodynamic changes
    ↑ Sympathetic nervous system activity
    ↑ Renal sodium retention
Markers of inflammation
    ↑ C-reactive protein
Abnormal uric acid metabolism
    ↑ Plasma uric acid concentration
    ↓ Renal uric acid clearance
Increased testosterone secretion (ovary)
Sleep-disordered breathing

---

role that insulin resistance seems to play in the pathophysiology of CAV suggests the opportunity for new therapeutic targets that increase insulin sensitivity while also ameliorating the associated proinflammatory state.

Clinical and pathologic features of cardiac allograft vasculopathy

The most common cause of retransplantation or death after heart transplantation is a rapidly progressive obliterative vascular disease involving the coronary arteries, termed "cardiac allograft vasculopathy" [6]. The characteristic pathologic features of CAV also have been observed in the vasculature of kidney, liver, and lung transplants that are chronically rejected, suggesting a similar mechanism for the disease process, regardless of the organ type [7–9]. Pathologic studies indicate that the lesions of CAV are characterized by diffuse fibrointimal proliferation composed of vascular smooth muscle cells and intercellular matrix and by a characteristic sparing of the internal elastic lamina that distinguishes it from native atherosclerosis (Figs. 1 and 2) [2]. The lesions are diffuse within the allograft, involving arteries, veins, and great vessels [10–12], but the disease is limited to the allograft [13]. Some observational studies suggest a correlation between CAV and acute rejection [14–16], but others have not confirmed a significant association [17,18]. Because of denervation of the transplanted heart, patients who have CAV typically are asymptomatic until they present with sudden death or congestive heart failure. There is a pressing need for greater understanding of the disease process, which might uncover targets for prevention and treatment. The metabolic consequences of insulin-resistance syndrome (IRS) are cluster of such potential targets.

Insulin-resistance syndrome in the pathophysiology of cardiac allograft vasculopathy

"Insulin-resistance syndrome" is a descriptive term describing the abnormalities and clinical syndromes that reflect a physiologic abnormality that increases the likelihood that one or more of the following abnormalities will be present: glucose intolerance, dyslipidemia, endothelial dysfunction, procoagulant factors, hemodynamic changes, markers of inflammation, abnormal uric acid metabolism, and increased testosterone secretion. The central physiologic abnormality is caused by impairment in the ability of insulin to stimulate glucose disposal and is known to vary sixfold in the

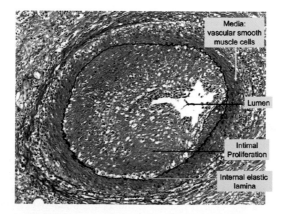

Fig. 1. Pathologic features of cardiac allograft vasculopathy. This histologic section is from the left anterior descending branch of the coronary artery of a patient who developed congestive cardiac failure 11 months after transplantation and died suddenly while being considered for retransplantation. It shows diffuse intimal proliferation (*blue arrow*) composed of smooth muscle and inflammatory cells and interstitial matrix sparing the intimal elastic lamina (*green arrow*). The medial layer (*yellow arrow*) is normal. The adventitial layer contains inflammatory cells. The result is a slitlike lumen (*black arrow*) that led to myocardial infarction and death.

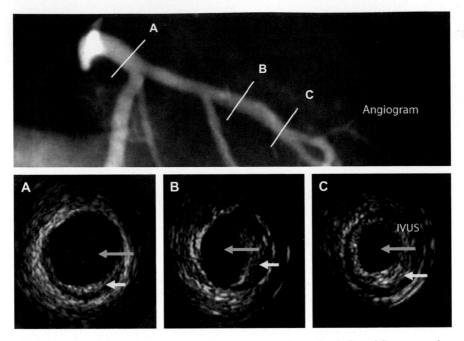

Fig. 2. (*Top panel*) A vessel appears normal on coronary angiography. A, B, and C correspond to the views in the bottom panel. (*Bottom panel A, B, C*) Intravascular ultrasound of the same vessel demonstrates considerable intimal thickening (*yellow arrow*), despite no relevant change in lumen volume can be detected, as seen also by normal angiogram (*green arrow*).

population at large [19]. When insulin-resistant individuals cannot secrete the amount of insulin needed to overcome the defect in insulin action, type 2 diabetes develops. Most of these individuals, however, are able to sustain the level of compensatory hyperinsulinemia required to maintain normal or nearly normal glucose tolerance. Although compensatory hyperinsulinemia can prevent the frank development of hyperglycemia, insulin-resistant/hyperinsulinemic individuals are at greatly increased risk for having some degree of glucose intolerance, a high plasma triglyceride (TG) level, a low high-density lipoprotein cholesterol (HDL-C) concentration, and essential hypertension, all of which arise as a consequence of the differential insulin sensitivity of various tissues. Because not all tissues share the defect in insulin action, the cost of secreting the amount of insulin needed to overcome insulin resistance, located primarily in muscle and adipose tissue, is the adverse impact of the compensatory hyperinsulinemia on tissues that retain normal insulin sensitivity. In the face of insulin resistance in muscle and adipose tissue, most other tissues in the body retain normal insulin sensitivity and can become victims of the compensatory hyperinsulinemia. For example, hyperinsulinemia acts on the normally insulin-sensitive kidney to decrease uric acid clearance and increase sodium retention, resulting in the increased uric acid concentration and salt sensitivity that occurs in insulin-resistant individuals [20]. Of particular relevance is the impact of hyperinsulinemia on the liver that normally is sensitive to insulin. This impact leads to the atherogenic lipoprotein phenotype that characterizes the insulin-resistant state [21] and also is responsible for the accumulation of liver fat that results in nonalcoholic fatty liver diseases [22]. Several population-based studies have demonstrated that hyperinsulinemia, both fasting and after glucose challenge, predicts the development of cardiovascular disease (CVD) in nondiabetic individuals [23,24]. It has been shown that insulin resistance, as quantified by a specific measure of insulin-mediated glucose uptake, is predictive of increased risk of CVD, and that this risk is present in one third of an apparently healthy population that has the greatest defect in insulin-mediated glucose disposal [25]. Although the evidence linking the atherogenic profile of insulin resistant/hyperinsulinemic individuals to increased CVD is the best established, consideration of the nonlipid CVD risk factors is important for improved understanding of how the multiple components of IRS might impact the biology of vascular diseases.

Observational studies throughout the past 3 decades of heart transplantation have reported consistently that hypertriglyceridemia is a major risk factor for CAV [26,27]. Evidence from clinical studies conducted over the past decade suggests that elevated TG is but one marker of insulin resistance in heart transplant recipients. The authors have demonstrated that CAV is accelerated in animal models of insulin resistance, independent of an alloimmune response [28]. It long has been recognized that heart transplant recipients have elevated levels of hemostatic and proinflammatory markers, mirroring the findings in nontransplanted insulin-resistant individuals [29]. The published data confirm that heart transplant recipients are insulin resistant and suggest that this state of impaired insulin action accelerates CAV.

The authors' group has demonstrated that the majority of nondiabetic long-term heart transplant recipients has impaired glucose tolerance and elevated plasma insulin concentrations, consistent with insulin resistance [27]. Importantly, patients who had a diagnosis of ischemic heart disease before transplantation had higher plasma glucose and insulin concentrations in response to oral glucose as well as higher fasting plasma TG, cholesterol, and low-density lipoprotein cholesterol (LDL-C) concentrations than did the normal age-matched controls. In addition, HDL-C concentrations were lower, and the ratio of cholesterol to HDL-C was higher than control values in patients who had a pretransplantation diagnosis of ischemic heart disease. Values for almost all variables were intermediate in patients who had a pretransplantation diagnosis of idiopathic cardiomyopathy, and in most instances these values differed significantly from the values in subjects who had ischemic heart disease before transplantation and from the values in normal subjects . Thus, cardiac transplant recipients are dyslipidemic, relatively glucose intolerant, and hyperinsulinemic compared with normal volunteers. This finding underscores the ongoing state of insulin resistance after

heart transplantation and its possible impact in poor cardiovascular outcomes in this patient population.

In addition to evidence for insulin resistance, a typical pattern of dyslipidemia—elevated TG and decreased high-density lipoprotein (HDL) concentration—was observed in these patients. The authors noted that these
abnormalities were most pronounced during the initial 3 months after transplantation and, although they became less marked over time, were still
demonstrable in the majority of patients 1 year after transplantation. The
mechanisms underlying the development of insulin resistance after transplantation are unclear but most likely are the consequence of genetic predisposition and the immunosuppressive drugs used to prevent acute rejection,
notably corticosteroids and calcineurin inhibitors such as cyclosporine and
tacrolimus. Although it is recognized that calcineurine inhibitors can impair
glucose metabolism [30], several studies in kidney and liver transplant recipients suggest that, among the immunosuppressive drugs, corticosteroids are
the major contributors to the development of IRS [31]. Additionally, cardiac
transplant recipients are known to demonstrate increased activation of the
sympathetic nervous system that generally is attributed to the state of cardiac denervation; however, the presence of insulin resistance and the compensatory hyperinsulinemia could further enhance sympathetic nervous
system activation [32].

Even before the introduction of cyclosporine as the primary immunosuppressive drug, the authors reported that elevated plasma TG concentration
was a major risk factor for CAV in heart transplant recipients whose major
immunosuppressive regimen consisted of corticosteroids [27]. Subsequent
studies in heart transplant recipients treated with cyclosporine A, including
one from Stanford University that found elevated TG and apolipoprotein B
levels, weight gain, and donor age to be independent predictors of CAV,
confirmed a significant correlation of hypertriglyceridemia with the development of CAV [33].

In addition to the studies conducted at the authors' institution, other retrospective, cross-sectional, and prospective studies have assessed the correlations of components of IRS and obesity with the incidence and risk of
developing CAV (Table 1).

In general, these studies have demonstrated that cardinal features of the
IRS, including hypertriglyceridemia, hyperinsulinemia, and elevated plasma
glucose levels, are associated with the presence of CAV by angiography and
intravascular ultrasound (IVUS). The authors have demonstrated that CAV
(defined as the presence of coronary artery intimal thickness > 0.3 mm) was
significantly correlated with many features of IRS, including plasma insulin
and glucose and insulin concentrations elevated in fasting and after glucose
challenge, elevated TG levels, and low plasma concentrations of HDL-C.
These markers of the IRS predicted the development of severe CAD by angiography as well as mortality from cardiovascular complications during
a 5-year follow-up period. Similarly, in a cross-sectional analysis of 606

Table 1
Studies assessing the correlations of components of insulin-resistance syndrome with the incidence and risk of developing cardiac allograft vasculopathy

Study	Component of insulin-resistance syndrome	N	Study design	Reference standard	Significant findings ($P < .05$)
Kato et al [75]	Glucose intolerance	151	Cross-sectional	Angiography IVUS	HbA1c (and δBMI) are associated with CAV by IVUS on multivariate analysis; HbA1c is associated with CAV by angiography on multivariate analysis.
Valantine et al [26]	Insulin resistance TG and HDL	66	Cross-sectional prospective	Angiography	High insulin and glucose levels are associated with increased risk of CAV; MIT > 0.3 mm are associated with higher levels of TG and lower levels of HDL.
Biadi et al [38]	Insulin resistance TG and HDL	98	Prospective	Angiography	TG:HDL ratio > 3.0 and high CRP are associated with threefold increase in risk of developing CAV and subsequent cardiovascular events.
Rickenbacher et al [33]	TG	116	Retrospective	Angiography IVUS	TG level and body weight are correlated with increased MIT at IVUS by multivariate regression; CAV progression at 1 year is associated with TG by regression.
Mehra et al [63]	TG	138	Cross-sectional prospective	IVUS	TG level is associated with increased risk of CAV by logistic regression.
Senechal et al [80]	Atherogenic triad (elevated fasting glucose, apolipoprotein B and small, dense low-density lipoprotein)	83	Cross-sectional	Angiography	25-fold increase in the risk of CAV is seen at angiography in the presence of the atherogenic triad by logistic regression.
Kapadia et al [44]	TG	93	Prospective	IVUS	TG level is associated with progression of donor-transmitted lesions at 1 year but not with development of new lesions.

Abbreviations: BMI, body mass index; CAV, cardiac allograft vasculopathy; CRP, C-reactive protein; HbA1c, hemoglobin A_{1c}; HDL, high-density lipoprotein; IVUS, intravascular ultrasound; MIT, maximal intimal thickness; TG, triglycerides.

renal transplant recipients, De Vries and colleagues [34] examined the relationship between IRS as a single entity and long-term allograft function. Among their study subjects, the presence of the IRS was highly correlated with impaired renal allograft function more than 1 year after transplantation. Multivariate analyses demonstrated that systolic blood pressure and TG contributed most to allograft dysfunction.

Many of the early studies focused predominantly on the role of hyperlipidemia and the impact of statins in blocking the development of CAV. Clinical trials using this approach indeed have documented amelioration of CAV progression and incidence and a survival benefit [35]. As demonstrated in a recent study by White and colleagues [36], however, an ongoing proinflammatory milieu persists despite the routine administration of statins. In this study, heart transplant recipients were found to have significant elevations in factor VIII, von Willebrand's factor, fibrinogen, plasminogen activator inhibitor I, and C-reactive protein, in addition to elevated plasma markers of vascular endothelial cell activation, such as surface vascular adhesion molecules, surface intercellular adhesion molecules, and E- and P-selectins. This proinflammatory milieu in heart transplant recipients has been reported in other studies and is entirely consistent with insulin resistance outside the transplantation setting. Although the pattern of lipid and lipoprotein abnormalities suggested that the heart transplant recipients enrolled in that study were insulin resistant, this factor was not evaluated. In a prospective cohort of 99 heart transplant recipients, the authors were able to demonstrate the clinical utility of a TG:HDL-C ratio greater than 3.0, an easily used marker of insulin resistance [37], to identify a group of patients with a higher prevalence of CAV [38]. Additionally, the presence of systemic inflammation, detected by elevated serum C-reactive protein levels, further refined the identification of patients who had CAV, and, combined with the TG:HDL ratio greater than 3.0, identified a subgroup of patients who had a threefold increased risk for subsequent cardiovascular events. Of note, in this series of patients, the authors found a significant correlation between markers of insulin resistance and systemic inflammation as detected by C-reactive protein, suggesting a pathophysiologic link between immunoinflammatory activation and insulin resistance.

In summary, most heart transplant recipients are markedly insulin resistant and demonstrate many of the features of compensatory hyperinsulinemia, including the atherogenic and proinflammatory profiles. The use of immunosuppressive drugs and genetic and environmental factors are major contributors to IRS, and the body of evidence suggests that insulin resistance in heart transplant recipients accelerates CAV.

Future therapeutic strategies for IRS treatment and prevention include peroxisome-proliferator-activated receptor gamma (PPAR-γ) agonists that act directly to improve insulin sensitivity. PPAR-γ is a nuclear transcription factor that regulates adipocytes differentiation, fatty acid and TG storage, and insulin-dependent glucose uptake [39]. A relatively new class of drug, thiazolidinediones, acts as an agonist of PPAR-γ, markedly improving cellular insulin sensitivity. Inhibitors of type-1 angiotensin receptors, commonly used antihypertensive agents, enhance PPAR-γ activity, potentially improving markers of insulin resistance [40]. Although there is no evidence that such an approach has any impact on CAV development, graft overexpression of angiotensin receptors predicted CAV [41] and the efficacy of a PPAR-γ agonist in reducing CAV in a rat model of heart transplantation [42]. These data provide a strong rationale for appropriately designed prospective studies to test the hypothesis that insulin resistance accelerates CAV.

Targeting individual components of insulin resistance syndrome for prevention of cardiac allograft vasculopathy

Hyperlipidemia

The epidemiologic data correlating elevated plasma concentrations of LDL and/or TG suggested potential therapeutic targets for preventing or slowing the progression of CAV [33]. Recent studies using intravascular ultrasound have shown a direct correlation between LDL plasma concentration and coronary intimal hyperplasia [43,44], even in patients largely treated with statins [45]. Further observational data from a recent multicenter study showed that high LDL-C was an independent risk factor for graft-related mortality and nonfatal major cardiac adverse events, albeit not significantly correlated with angiographic coronary lesions [46].

Because the immunosuppressive drugs routinely used in the management of patients after transplantation induce dyslipidemia, the question has been raised as to which of these agents is most atherogenic. Although the mechanism is unclear, calcineurin inhibitors seem to have a greater impact than corticosteroids for increasing cholesterol absorption [47], with no apparent difference seen between the two calcineurin inhibitors (cyclosporine and tacrolimus) [48]. Other studies, however, have found that plasma concentrations of HDL-C were significantly higher in cyclosporine-treated patients [49]. The discordance of the data between immunosuppression levels and dyslipidemia make it unlikely that reduction of immunosuppressive agents alone will address the control of hyperlipidemia and CAV adequately.

Further complicating the issue of hyperlipidemia and CAV is the observation that sirolimus and everolimus, mammalian target of rapamycin (mTOR) inhibitors, cause profound hypercholesterolemia and hypertriglyceridemia [48]. This new class of immunosuppressive drugs, however, has been shown to reduce the progression of coronary artery intimal thickening, a marker of CAV detected by IVUS, and to decrease the incidence of major adverse cardiovascular events [50,51]. This beneficial effect of mTOR inhibitors was observed despite the high cholesterol and TG levels in patients receiving statins to lower plasma lipid concentrations. Experimental models suggest that the increase in circulating lipids is overcome by decreased deposition in the vascular wall in animals simultaneously treated with mTOR inhibitors and statins (Corsini and colleagues, personal communication, 2007).

Routine statin therapy, started immediately after heart transplantation, has become the main prevention strategy for CAV, based on two randomized, controlled trials [35,52]. In a 12-month randomized study of 97 patients, those who received pravastatin in addition to immunosuppression early after cardiac transplantation had significantly lower mean cholesterol, LDL-C, and TG levels; higher HDL-C levels; less frequent cardiac rejection; better survival; and a lower incidence of CAV when compared with a control group who did not receive a statin [52]. A 4-year prospective study of 72 heart transplant recipients showed that those treated with simvastatin had significantly improved survival and a lower incidence of CAV than the control group who received dietary therapy but no statin [35]. In addition to the data from randomized, clinical trials, the benefit of statins also has been demonstrated in several registries reporting real-life clinical practice. In these studies, a survival benefit of statin therapy, apparently independent of cholesterol plasma levels, has been reported [53,54]. Both studies, however, report a rate of creatinine kinase elevation greater than seen in the general population, indicating the need for caution because the interaction of statins with cyclosporine might increase the risk of creatinine kinase elevation and rhabomyolisis. Among the different statins available, fluvastatin has been shown not to interact significantly with cyclosporine and to improve cardiovascular prognosis in kidney transplantation with an appropriate safety profile [55]. Preliminary data suggest that when statins are not tolerated or are ineffective, the use of ezetimibe, an intestinal cholesterol absorption inhibitor, can decrease LDL-C effectively [56]. This specific mechanism may be particularly effective in antagonizing the increase in cholesterol absorption induced by calcineurin inhibitors [47]. Whether LDL-C reduction obtained by a mechanism of action different from statins has any protective effect on prognosis or CAV development remains to be proven.

Hypertension

Hypertension is a common finding after heart transplantation. According to the data reported by the registry of the International Society for Heart and Lung Transplantation, 76% of patients are hypertensive 1 year after transplantation, and 94% are hypertensive at 5 years [3].

Postoperative hypertension after heart transplantation has been associated significantly with the onset of angiographic CAV [57]. There is evidence that hypertension is a consequence of both immunosuppressive therapy, particularly calcineurine antagonists, and the denervation of cardiac volume- and chemo-receptors [58]. Among the calcineurin inhibitors, there is an indication that tacrolimus may be associated with less hypertension than is cyclosporine [46,59,60]. Posttransplantation hypertension associated with calcineurin inhibitors can be managed effectively with antihypertensive therapy, but it may require use of more than one antihypertensive agent. Angiotensin-converting enzyme (ACE) inhibition normalizes blood pressure and fluid homeostasis in heart transplant recipients receiving cyclosporine, prednisone, and azathioprine. This normalization suggests that posttransplantation hypertension is related to an inability to suppress the renin–angiotensin–aldosterone system when patients become hypovolemic [61].

Posttransplantation hypertension associated with calcineurin inhibitors can be managed effectively with antihypertensive therapy but may require use of more than one antihypertensive agent. Indeed, antihypertensive medication has been associated with improved measures of CAV. In 57 cardiac transplant recipients followed angiographically after randomization to diltiazem or no calcium-channel blocker, the average coronary artery diameter at 2 years was similar to baseline in the diltiazem group but was significantly smaller in those not receiving a calcium-channel blocker; the difference between the groups was significant [62]. Similarly, in 32 cardiac transplant recipients, intimal thickness at 1 year measured by IVUS was significantly greater in the untreated control group than in those who received calcium-channel blockers, ACE inhibitors, or both [63]. These promising results from small, randomized studies are supported by data from two observational studies in which the use of ACE inhibitors was associated with less progression of plaque volume measured by IVUS [64]. This protective effect was most evident if ACE inhibitors were used in combination with calcium-channel blockers and was independent of blood pressure levels [65].

Diabetes

More than 30% of adult heart recipients are diabetic 1 year after transplantation, and more than half of them developed diabetes after the transplantation because of immunosuppressive therapy [3,66–68]. The risk factors for new-onset diabetes include pretransplantation blood glucose levels higher than 5.6 mmol/L, a family history of diabetes, and pretransplantation overweight (which seems to be the most important pretransplantation risk factor [69]), the need for insulin on the second day after transplantation, and immunosuppressive drugs [68], particularly calcineurin inhibitors and corticosteroids [48]. More recently, it also has been suggested that asymptomatic cytomegalovirus infection may predispose a patient to the onset of diabetes after transplantation [70].

The immunosuppressive agents vary considerably in their diabetogenicity [48]. Indeed, the type of immunosuppressive regimen used (steroids, cyclosporine, or tacrolimus) was found to explain 74% of the variability in the incidence of new-onset diabetes after transplantation reported in different studies. Corticosteroids are associated with the greatest risk of developing new-onset diabetes after transplantation, with rates as high as 46% reported in kidney transplant recipients receiving high-dose prednisolone [71]. Higher doses of prednisolone also have been found to be a risk factor for the development of new-onset diabetes in heart transplant recipients [68,72]. Among the calcineurine antagonists, tacrolimus has been reported to predispose recipients to new-onset diabetes more frequently than does cyclosporine [48,73]. Results from randomized studies in heart recipients are inconsistent regarding the diabetogenic effect of tacrolimus, however. For example, a European-based trial in heart transplant recipients reported a 20% incidence of new-onset diabetes with tacrolimus, compared with 10% in the cyclosporine arm. This finding contrasts with data from a similar United States–based trial reporting that tacrolimus was associated only with worse glycemic control, not with an increase in new-onset diabetes [60,74].

Discrepancies between studies may be explained in part by the variability in criteria used for diagnosis of diabetes, the degree of glycemic control obtained with antidiabetic therapy, and the presence of diabetes-related complications. In particular, a study from the authors' group found that hemoglobin A_{1c}, a marker of glycemic control, was associated with the severity of CAV, independently of the cumulative doses of diabetogenic immunosuppressive drugs and of the presence of diabetes before transplantation [75]. In a retrospective analysis of all 20,000 patients who underwent heart transplantation in the United States between 1995 and 2005, posttransplantation survival was affected not by diabetes per se but by the presence of diabetes-related complications, such as obesity, cerebrovascular accident, and peripheral arterial disease. Compared with nondiabetic patients, diabetic patients had only a slightly increased incidence of CAV but much greater renal dysfunction, irrespective of diabetes-related complications [76]. Additionally, in a single-center report, only pretransplantation diabetes, not diabetes occurring after transplantation, seemed to impact survival [77]. Despite the discordances between these observational studies, these data taken together suggest that the duration of diabetes and lack of aggressive glycemic control negatively impact long-term graft survival. This hypothesis also is supported by the experimental evidence showing that metformin treatment prevents CAV development in a diabetic rat model [28]. Randomized, controlled trials are needed to determine the effect of antidiabetic therapy on CAV development and on prognosis.

Summary

The ability of insulin to stimulate glucose disposal, as measured by the steady-state plasma glucose (SSPG) concentration, varies widely in apparently healthy individuals, and those at the upper tertile of the normal continuum of SSPG are at increased risk of CVD. Most heart transplant recipients are markedly insulin resistant and demonstrate many of the features of compensatory hyperinsulinemia, including the atherogenic and proinflammatory profile and the clinical signs of the metabolic syndrome. Multiple lines of evidence suggest that insulin resistance in heart transplant recipients contributes significantly to the development of CAV. Immuno-suppressive drugs, in particular corticosteroids and calcineurin inhibitors, seem to play a major role in the predisposition to insulin resistance. Reduction of these immunosuppressive agents, an approach that has been effective in kidney transplant recipients, is a first step toward ameliorating the negative clinical impact of insulin resistance, for reducing obesity, fasting insulin, and apolipoprotein B concentrations [78]. Nevertheless, the authors believe that a more aggressive approach directed at close monitoring and treatment of the metabolic abnormalities associated with IRS is necessary to prevent CAV and improve long-term prognosis. In addition, specific therapies such as the thiazolidinedione compounds and metformin, shown to be effective in correcting insulin resistance and improving cardiovascular prognosis in the general population [79] and in experimental models [28,42], offer new and promising therapeutic targets for CAV prevention that warrant testing in randomized, controlled trials. If well designed, such trials undoubtedly will further the understanding of the pathophysiology of CAV.

References

[1] Costanzo M, Naftel D, Pritzker M, et al. Heart transplant coronary artery disease detected by coronary angiography: a multiinstitutional study of preoperative donor and recipient risk factor. J Heart Lung Transplant 1998;17:744–53.

[2] Billingham M. Hystopathology of graft coronary disease. J Heart Lung Transplant 1992;11: S38–44.

[3] Taylor DO, Edwards LB, Boucek MM, et al. Registry of the International Society for Heart and Lung Transplantation: twenty-third official adult heart transplantation report–2006. J Heart Lung Transplant 2006;25(8):869–79.

[4] Valantine HA. Cardiac allograft vasculopathy: central role of endothelial injury leading to transplant "atheroma". Transplantation 2003;76(6):891–9.

[5] Mehra M. Contemporary concepts in prevention and treatment of cardiac allograft vasculopathy. Am J Transplant 2006;6(6):1248–56.

[6] Valantine HA, Schroeder JS. Recent advances in cardiac transplantation. N Engl J Med 1995;333(10):660–1.

[7] Tufveson G, Johnsson C. Chronic allograft dysfunction–chronic rejection revisited. Transplantation 2000;70(3):411–2.

[8] Blakolmer K, Jain A, Ruppert K, et al. Chronic liver allograft rejection in a population treated primarily with tacrolimus as baseline immunosuppression: long-term follow-up and evaluation of features for histopathological staging. Transplantation 2000;69(11): 2330–6.

[9] Girgis RE, Tu I, Berry GJ, et al. Risk factors for the development of obliterative bronchiolitis after lung transplantation. J Heart Lung Transplant 1996;15(12):1200–8.

[10] Liu G, Butany J. Morphology of graft arteriosclerosis in cardiac transplant recipients. Hum Pathol 1992;23(7):768–73.

[11] Oni AA, Ray J, Hosenpud JD. Coronary venous intimal thickening in explanted cardiac allografts. Evidence demonstrating that transplant coronary artery disease is a manifestation of a diffuse allograft vasculopathy. Transplantation 1992;53(6):1247–51.

[12] Higuchi ML, Benvenuti LA, Demarchi LM, et al. Histological evidence of concomitant intramyocardial and epicardial vasculitis in necropsied heart allografts: a possible relationship with graft coronary arteriosclerosis. Transplantation 1999;67(12):1569–76.

[13] Russell ME, Fujita M, Masek MA, et al. Cardiac graft vascular disease. Nonselective involvement of large and small vessels. Transplantation 1993;56(6):1599–601.

[14] Rose EA, Smith CR, Petrossian GA, et al. Humoral immune responses after cardiac transplantation: correlation with fatal rejection and graft atherosclerosis. Surgery 1989;106(2): 203–7 [discussion: 207–8].

[15] Hauptman PJ, Nakagawa T, Tanaka H, et al. Acute rejection: culprit or coincidence in the pathogenesis of cardiac graft vascular disease? J Heart Lung Transplant 1995;14(6 Pt 2):S173–80.

[16] Caforio AL, Tona F, Fortina AB, et al. Immune and nonimmune predictors of cardiac allograft vasculopathy onset and severity: multivariate risk factor analysis and role of immunosuppression. Am J Transplant 2004;4(6):962–70.

[17] Gao SZ, Schroeder JS, Hunt SA, et al. Influence of graft rejection on incidence of accelerated graft coronary artery disease: a new approach to analysis. J Heart Lung Transplant 1993; 12(6 Pt 1):1029–35.

[18] Costanzo MR. The role of histoincompatibility in cardiac allograft vasculopathy. J Heart Lung Transplant 1995;14(6 Pt 2):S180–4.

[19] Yeni-Komshian H, Carantoni M, Abbasi F, et al. Relationship between several surrogate estimates of insulin resistance and quantification of insulin-mediated glucose disposal in 490 healthy nondiabetic volunteers. Diabetes Care 2000;23(2):171–5.

[20] Facchini F, Chen YD, Hollenbeck CB, et al. Relationship between resistance to insulin-mediated glucose uptake, urinary uric acid clearance, and plasma uric acid concentration. JAMA 1991;266(21):3008–11.

[21] Castelli W. Lipoproteins and cardiovascular disease: biological basis and epidemiological studies. Value Health 1998;1(2):105–9.

[22] Saadeh S, Younossi ZM. The spectrum of nonalcoholic fatty liver disease: from steatosis to nonalcoholic steatohepatitis. Cleve Clin J Med 2000;67(2):96–7, 101–4.

[23] Despres JP, Lamarche B, Mauriege P, et al. Hyperinsulinemia as an independent risk factor for ischemic heart disease. N Engl J Med 1996;334(15):952–7.

[24] Zavaroni I, Bonini L, Gasparini P, et al. Hyperinsulinemia in a normal population as a predictor of non-insulin-dependent diabetes mellitus, hypertension, and coronary heart disease: the Barilla factory revisited. Metabolism 1999;48(8):989–94.

[25] Facchini F, Reaven G. Resistance to insulin-mediated glucose disposal as a predictor of cardiovascular disease. J Clin Endocrinol Metab 1998;83:2773–6.

[26] Valantine H, Rickenbacker P, Kemna M, et al. Metabolic abnormalities characteristic of dysmetabolic syndrome predict the development of transplant coronary artery disease: a prospective study. Circulation 2001 2001;103(17):2144–52.

[27] Kemna MS, Valantine HA, Hunt SA, et al. Metabolic risk factors for atherosclerosis in heart transplant recipients. Am Heart J 1994;128(1):68–72.

[28] Cantin B, Zhu D, Wen P, et al. Reversal of diabetes-induced rat graft transplant coronary artery disease by metformin. J Heart Lung Transplant 2002;21(6):637–43.

[29] de Lorgeril M, Dureau G, Boissonnat P, et al. Platelet function and composition in heart transplant recipients compared with nontransplanted coronary patients. Arterioscler Thromb 1992;12(2):222–30.

[30] Keogh A. Calcineurin inhibitors in heart transplantation. J Heart Lung Transplant 2004; 23(5 Suppl):S202–6.

[31] Jindal RM, Sidner RA, Milgrom ML. Post-transplant diabetes mellitus. The role of immunosuppression. Drug Saf 1997;16(4):242–57.

[32] Grassi G, Dell'Oro R, Quarti-Trevano F, et al. Neuroadrenergic and reflex abnormalities in patients with metabolic syndrome. Diabetologia 2005;48(7):1359–65.

[33] Rickenbacher PR, Kemna MS, Pinto FJ, et al. Coronary artery intimal thickening in the transplanted heart. An in vivo intracoronary ultrasound study of immunologic and metabolic risk factors. Transplantation 1996;61(1):46–53.

[34] de Vries AP, Bakker SJ, van Son WJ, et al. Insulin resistance as putative cause of chronic renal transplant dysfunction. Am J Kidney Dis 2003;41(4):859–67.

[35] Wenke K, Meiser B, Thiery J, et al. Simvastatin reduces graft vessel disease and morality after heart transplantation. Circulation 1997;96:1398–402.

[36] White M, Ross H, Haddad H, et al. Subclinical inflammation and prothrombotic state in heart transplant recipients: impact of cyclosporin microemulsion vs. tacrolimus. Transplantation 2006;82(6):763–70.

[37] McLaughlin T, Abbasi F, Cheal K, et al. Use of metabolic markers to identify overweight individuals who are insulin resistant. Ann Intern Med 2003;139:802–9.

[38] Biadi O, Potena L, Fearon WF, et al. Interplay between systemic inflammation and markers of insulin resistance in cardiovascular prognosis after heart transplantation. J Heart Lung Transplant 2007;26(4):324–30.

[39] Ferre' P. The biology of peroxisome proliferator-activated receptors. Relationship with lipid metabolism and insulin sensitivity. Diabetes 2004;53(Suppl 1):S43–50.

[40] Schupp M, Janke J, Clasen R, et al. Angiotensin type 1 receptor blockers induce peroxisome proliferator-activated receptor gamma activity. Circulation 2004;109:2054–7.

[41] Yousufuddin M, Haji S, Starling R, et al. Cardiac angiotensin II receptors as predictors of transplant coronary artery disease following heart transplantation. Eur Heart J 2004;25: 377–85.

[42] Kosuge H, Haraguchi G, Koga N, et al. Pioglitazone prevents acute and chronic cardiac allograft rejection. Circulation 2006;113:2613–22.

[43] Pethig K, Klauss V, Heublein B, et al. Progression of cardiac allograft vascular disease as assessed by serial intravascular ultrasound: correlation to immunological and non-immunological risk factors. Heart 2000;84(5):494–8.

[44] Kapadia S, Nissen S, Ziada K, et al. Impact of lipid abnormalities in development and progression of transplant coronary disease: a serial intravascular ultrasound study. J Am Coll Cardiol 2001;38:206–13.

[45] Potena L, Grigioni F, Ortolani P, et al. Relevance of cytomegalovirus infection and coronary-artery remodeling in the first year after heart transplantation: a prospective three-dimensional intravascular ultrasound study. Transplantation 2003;75(6):839–43.

[46] Kobashigawa J, Starling R, Mehra M, et al. Multicenter retrospective analysis of cardiovascular risk factors affecting long-term outcome of de novo cardiac transplant recipients. J Heart Lung Transplant 2006;25:1063–9.

[47] Zawaideh MA, Ghishan FK, Molmenti EP. Regulation of cholesterol homeostasis in solid organ transplantation. Transplantation 2006;81(3):316–7.

[48] Lindenfeld J, Miller G, Shakar S, et al. Drug therapy in the heart transplant recipient. Part II: immunosuppressive drugs. Circulation 2004;110(25):3858–65.

[49] Taylor D, Barr M, Radovancevic B, et al. A randomized multicenter comparison of tacrolimus and cyclosporine immunosuppressive regimens in cardiac transplantation: decreased hyperlipidemia and hypertension with tacrolimus. J Heart Lung Transplant 1999;18: 336–45.

[50] Eisen HJ, Tuzcu EM, Dorent R, et al. Everolimus for the prevention of allograft rejection and vasculopathy in cardiac-transplant recipients. N Engl J Med 2003;349(9):847–58.

[51] Keogh A, Richardson M, Ruygrok P, et al. Sirolimus in de novo heart transplant recipients reduces acute rejection and prevents coronary artery disease at 2 years: a randomized clinical trial. Circulation 2004;110(17):2694–700.

[52] Kobashigawa JA, Katznelson S, Laks H, et al. Effect of pravastatin on outcomes after cardiac transplantation. N Engl J Med 1995;333(10):621–7.

[53] Wu H, Ballantyne C, Short B, et al. Statin use and risks of death or fatal rejection in the heart transplant lipid registry. Am J Cardiol 2004;95:367–72.

[54] Grigioni F, Carigi S, Potena L, et al. Long-term safety and effectiveness of statins for heart transplant recipients in routine clinical practice. Transplant Proc 2006;38(5):1507–10.

[55] Holdaas H, Fellstrom B, Cole E, et al. Long-term cardiac outcomes in renal transplant recipients receiving fluvastatin: the ALERT extension study. Am J Transplant 2005;5(12): 2929–36.

[56] Patel AR, Ambrose MS, Duffy GA, et al. Treatment of hypercholesterolemia with ezetimibe in cardiac transplant recipients. J Heart Lung Transplant 2007;26(3):281–4.

[57] Radovancevic B, Poindexter S, Birovijev S, et al. Risk factors for development of accelerated coronary artery disease in cardiac transplant recipients. Eur J Cardiothorac Surg 1990;4: 309–13.

[58] Ciarka A, Najem B, Cuylits N, et al. Effects of peripheral chemoreceptors deactivation on sympathetic activity in heart transplant recipients. Hypertension 2005;45(5):894–900.

[59] Klauss V, Koning A, Spes C, et al. Cyclosporine versus tacrolimus (FK 506) for prevention of cardiac allograft vasculopathy. Am J Cardiol 2000;85:266–9.

[60] Grimm M, Rinaldi M, Yonan NA, et al. Superior prevention of acute rejection by tacrolimus vs. cyclosporine in heart transplant recipients—a large European trial. Am J Transplant 2006;6(6):1387–97.

[61] Braith RW, Mills RM, Wilcox CS, et al. High-dose angiotensin-converting enzyme inhibition restores body fluid homeostasis in heart-transplant recipients. J Am Coll Cardiol 2003;41(3):426–32.

[62] Schroeder JS, Gao SZ, Alderman EL, et al. A preliminary study of diltiazem in the prevention of coronary artery disease in heart-transplant recipients. N Engl J Med 1993;328(3): 164–70.

[63] Mehra MR, Ventura HO, Smart FW, et al. An intravascular ultrasound study of the influence of angiotensin-converting enzyme inhibitors and calcium entry blockers on the development of cardiac allograft vasculopathy. Am J Cardiol 1995;75(12):853–4.

[64] Bae JH, Rihal CS, Edwards BS, et al. Association of angiotensin-converting enzyme inhibitors and serum lipids with plaque regression in cardiac allograft vasculopathy. Transplantation 2006;82(8):1108–11.

[65] Erinc K, Yamani MH, Starling RC, et al. The effect of combined angiotensin-converting enzyme inhibition and calcium antagonism on allograft coronary vasculopathy validated by intravascular ultrasound. J Heart Lung Transplant 2005;24(8):1033–8.

[66] Nieuwenhuis MG, Kirkels JH. Predictability and other aspects of post-transplant diabetes mellitus in heart transplant recipients. J Heart Lung Transplant 2001;20(7):703–8.

[67] Hathout EH, Chinnock RE, Johnston JK, et al. Pediatric post-transplant diabetes: data from a large cohort of pediatric heart-transplant recipients. Am J Transplant 2003;3(8):994–8.

[68] Depczynski B, Daly B, Campbell LV, et al. Predicting the occurrence of diabetes mellitus in recipients of heart transplants. Diabet Med 2000;17(1):15–9.

[69] Kahn J, Rehak P, Schweiger M, et al. The impact of overweight on the development of diabetes after heart transplantation. Clin Transplant 2006;20(1):62–6.

[70] Hjelmesaeth J, Sagedal S, Hartmann A, et al. Asymptomatic cytomegalovirus infection is associated with increased risk of new-onset diabetes mellitus and impaired insulin release after renal transplantation. Diabetologia 2004;47(9):1550–6.

[71] Gunnarsson R, Lundgren G, Magnusson G, et al. Steroid diabetes—a sign of overtreatment with steroids in the renal graft recipient? Scand J Urol Nephrol Suppl 1980;54:135–8.

[72] Wilkinson A, Davidson J, Dotta F, et al. Guidelines for the treatment and management of new-onset diabetes after transplantation. Clin Transplant 2005;19(3):291–8.

[73] Heisel O, Heisel R, Balshaw R, et al. New onset diabetes mellitus in patients receiving calcineurin inhibitors: a systematic review and meta-analysis. Am J Transplant 2004;4(4):583–95.

[74] Kobashigawa JA, Miller LW, Russell SD, et al. Tacrolimus with mycophenolate mofetil (MMF) or sirolimus vs. cyclosporine with MMF in cardiac transplant patients: 1-year report. Am J Transplant 2006;6(6):1377–86.

[75] Kato T, Chan MC, Gao SZ, et al. Glucose intolerance, as reflected by hemoglobin A1c level, is associated with the incidence and severity of transplant coronary artery disease. J Am Coll Cardiol 2004;43(6):1034–41.

[76] Russo MJ, Chen JM, Hong KN, et al. Survival after heart transplantation is not diminished among recipients with uncomplicated diabetes mellitus: an analysis of the United Network of Organ Sharing database. Circulation 2006;114(21):2280–7.

[77] Klingenberg R, Gleissner C, Koch A, et al. Impact of pre-operative diabetes mellitus upon early and late survival after heart transplantation: a possible era effect. J Heart Lung Transplant 2005;24(9):1239–46.

[78] Lemieux I, Houde I, Pascot A, et al. Effects of prednisone withdrawal on the new metabolic triad in cyclosporine-treated kidney transplant patients. Kidney Int 2002;62(5):1839–47.

[79] Erdmann E, Dormandy JA, Charbonnel B, et al. The effect of pioglitazone on recurrent myocardial infarction in 2,445 patients with type 2 diabetes and previous myocardial infarction: results from the PROactive (PROactive 05) Study. J Am Coll Cardiol 2007;49(17): 1772–80.

[80] Senechal M, Lemieux I, Beucler I, et al. Features of the metabolic syndrome of "hypertriglyceridemic waist" and transplant coronary artery disease. J Heart Lung Transplant 2005;24(7):819–26.

ELSEVIER
SAUNDERS

Endocrinol Metab Clin N Am
36 (2007) 983–998

ENDOCRINOLOGY
AND METABOLISM
CLINICS
OF NORTH AMERICA

Endocrine Complications of Hematopoietic Stem Cell Transplantation

Wassim Chemaitilly, MD[a], Charles A. Sklar, MD[b],*

[a]Department of Pediatrics, Schneider Children's Hospital, 269-01 76th Avenue,
New Hyde Park, NY 11040, USA
[b]Department of Pediatrics, Memorial-Sloan-Kettering Cancer Center,
New York, NY 100021, USA

Advances in hematopoietic stem cell transplantation (HSCT) have resulted in broader indications for this therapeutic modality in both malignant diseases, such as leukemia, and nonmalignant conditions such as immunodeficiency disorders, aplastic anemia, thalassemia major and sickle cell disease [1]. In autologous HSCT, healthy hematopoietic stem cells are harvested, stored and reinfused, after cytoreduction, to the same individual (ie, the patient is his or her own donor). This treatment modality is particularly useful in situations where delivering enough chemotherapy to treat the underlying malignancy would otherwise be hampered by bone marrow toxicity [2]. In allogeneic HSCT, healthy hematopoietic stem cells are harvested from a separate, related or unrelated, ideally human leukocyte antigen (HLA)-matched donor, and used to replace the patient's own abnormal hematopoietic stem cells [2]. Conditioning regimens for HSCT often combine total body irradiation (TBI) and high-dose chemotherapy, although regimens that employ chemotherapy alone increasingly are being used to reduce the exposure of patients to radiotherapy and its adverse effects. Individuals successfully treated with HSCT are, therefore, at risk of developing long-term complications as a result of drug and radiation toxicity, as are those treated with allogeneic HSCT as a consequence of graft versus host disease (GvHD). Endocrine complications are among the most prevalent late effects observed in HSCT recipients [3]. This article focuses on the late endocrine abnormalities that are most commonly observed following

---

* Corresponding author.
E-mail address: sklarc@mskcc.org (C.A. Sklar).

endo.theclinics.com

successful HSCT, with a special emphasis on pediatric HSCT recipients, for whom long-term follow-up data are increasingly available.

Growth failure and growth hormone deficiency

Growth failure, including impaired linear growth during childhood and adolescence and reduced adult heights frequently are observed in childhood cancer survivors treated with HSCT. There are many factors, both endocrine and nonendocrine, that contribute to growth failure following HSCT [4–8]. Patient characteristics (eg, young age), treatment variables (eg, TBI, prior cranial radiation), and post-treatment complications such as chronic GvHD are the main determinants of abnormal growth [8]. They can create a situation detrimental to linear growth by inducing poor nutritional conditions, growth hormone (GH) deficiency and/or skeletal dysplasia (secondary to the exposure of the growth plate to radiation toxicity). The current knowledge of the impact of HSCT on the hypothalamic-pituitary-GH axis is derived primarily from the study of pediatric cohorts. Data pertaining to the GH status of individuals treated with HSCT during adulthood remain limited [9,10].

Impact of the use of chemotherapy in hematopoietic stem cell transplantation conditioning regimens

Preparative regimens that employ chemotherapy alone increasingly are being used to reduce the exposure of patients to radiotherapy and its adverse effects. Examples include the use of cyclophosphamide for aplastic anemia, high doses of cyclophosphamide and busulfan, and, more recently, fludarabine and busulfan [11] in preparation for HSCT. Children treated with cyclophosphamide for aplastic anemia appear to grow normally, so long as they do not develop a significant complication (eg, GvHD, liver dysfunction) after transplantation [12–15]. The consequences on growth of pretransplant conditioning regimens combining high doses of busulfan and cyclophosphamide remain controversial. Most authors have not found evidence of sustained growth failure in the patients who received such conditioning regimens in the absence of significant post-transplant complications [5,12–16]. Growth failure, possibly caused by GH deficiency, has been reported by some authors, however [17–19]. More studies with additional adult height data are needed for a better understanding of the impact of this conditioning regimen on linear growth and on the hypothalamic-pituitary-GH axis.

Data pertaining to the impact of chemotherapy-based preparative regimes on the hypothalamic-GH axis in adult recipients of HSCT are quite limited. Reporting on a cohort of 40 adult HSCT recipients whose conditioning regimen combined cyclophosphamide and busulfan, Tauchmanova and colleagues [10] showed that a significant proportion (38%) of those individuals who suffered from chronic GvHD had low insulin growth factor-1 (IGF-1) levels. The significance of these findings is not clear, because the authors did not provide any clinical information specifically pertaining to these individuals;

nonetheless the subject deserves further investigation, given the potential benefits of GH replacement in adults who have severe GH deficiency [20].

Impact of the use of radiotherapy in hematopoietic stem cell transplantation conditioning regimens

Total lymphoid irradiation

Linear growth seems to be altered in patients treated for aplastic anemia with cyclophosphamide plus total lymphoid irradiation (TLI), but to a lesser extent than in patients treated with TBI [21,22]. As expected, there does not seem to be an association between the use of TLI and the occurrence of GH deficiency [22].

Total body irradiation

Total body irradiation, when administered during childhood, alters linear growth. The loss of growth potential is more severe in patients treated with single-dose irradiation when compared with those treated with fractionated TBI, despite the fact that the total dose of irradiation is higher in the latter group [12,23,24]. These results indicate that both the total dose and dose per fraction are likely important determinants of the height outcome following HSCT [25,26]. The age at the time that TBI is administered is also critical. Patients treated with TBI at a young age, and who have many years of linear growth ahead of them, suffer a greater height loss than those treated at an older age, and indeed, younger age at the time of HSCT has been the most cited risk factor for short adult stature [5–7,27–33].

TBI can alter linear growth by various mechanisms, including the induction of GH deficiency and the development of skeletal dysplasia [34]. An increased incidence of GH deficiency after TBI in childhood has been reported in several studies [6,35–38]. The observed GH deficiency, however, could be a transient effect; some patients, diagnosed as GH deficient in childhood, had normal GH responses when retested in adulthood [22,32].

GH replacement therapy is indicated in patients with documented GH deficiency who have been in remission for more than a year, and who demonstrate clinical evidence of impaired linear growth and/or poor height prognosis. Although GH replacement does not appear to increase the risk of disease recurrence or death in survivors of childhood cancer, there may be a small increased risk of developing second tumors [30,39]. The impact of GH replacement on the final heights achieved by pediatric HSCT recipients treated with TBI has been difficult to assess. The most recent long-term follow up data suggest that height stabilization, rather than catch-up growth, is the most frequently observed outcome following GH replacement in this population [24,30,33,36,38,40]. Furthermore, the effect of GH treatment seems to vary according to patient characteristics. Thus, younger patients are likely to respond better to GH therapy. For instance, Sanders and colleagues [30] reported a beneficial effect of GH replacement in pediatric HSCT recipients treated with fractionated TBI. This, however, was only evident for those treated with HSCT before the age of 10 years. Couto-Silva and colleagues

[29] reported similar findings, as they demonstrated a significant reduction of the height loss by GH replacement for children treated with TBI between the ages of 4 and 8 years. The response to GH therapy could be limited as the main target of GH action, the growth plate, already may have suffered significant damage by the time GH treatment is initiated [35].

Skeletal dysplasia remains an important determinant of the loss of growth potential. Of note, disproportionate growth has been reported by some authors, with spinal growth being more impaired than growth of the legs following TBI [22,32,33,35]. Irradiation of the long bones also may contribute to some extent to the height loss after TBI [27].

Data pertaining to the GH status of individuals treated with HSCT during adulthood and whose conditioning regimen included TBI remain scarce. Reporting on a cohort of 20 adult HSCT recipients (11 of whom were treated with TBI), Kauppila and colleagues [9] showed that five individuals had low levels of GH in response to stimulation with growth hormone releasing hormone (GHRH). The GH response, however, did not correlate with any particular patient characteristic or treatment variable. Again, the clinical significance of these findings remains unclear, but the subject deserves further investigation.

Other risk factors affecting linear growth in hematopoietic stem cell transplantation recipients

Exposure to cranial radiotherapy before hematopoietic stem cell transplantation

Hypothalamic and/or pituitary damage in HSCT recipients also can be caused by exposure to prior cranial irradiation, which has been cited as an important risk factor for poor growth after transplantation [5,24,30–32,38,40,41]. Furthermore, prior cranial radiotherapy has been associated with a higher incidence of central precocious puberty, a condition that can alter an individual's growth potential further by causing early bone maturation and premature epiphyseal fusion [42].

Chronic graft versus host disease

The treatment of chronic GvHD usually involves the use of high-dose glucocorticoids, which are associated with impaired skeletal growth. Catch-up growth does not always occur after recovery from chronic GvHD, as the primary disease and the previous treatments may have altered the patient's growth potential irreversibly [14,34].

Disturbances of the other hypothalamic–pituitary axes

Corticotropin deficiency

Corticotropin (ACTH) deficiency has been shown to be very rare in both pediatric and adult recipients of HSCT [9,37]. A higher incidence (up to

24%) of ACTH deficiency was reported by Sanders and colleagues [12] in patients exposed to TBI, but the authors had based their conclusions on subnormal levels of 11-deoxycortisol (Compound S) after metyrapone stimulation, a method which is subject to a great deal of variability.

Thyrotropin deficiency

Central hypothyroidism is a rare complication following HSCT [24,37]. The surprisingly high incidence of hidden thyrotropin (TSH) deficiency following TBI that was reported by Rose and colleagues [43] (reaching 20% 4 years after HSCT) was based on abnormal responses to the TSH-releasing hormone (TRH) stimulation test and on abnormal nocturnal TSH levels, despite normal levels of free T4. The clinical relevance of these findings is unclear, and the benefit of thyroxine replacement therapy in such patients has not been established. Of note, in a report on 37 euthyroid cranially irradiated adult cancer survivors, Darzy and Shalet [44] suggested that the abnormalities of TSH dynamics noted after cranial irradiation were a reflection of subtle functional disturbances in TSH secretion that did not appear to be clinically meaningful.

Disorders of gonadotropin secretion

Hypogonadotropic hypogonadism is distinctly uncommon in the context of HSCT [24,37]. On the other hand, cases of central precocious puberty following HSCT in patients who received prior cranial irradiation have been reported [42]. This premature activation of the hypothalamic-pituitary-gonadotropin axis is thought to be triggered by the disruption of the inhibitory influence of the cortex secondary to the brain's exposure to radiation. Central precocious puberty can worsen the height outcome of these patients who often have coexistent GH deficiency [42].

Thyroid dysfunction

Several thyroid abnormalities have been described following HSCT. These include therapy-induced primary hypothyroidism, autoimmune thyroid disease, and thyroid neoplasms.

Therapy-induced primary hypothyroidism

Individuals exposed to radiotherapy
The incidence of primary thyroid dysfunction has varied greatly from series to series, owing to differences in the type of treatments delivered and the duration of follow-up. The overall incidence of hypothyroidism has been greater following single-dose TBI (23% to 73%) compared with that seen after fractionated TBI (10% to 28%) [32,37,45–49]. Moreover,

the longer the follow-up time, the higher the incidence of impaired thyroid function [50]. Additionally, younger age at HSCT has been shown to increase the risk of hypothyroidism in some series [51,52]. Along similar lines, Al-Fiar and colleagues [52] reported a lower prevalence of hypothyroidism (8.9%) in adult HSCT recipients when compared with pediatric HSCT recipients. Most patients develop a mild, compensated primary hypothyroidism that may be transient and can resolve spontaneously [48].

Individuals conditioned without radiation

Mildly elevated TSH levels have been reported following cytoreduction with busulfan and cyclophosphamide [10,15,18,48,50,52,53]. Slatter and colleagues [54] described more severe cases of primary hypothyroidism in a series of 83 subjects with various types of immunodeficiency who received cyclophosphamide plus busulfan as conditioning for a HSCT.

Autoimmune thyroid disease

There are several reports of the occurrence of autoimmune thyroid disease in HSCT recipients [10,54–57]. For example, in a report on a cohort of 721 adult HSCT recipients, Au and colleagues [56] described 10 cases of autoimmune thyroid disease. Five subjects presented with hyperthyroidism; three developed hypothyroidism, and two had sequential hyperthyroidism followed by hypothyroidism. All patients were clinically symptomatic, and all had elevated titers of antithyroglobulin antibodies [56]. Sklar and colleagues [57] reported three cases of autoimmune hyperthyroidism following pediatric HSCT; all had raised T4 and/or T3 levels and suppressed TSH levels, while two subjects had elevated levels of the antibody to the TSH receptor. In two cases, radioactive iodine was necessary to correct the hyperthyroidism, while in the third case, the condition spontaneously resolved over a 6-month period. All three HSCT donors consequently were found to have elevated levels of TSH receptor antibody. The adoptive transfer of abnormal clones of T or B cells from donor to recipient could be responsible for the development of autoimmune thyrotoxicosis-observed HSCT [55–58].

Thyroid neoplasms

Thyroid neoplasms, both benign and malignant. can develop following irradiation of the thyroid gland [30,32,46,59–62]. Reporting on a series of 113 pediatric HSCT patients, Cohen and colleagues [63] showed that the incidence of thyroid carcinoma was higher than in the general population, with eight cases diagnosed between 3.1 and 15.7 years after transplant. Given the length of the latency period between radiation and the appearance of thyroid neoplasms, the number of affected individuals almost certainly will increase with increasing follow-up time after HSCT.

Gonadal and reproductive dysfunction

Males

The impact of chemotherapy

Young boys and adolescent males who receive standard-dose cyclophosphamide alone (200 mg/kg) as therapy for aplastic anemia appear to retain normal Leydig cell function. Most are reported to have normal plasma concentrations of luteinizing hormone (LH) and testosterone and to enter and progress normally through puberty. In a study by Sanders and colleagues [64], all 28 boys who received that conditioning regimen achieved a normal pubertal development. Leydig cell function appears to be preserved in most adult males following similar exposures [10,15,18,53].

Standard-dose cyclophosphamide alone (200 mg/kg) used for aplastic anemia has been associated with some degree of germ cell damage, which may be more common in males treated during or after puberty compared with males treated before the onset of puberty. Sanders and colleagues [46] reported normal plasma concentrations of follicle-stimulating hormone (FSH) in most males who were treated before puberty, whereas FSH levels were increased in nearly half the males who were treated during or after puberty. Nonetheless, semen analyses have been normal in approximately two thirds of the males, and a sizeable number of males, including 18 who were prepubertal at transplant, have fathered normal children after treatment with high-dose cyclophosphamide [46,64,65].

The combination of busulfan and cyclophosphamide does appear to cause damage to the germinal epithelium in most male patients. Recovery of spermatogenesis seems to occur more frequently in patients receiving lower doses of cyclophosphamide (120 mg/kg) than in those treated with higher doses of cyclophosphamide (200 mg/kg) [66]. Anserini and colleagues [67] showed that recovery of some spermatogenetic activity also occurred in 50% of cases in the latter group, but semen quality was impaired. Overall, the ultimate effect of this treatment on male fertility remains to be determined.

In a report on 32 adult recipients of HSCT, Kyriacou and colleagues [68] showed that both Leydig cell and germ cell functions were impaired after treatment with a nonmyeloablative conditioning regimen that combined fludarabine, melphalan, and CAMPATH-1H. Their data, however, were based solely on hormonal indices and did not include the results of semen analyses.

The impact of total body irradiation

Leydig cell function generally is preserved in males treated with TBI-based preparative regimens, both single dose and fractionated, regardless of the age at treatment, so long as the total cumulative dose of radiotherapy to the testis (including testicular irradiation before HSCT) is less than 2000 cGy [12,36,46,69]. On the other hand, many patients treated with higher doses of testicular radiotherapy (2000 to 2400 cGy range) go on to develop Leydig cell insufficiency and require androgen replacement therapy [69].

Germ cell dysfunction is present in essentially all males treated with TBI, and azoospermia generally is observed during the first few years after TBI [65]. The effect of TBI on germ cells seems, however, to vary according to the length of follow-up and the age at treatment. In a recent report on 39 HSCT recipients (mean age at study 34 years; seen on average 9 years after HSCT; 82% treated with TBI), Rovo and colleagues [70] showed that while all subjects had some degree of germ cell dysfunction, 28% of them had detectable spermatozoa in their ejaculate. Of the 11 patients who showed some evidence of spermatogenesis, seven had been treated with TBI. Factors associated with the persistence of spermatogenetic activity included younger age at HSCT (less than 25 years), longer time interval since HSCT ,and absence of chronic GvHD [70]. In a similar-sized but slightly older cohort (35 patients, including 33 treated with TBI; mean age at study 38 years), Savani and colleagues [71] reported a lower percentage of HSCT recipients with evidence of spermatogenetic activity (14%) and confirmed the association between preservation of spermatogenesis and younger age at HSCT (no more than 30 years) and longer follow-up interval. A few men have been reported to father a child following TBI [65–72].

In a report on 30 pediatric HSCT survivors, of whom 25 were treated with TBI, Ishiguro and colleagues [72] showed that the nine patients for whom gonadal shielding was used during TBI had better preserved testicular growth, reflected by a significantly higher testicular size when compared with individuals treated with TBI without gonadal shielding. Additional long-term follow-up data are required to determine the definitive impact of this intervention on fertility. In the meantime, semen banking before HSCT remains the gold standard for preservation of fertility in sexually mature male HSCT recipients [73].

Females

The impact of chemotherapy

Following transplant for aplastic anemia with high-dose cyclophosphamide during childhood and adolescence, ovarian function has remained normal in females treated before and after the onset of puberty [46,74]. Sanders and colleagues [74] have observed numerous pregnancies and normal offspring in their cohort treated with cyclophosphamide alone. Data from patients treated with high-dose alkylating agents for other indications, however, suggest that these subjects may be at increased risk of an early menopause later in life [75,76].

Females treated with busulfan and cyclophosphamide are at very high risk of developing ovarian failure [8,15,19,53]. This has been observed in patients treated before and after pubertal development. It is characterized by menopausal levels of LH and FSH, delayed or arrested puberty, and amenorrhea. Recovery of function has been recorded only rarely, but the follow-up time has been relatively brief for most of the patients. Most young girls treated with the combination of busulfan and cyclophosphamide will require long-term hormonal replacement therapy.

The impact of total body irradiation

Patient age at the time of TBI appears to be a critical variable in determining the outcome of ovarian function [77]. Approximately 50% of prepubertal girls given fractionated TBI will enter puberty spontaneously and achieve menarche at a normal age [42,49,78]. On the other hand, ovarian failure is seen in essentially all patients who are greater than age 10 years at the time they are treated with TBI [42,74,77,78]. Recovery of ovarian function has been documented in a small number of women who have received TBI [65,79,80]. Thus, in a recent report from the bone marrow transplant survivor group, Carter and colleagues [80] showed that out of 292 female study participants, five women treated with TBI reported a pregnancy after HSCT. Preliminary data from Nakagawa and colleagues [81] suggest that gonadal shielding during TBI may help preserve ovarian function, reflected by the resumption of menstrual activity after HSCT in two out of the three subjects included in the study. The small number of cases in this study and absence of fertility/pregnancy outcome data, however, mandate further evaluation of the impact of this intervention.

In terms of pregnancy outcomes, Sanders and colleagues [65] reported a high rate of spontaneous abortions in women who were treated with TBI when they were prepubertal, while in women treated with TBI at an older age, the small numbers of pregnancies were associated with an increased risk of delivery of premature and low birth weight infants. In contrast to these findings, none of the five women treated with TBI reported by Carter and colleagues had a miscarriage after HSCT.

Exposure to TBI may have consequences on uterine function that may contribute to the higher incidence of pregnancy complications reported by some. Holm and colleagues [82] and Bath and colleagues [83] demonstrated that the uterine volume of patients treated with TBI is smaller than in normal controls and in cancer survivors treated exclusively with chemotherapy. Moreover, the blood supply to the uterus may be decreased significantly after TBI [82,83].

Effects on bone density

Survivors of HSCT appear to be at increased risk for the development of reduced bone density in later life [84–88]. The incidence of osteopenia was close to 50% 4 to 6 years following bone marrow transplantation (BMT) in reports on adult HSCT recipients by Schimmer and colleagues [87] and Kerschan-Schindl and colleagues [88]. Both the therapies employed to treat these malignancies and various treatment-related complications appear to interfere with normal bone accretion [89]. Risk factors for reduced bone mineral density in survivors of HSCT include treatment with glucocorticoids for chronic GvHD, prior cranial irradiation (most likely a surrogate for GH deficiency), and sex hormone insufficiency [84,90,91]. The underlying mechanisms of post-HSCT osteoporosis remain unclear. Lee and colleagues [92] suggested that impaired differentiation of bone marrow stroma cells into osteoblasts may explain post-HSCT osteoporosis partly. The progressive increase in bone resorption during the immediate post-HSCT period was related to steroid dose and increased bone marrow interleukin-6 levels [93]. The latter is a potent stimulator of bone resorption in vivo, and is also known to be involved in postmenopausal osteoporosis [92]. More recently, Kerschan-Schindl and colleagues [88] suggested that the higher bone resorption rate could be related to increased levels of osteoprotegerin-ligand of receptor activator of nuclear factor-kappa-B (RANK-L) complexes in individuals treated with HSCT.

Periodic bone mineral density studies are recommended in HSCT survivors, given the risk of osteoporosis. Dual-energy radiograph absorptiometry (DEXA) is the most widely used tool for measuring bone mineral density. Its results, however, should be interpreted according to age, pubertal stage, and height in the pediatric population. Failure to take these elements into account may result in overdiagnosing osteoporosis [86].

Preventive measures (eg, supplementation with calcium and vitamin D, smoking cessation, weight-bearing exercise) should be encouraged in all individuals with low or borderline bone mineral density. Therapeutic interventions (eg, bisphosphonates) may prove beneficial for those with abnormally reduced bone density despite appropriate and timely replacement of hormonal deficits (eg, sex hormones), but long-term follow-up data are not available.

Disorders of glucose homeostasis

Several authors have reported an increased risk of insulin resistance and metabolic syndrome (insulin resistance, glucose intolerance, dyslipidemia, and hypertension) in patients who have undergone HSCT [94–101]. Exposure to TBI has emerged consistently as a significant risk factor for insulin resistance [31,95,97,98,102,103]. Furthermore, in a recent report from the Bone Marrow Transplant Survivor Study, Baker and colleagues [103] demonstrated a significant association between the occurrence of diabetes mellitus and exposure to TBI, a correlation that persisted even after adjusting for age and body mass index. Some authors have suggested that the incidence of both type 1 (ie, insulinopenia) and type 2 (ie, insulin resistance) diabetes mellitus may be increased following TBI [96]. The heterogeneity of the populations included in the published studies, the diversity of the treatments they received, and the differences in the time intervals since the completion of cancer treatments all make interpretation of the findings difficult [95,97]. More studies are needed to clarify the true incidence of the metabolic syndrome and to better understand the possible mechanisms involved.

Summary

Endocrine complications are highly prevalent following HSCT. Linear growth can be severely affected in recipients of pediatric HSCT as a result of skeletal dysplasia, GH deficiency, and exposure to glucocorticoids. The impact of HSCT on the hypothalamic-GH axis in adults requires further investigation. Periodic evaluation of thyroid function and bone mineral density should be part of the follow-up care of individuals treated with HSCT given the high incidence of thyroid dysfunction and osteopenia/osteoporosis after HSCT. Fertility issues are common after HSCT, and new strategies aiming at the preservation of reproductive potential of patients need to be considered. Disorders of glucose homeostasis increasingly are reported following HSCT; more studies are required to investigate the prevalence, pathogenesis, and long-term impact of these disorders on the health status of HSCT survivors.

References

[1] Thomas ED. History of haemopoietic cell transplantation. Br J Haematol 1999;105: 330–9.

[2] Fisher VL, Abramovitz LZ. A brief overview of hemaotopoietic stem-cell transplantation. In: Kline RM, editor. Pediatric hematopoietic stem cell transplantation. New York: Informa Healthcare; 2006. p. 601–2.

[3] Hows JM, Passweg JR, Tichelli A, et al. Comparison of long-term outcomes after allogeneic hematopoietic stem cell transplantation from matched sibling and unrelated donors. Bone Marrow Transplant 2006;38:799–805.

[4] Boulad F, Sands S, Sklar C. Late complications after BMT in children and adolescents. Curr Probl Pediatr 1998;28:277–97.

[5] Cohen A, Rovelli A, Bakker B, et al. Final height of patients who underwent bone marrow transplantation for hematological disorders during childhood: a study by the Working Party for Late Effects-EBMT. Blood 1999;93:4109–15.

[6] Clement-De Boers A, Oostdijk W, Van Weel-Sipman MH, et al. Final height and hormonal function after bone marrow transplantation in children. J Pediatr 1996;129:544–50.

[7] Frisk P, Arvidson J, Gustafsson J, et al. Pubertal development and final height after autologous bone marrow transplantation for acute lymphoblastic leukemia. Bone Marrow Transplant 2004;33:205–10.

[8] Sklar C. Growth and endocrine disturbances after bone marrow transplantation in childhood. Acta Paediatr 1995;411:57–61.

[9] Kauppila M, Koskinen P, Irjala K, et al. Long-term effects of allogeneic bone marrow transplantation (BMT) on pituitary, gonad, thyroid, and adrenal function in adults. Bone Marrow Transplant 1998;22:331–7.

[10] Tauchmanova L, Selleri C, Rosa GD, et al. High prevalence of endocrine dysfunction in long-term survivors after allogeneic bone marrow transplantation for hematologic diseases. Cancer 2002;95:1076–84.

[11] de Lima M, Couriel D, Thall PF, et al. Once-daily intravenous busulfan and fludarabine: clinical and pharmacokinetic results of a myeloablative, reduced-toxicity conditioning regimen for allogeneic stem cell transplantation in AML and MDS. Blood 2004;104: 857–64.

[12] Sanders JE, Pritchard S, Mahoney P, et al. Growth and development following marrow transplantation for leukemia. Blood 1986;68:1129–35.

[13] Giorgiani G, Bozzola M, Locatelli F, et al. Role of busulfan and total body irradiation on growth of prepubertal children receiving bone marrow transplantation and results of treatment with recombinant human growth hormone. Blood 1995;86:825–31.

[14] Adan L, de Lanversin M-L, Thalassinos C, et al. Growth after bone marrow transplantation in young children conditioned with chemotherapy alone. Bone Marrow Transplant 1997;19:253–6.

[15] Afify A, Shaw PJ, Clavano-Harding A, et al. Growth and endocrine function in children with acute myeloid leukaemia after bone marrow transplantation using busulfan/cyclophosphamide. Bone Marrow Transplant 2000;25:1087–92.

[16] Lähteenmäki PM, Chakrabarti S, Cornish JM, et al. Outcome of single-fraction total body irradiation-conditioned stem cell transplantation in younger children with malignant disease, comparison with a busulfan–cyclophosphamide regimen. Acta Oncol 2004;43: 196–203.

[17] Sanders JE. Growth and development after bone marrow transplantation. In: Forman SJ, Blume KG, Thomas ED, editors. Bone marrow transplantation. Boston: Blackwell Scientific Publications; 1994. p. 527–37.

[18] Bakker B, Oostdijk W, Bresters D, et al. Disturbances of growth and endocrine function after busulfan-based conditioning for haematopoietic stem cell transplantation during infancy and childhood. Bone Marrow Transplant 2004;33:1049–56.

[19] De Sanctis V. Growth and puberty and its management in thalassemia. Horm Res 2002;58: 72–9.

[20] Molitch ME, Clemmons DR, Malozowski S, et al, Endocrine Society's Clinical Guidelines Subcommittee. Evaluation and treatment of adult growth hormone deficiency: an Endocrine Society clinical practice guideline. J Clin Endocrinol Metab 2006;91:1621–34.

[21] Bushhouse S, Ramsay NKC, Pescovitz OH, et al. Growth in children following irradiation for bone marrow transplantation. Am J Pediatr Hematol Oncol 1989;11:134–40.

[22] Couto-Silva AC, Trivin C, Esperou H, et al. Changes in height, weight, and plasma leptin after bone marrow transplantation. Bone Marrow Transplant 2000;26:1205–10.

[23] Brauner R, Fontoura M, Zucker JM, et al. Growth and growth hormone secretion after bone marrow transplantation. Arch Dis Child 1993;68:458–63.

[24] Thomas BC, Stanhope R, Plowman PN, et al. Growth following single-fraction and fractionated total body irradiation for bone marrow transplantation. Eur J Pediatr 1993;152: 888–92.

[25] Wither HR. Biologic basis for altered fractionation schemes. Cancer 1985;55:2086–95.

[26] Yahalom J, Fuks ZY. Strategies for the use of total body irradiation as a systemic therapy in leukemia and lymphoma. In: Armitage JO, Antman KH, editors. High-dose chemotherapy. Baltimore (MD): Williams and Wilkins; 1992. p. 61–83.

[27] Bakker B, Oostdijk W, Geskus RB, et al. Patterns of growth and body proportions after total body irradiation and hematopoietic stem cell transplantation during childhood. Pediatr Res 2006;59:259–64.

[28] Bakker B, Massa GG, Oostdijk W, et al. Pubertal development and growth after total-body irradiation and bone marrow transplantation for haematological malignancies. Eur J Pediatr 2000;159:31–7.

[29] Couto-Silva AC, Trivin C, Esperou H, et al. Final height and gonad function after total body irradiation during childhood. Bone Marrow Transplant 2006;38:427–32.

[30] Sanders JE, Guthrie KA, Hoffmeister PA, et al. Final adult height of patients who received hematopoietic cell transplantation in childhood. Blood 2005;105:1348–54.

[31] Shalitin S, Philip M, Stein J, et al. Endocrine dysfunction and parameters of the metabolic syndrome after bone marrow transplantation during childhood and adolescence. Bone Marrow Transplant 2006;37:1109–17.

[32] Holm K, Nysom K, Rasmussen MH, et al. Growth, growth hormone, and final height after BMT. Possible recovery of irradiation-induced growth hormone insufficiency. Bone Marrow Transplant 1996;18:163–70.

[33] Chemaitilly W, Boulad F, Heller G, et al. Final height in pediatric patients after hyperfractionated total body irradiation and stem cell transplantation. Bone Marrow Transplant 2007;40:29–35.

[34] Brennan BMD, Shalet MS. Endocrine late effects after bone marrow transplantation. Br J Haematol 2002;118:56–66.

[35] Brauner R, Adan L, Souberbielle JC, et al. Contribution of growth hormone deficiency to the growth failure that follows bone marrow transplantation. J Pediatr 1997;130:785–92.

[36] Papadimitrou A, Uruena M, Stanhope R, et al. Growth hormone treatment of growth failure secondary to total body irradiation and bone marrow transplantation. Arch Dis Child 1991;66:689–92.

[37] Ogilvy-Stuart AL, Clark DJ, Wallace WHB, et al. Endocrine deficit after fractionated total body irradiation. Arch Dis Child 1992;67:1107–10.

[38] Huma Z, Boulad F, Black P, et al. Growth in children after bone marrow transplantation for acute leukemia. Blood 1995;86:819–24.

[39] Sklar CA, Mertens AC, Mitsby P, et al. Risk of disease recurrence and second neoplasms in survivors of childhood cancer treated with growth hormone: a report from the childhood cancer survivor study. J Clin Endocrinol Metab 2002;87:3136–41.

[40] Wingard JR, Plotnick LP, Freemer CS, et al. Growth in children after bone marrow transplantation: busulfan plus cyclophosphamide versus cyclophosphamide plus total body irradiation. Blood 1992;79:1068–73.

[41] Bozzola M, Giorgiani G, Locatelli F, et al. Growth in children after bone marrow transplantation. Horm Res 1993;39:122–6.

[42] Sarafoglou K, Boulad F, Gillio A, et al. Gonadal function after bone marrow transplantation for acute leukemia during childhood. J Pediatr 1997;130:210–6.

[43] Rose SR, Lustig RH, Pituksheewanont P, et al. Diagnosis of hidden central hypothyroidism in survivors of childhood cancer. J Clin Endocrinol Metab 1999;84:4472–9.

[44] Darzy KH, Shalet SM. Circadian and stimulated thyrotropin secretion in cranially irradiated adult cancer survivors. J Clin Endocrinol Metab 2005;90:6490–7.

[45] Thomas O, Mahe M, Campion L, et al. Long-term complications of total body irradiation in adults. Int J Radiat Oncol Biol Phys 2001;49:125–31.

[46] Sanders JE. The impact of marrow transplant preparative regimens on subsequent growth and development. The Seattle Marrow Transplant Team. Semin Hematol 1991;28:244–9.

[47] Thomas BC, Stanhope R, Plowman PN, et al. Endocrine function following single fraction and fractionated total body irradiation for bone marrow transplantation in childhood. Acta Endocrinol 1993;128:508–12.

[48] Boulad F, Bromley M, Black P, et al. Thyroid dysfunction following bone marrow transplantation using hyperfractionated radiation. Bone Marrow Transplant 1995;15:71–6.

[49] Sklar CA, Kim TH, Ramsay NKC. Thyroid dysfunction among long-term survivors of bone marrow transplantation. Am J Med 1982;73:688–94.

[50] Berger C, Le-Gallo B, Donadieu J, et al. Late thyroid toxicity in 153 long-term survivors of allogeneic bone marrow transplantation for acute lymphoblastic leukaemia. Bone Marrow Transplant 2005;35:991–5.

[51] Ishiguro H, Yasuda Y, Tomita Y, et al. Long-term follow-up of thyroid function in patients who received bone marrow transplantation during childhood and adolescence. J Clin Endocrinol Metab 2004;89:5981–6.

[52] Al-Fiar FZ, Colwill R, Lipton JH, et al. Abnormal thyroid stimulating hormone (TSH) levels in adults following allogeneic bone marrow transplants. Bone Marrow Transplant 1997;19:1019–22.

[53] Michel G, Socie G, Gebhard F, et al. Late effects of allogeneic bone marrow transplantation for children with acute myeloblastic leukemia in first complete remission: the impact of conditioning regimen without total-body irradiation—a report from the Société Française de Greffe de Moelle. J Clin Oncol 1997;15:2238–46.

[54] Slatter MA, Gennery AR, Cheetham TD, et al. Thyroid dysfunction after bone marrow transplantation for primary immune deficiency without the use of total body irradiation. Bone Marrow Transplant 2004;33:949–53.

[55] Karthaus M, Gabrysiak T, Brabant G, et al. Immune thyroiditis after transplantation of allogeneic CD34+ selected peripheral blood cells. Bone Marrow Transplant 1997;20:697–9.

[56] Au WY, Lie AKW, Kung AWC, et al. Autoimmune thyroid dysfunction after hematopoietic stem cell transplantation. Bone Marrow Transplant 2005;35:383–8.

[57] Sklar C, Boulad F, Small T, et al. Endocrine complications of pediatric stem cell transplantation. Front Biosci 2001;6:G17–22.

[58] Holland FJ, McConnon JK, Volpé R, et al. Concordant Graves' disease after bone marrow transplantation: implications for pathogenesis. J Clin Endocrinol Metab 1991;72:837–40.

[59] Ron E, Lubin JH, Shore RE, et al. Thyroid cancer after exposure to external radiation: a pooled analysis of seven studies. Radiat Res 1995;141:259–77.

[60] Tucker MA, Jones PH, Boice JD Jr, et al. Therapeutic radiation at a young age is linked to secondary thyroid cancer. Cancer Res 1991;51:2885–8.

[61] Acharya S, Sarafoglou K, LaQuaglia M, et al. Thyroid neoplasms after therapeutic radiation for malignancies during childhood and adolescence. Cancer 2003;97:2397–403.

[62] Uderzo C, van Lint MT, Rovelli A, et al. Papillary thyroid carcinoma after total body irradiation. Arch Dis Child 1994;71:256–8.

[63] Cohen A, Rovelli A, van Lint MT, et al. Secondary thyroid carcinoma after allogeneic bone marrow transplantation during childhood. Bone Marrow Transplant 2001;28:1125–8.

[64] Sanders JE. Endocrine complications of high-dose therapy with stem cell transplantation. Pediatr Transplant 2004;8(Suppl 5):39–50.

[65] Sanders JE, Hawley J, Levy W, et al. Pregnancies following high-dose cyclophosphamide with or without high-dose busulfan or total-body irradiation and bone marrow transplantation. Blood 1996;87:3045–52.

[66] Grigg AP, McLachlan R, Zajac J, et al. Reproductive status in long-term bone marrow transplant survivors receiving busulfan–cyclophosphamide (120mg/kg). Bone Marrow Transplant 2000;26:1089–95.

[67] Anserini P, Chiodi S, Costa M, et al. Semen analysis following allogeneic bone marrow transplantation. Additional data for evidence-based counseling. Bone Marrow Transplant 2002;30:447–51.

[68] Kyriacou C, Kottaridis PD, Eliahoo J, et al. Germ cell damage and Leydig cell insufficiency in recipients of nonmyeloablative transplantation for haematological malignancies. Bone Marrow Transplant 2003;31:45–50.

[69] Sklar CA, Robison LL, Nesbit ME, et al. Effects of radiation on testicular function in long-term survivors of childhood acute lymphoblastic leukemia: a report from the Children's Cancer Study Group. J Clin Oncol 1990;8:1981–7.

[70] Rovo A, Tichelli A, Passweg JR, et al. Spermatogenesis in long-term survivors after allogeneic hematopoietic stem cell transplantation is associated with age, time interval since transplantation, and apparently absence of chronic GvHD. Blood 2006;108:1100–5.

[71] Savani BN, Kozanas E, Shenoy A, et al. Recovery of spermatogenesis after total body irradiation. Blood 2006;108:4292–3.

[72] Ishiguro H, Yasuda Y, Tomita Y, et al. Gonadal shielding to irradiation is effective in protecting testicular growth and function in long-term survivors of bone marrow transplantation during childhood or adolescence. Bone Marrow Transplant 2007;39:483–90.

[73] Chatterjee R, Kottaridis PD. Treatment of gonadal damage in recipients of allogeneic or autologous transplantation for haematological malignancies. Bone Marrow Transplant 2002;30:629–35.

[74] Sanders JE, Buckner CD, Amos D, et al. Ovarian function following marrow transplantation for aplastic anemia or leukemia. J Clin Oncol 1988;6:813–8.

[75] Byrne J, Fears TR, Gail MH, et al. Early menopause in long-term survivors of cancer during adolescence. Am J Obstet Gynecol 1992;166:788–93.

[76] Sklar CA, Mertens AC, Mitby P, et al. Premature menopause in survivors of childhood cancer: a report from the Childhood Cancer Survivor Study. J Natl Cancer Inst 2006;98:890–6.

[77] Mertens AC, Ramsay NKC, Kouris S, et al. Patterns of gonadal dysfunction following bone marrow transplantation. Bone Marrow Transplant 1998;22:345–50.

[78] Matsumoto M, Shinohara O, Ishiguro H, et al. Ovarian function after bone marrow transplantation performed before menarche. Arch Dis Child 1999;80:452–4.

[79] Salooja N, Szydio RM, Socle G, et al. Pregnancy outcomes after peripheral blood or bone marrow transplantation: a retrospective study. Lancet 2001;358:271–6.

[80] Carter A, Robison LL, Francisco L, et al. Prevalence of conception and pregnancy outcomes after hematopoietic stem cell transplantation: report from the bone marrow transplant survivor study. Bone Marrow Transplant 2006;37:1023–9.

[81] Nakagawa K, Kanda Y, Yamashita H, et al. Preservation of ovarian function by ovarian shielding when undergoing total body irradiation for hematopoietic stem cell transplantation: a report of two successful cases. Bone Marrow Transplant 2006;37:583–7.

[82] Holm K, Nysom K, Brocks V, et al. Ultrasound B—mode changes in the uterus and ovaries and Doppler changes in the uterus after total body irradiation and allogeneic bone marrow transplantation in childhood. Bone Marrow Transplant 1999;23:259–63.

[83] Bath LE, Critchley HOD, Chambers SE, et al. Ovarian and uterine characteristics after total body irradiation in childhood and adolescence: response to sex steroid replacement. Br J Obstet Gynaecol 1999;106:1265–72.

[84] Aisenberg J, Hsieh K, Kalaitzoglou G, et al. Bone mineral density (BMD) in long-term survivors of childhood cancer. J Pediatr Hematol Oncol 1998;20:241–5.

[85] Bhatia S, Ramsay NKC, Weisdorf D, et al. Bone mineral density in patients undergoing bone marrow transplantation for myeloid malignancies. Bone Marrow Transplant 1998; 22:87–90.

[86] Nysom K, Holm K, Michaelsen KF, et al. Bone mass after allogeneic bone marrow transplantation for childhood leukaemia or lymphoma. Bone Marrow Transplant 2000;25: 191–6.

[87] Schimmer AD, Mah K, Bordeleau L, et al. Decreased bone mineral density is common after autologous blood or marrow transplantation. Bone Marrow Transplant 2001;28:387–91.

[88] Kerschan-Schindl K, Mitterbauer M, Füreder W, et al. Bone metabolism in patients more than five years after bone marrow transplantation. Bone Marrow Transplant 2006;34: 491–6.

[89] Cohen A, Shane E. Osteoporosis after solid organ and bone marrow transplantation. Osteoporos Int 2003;14:617–30.

[90] Stern JM, Chesnut CH 3rd, Bruemmer B, et al. Bone density loss during treatment of chronic GVHD. Bone Marrow Transplant 1996;17:395–400.

[91] Gilsanz V, Carlson ME, Roe TF, et al. Osteoporosis after cranial irradiation for acute lymphoblastic leukemia. J Pediatr 1990;117:238–44.

[92] Lee WY, Cho SW, Oh ES, et al. The effect of bone marrow transplantation on the osteoblastic differentiation of human bone marrow stromal cells. J Clin Endocrinol Metab 2002;87:329–35.

[93] Lee WY, Kang MI, Oh ES, et al. The role of cytokines in the changes in bone turnover following bone marrow transplantation. Osteoporos Int 2002;13:62–8.

[94] Smedmyr B, Wilbell L, Simonsson B, et al. Impaired glucose tolerance after autologous bone marrow transplantation. Bone Marrow Transplant 1990;6:89–92.

[95] Lorini R, Cortona L, Scaramuzza A, et al. Hyperinsulinemia in children and adolescents after bone marrow transplantation. Bone Marrow Transplant 1995;15:873–7.

[96] Taskinen M, Saarinen-Pihkala UM, Hovi L, et al. Impaired glucose tolerance and dyslipidaemia as late effects after bone marrow transplantation in childhood. Lancet 2000;356: 993–7.

[97] Traggiai C, Stanhope R, Nussey S, et al. Diabetes mellitus after bone marrow transplantation during childhood. Med Pediatr Oncol 2003;40:128–9.

[98] Hoffmeister PA, Storer BE, Sanders JE. Diabetes mellitus in long-term survivors of pediatric hematopietic cell transplantation. J Pediatr Hematol Oncol 2004;26:81–90.

[99] d'Annunzio G, Bonetti F, Locatelli F, et al. Insulin resistance in children and adolescents after bone marrow transplant for malignancies. Haematologica 2006;91:20–1.

[100] Chatterjee R, Palla K, McGarrigle HH, et al. Syndrome X in adult female recipients of bone marrow transplantation for haematological malignancies. Bone Marrow Transplant 2005; 35:209–10.

[101] Higgins K, Noon C, Davies M, et al. Features of the metabolic syndrome present in survivors of bone marrow transplantation in adulthood. Bone Marrow Transplant 2005;36: 279–80.

[102] Neville KA, Cohn RJ, Steinbeck KS, et al. Hyperinsulinemia, impaired glucose tolerance and diabetes mellitus in survivors of childhood cancer: prevalence and risk factors. J Clin Endocrinol Metab 2006;91:4401–7.

[103] Baker KS, Ness KK, Steinberger J, et al. Diabetes, hypertension, and cardiovascular events in survivors of hematopoietic stem cell transplantation: a report from the bone marrow transplant survivor study. Blood 2007;109:1765–72.

ELSEVIER
SAUNDERS

Endocrinol Metab Clin N Am
36 (2007) 999–1013

ENDOCRINOLOGY
AND METABOLISM
CLINICS
OF NORTH AMERICA

Pancreatic Islet Cell Transplant for Treatment of Diabetes

Paolo Fiorina, MD, PhD[a,b,d], Antonio Secchi, MD[a,c,*]

[a]*Transplantation Medicine, San Raffaele Scientific Institute, Via Olgettina 60, 20132 Milan, Italy*
[b]*Transplantation Research Center, Children's Hospital-Brigham and Women's Hospital, Harvard Medical School, 221 Longwood Avenue, Boston, MA 02115, USA*
[c]*Universita' Vita-Salute, Via Olgettina 58, 20132 Milan, Italy*
[d]*Harvard Stem Cell Institute, 1350 Massachusetts Avenue, Boston, MA 02115, USA*

Insulin treatment, the master treatment for patients affected by type 1 diabetes mellitus, cannot prevent chronic complications related to diabetes fully, and intensive insulin treatment to improve metabolic control increases the risk of fatal hypoglycemic episodes [1–4]. The hypothesis that replacement of the endocrine pancreas by transplanting fragments of insulin-producing tissue could be helpful is not novel [5]. Pancreatic fragments indeed can produce their own insulin with closely controlled and finely timed insulin release.

History of islet transplantation

The history of islets transplantation is fascinating, and Paul E. Lacy [6] can be considered the man who made it happen. He invented islet transplantation and the first method to isolate islet from rodent pancreata. In 1972, a terrific breakthrough was reported when Ballinger and Lacy [7] performed the first islet isografts from normal rats, reversing streptozotocin-induced diabetes in rats.

The authors thank JDRF, JDRF-Telethon, NIH, ITN, and many other funding agencies for providing financial support for most of their studies. Paolo Fiorina is receiving an AST/JDRF Faculty grant.

* Corresponding author. Transplantation Medicine, San Raffaele Scientific Institute, Via Olgettina 60, 20132 Milan, Italy.

E-mail address: antonio.secchi@hsr.it (A. Secchi).

During the 1980s, different reports suggested for the very first time the feasibility of islet transplantation in people by transplanting autologous islet transplantation in patients who had painful and chronic pancreatitis and who underwent total pancreatectomy for pain relief [8]. This approach confirms that islet isolation could sustain in the long-term normoglycemia. In 1986, a big step in the field of islet transplantation was done, when Camillo Ricordi invented the chamber to automatically isolate islets. Ricordi [9] showed that it was possible to digest the pancreas with the help of collagenase and to process the pancreas with a gradient procedure. A cannula is placed in the pancreatic duct to allow collagenase to distend the organ, which is digested thereafter in the Ricordi Chamber into fragments of decreasing sizes. Cooling and washing served to protect islets during the procedure. A density gradient was used to separate the small islet from the exocrine tissues and nonislet tissue [10,11]. The Miami Center for Islets Transplantation performed a first series of six successful islet allograft transplantations in people in the 1990s, with long-term insulin independence [12,13].

Thereafter, the use of endotoxin-free reagents has been introduced [14,15], and the Islet Transplantation Registry (ITR) was born in Giessen, Germany. Despite all the effort, the overall rates of success reported for islet transplantation (considering insulin independence) was less than 10% as reported by the ITR newsletter of June 2001. From collaboration between the Milan, Italy, and the Giessen group, the idea of partial function appeared in literature [16], showing that the restoration of partial islet function could contribute to improve hypoglycemia awareness and ameliorate insulin resistance with beneficial effects on glucose metabolic control [16].

In 2000, Shapiro and colleagues [17] reported 100% insulin independence in seven type 1 diabetic patients who received islet allografts. Induction patients received anti-IL2r drug (daclizumab), and steroids were banned from the induction. In 2003, the first paper showing a clear positive and beneficial effect of transplanted islets on kidney function was published by Fiorina and colleagues [18].

In September 2006, the report from the International Trial of the Edmonton Protocol was published in the *New England Journal of Medicine* [19], confirming that insulin independence can be achieved in more than 50% of transplanted patients. This study showed that more than 80% of the patients showed the restoration of endogenous C peptide production for more than 2 years with a positive impact on glycated hemoglobin levels and very few adverse events. More trials are on the way confirming the excitement for this procedure.

Metabolic effects of islet transplantation

Several studies have shown that islet transplantation is capable of leading to full insulin independence [17,19–22]. Rates have ranged from 60% to 90%, according to different reports. The endogenous secretion of insulin from the transplanted islets induces a near normalization of glucose homeostasis [17,19–22]. Several metabolic studies were performed during the state of insulin independence with the aim to evaluate the fine tuning of endogenous insulin secretion in these patients and to study the potential influence of immunosuppressant agents [23]. Contrary to what was observed in the model of systemic drained pancreas transplantation, in which insulin was secreted in the general circulation instead of the portal circulation, in the model of intrahepatic islet transplantation, insulin was secreted intrahepatically and cleaved by the liver, thereby avoiding peripheral hyperinsulinemia and mimicking physiological insulin secretion [16]. Metabolic studies have shown that functioning islet grafts normalize basal hepatic glucose output, ameliorate insulin action, and normalize the plasma concentration of amino acids [16]. Despite several studies, it is unknown the real number of islets required to restore euglycemia, because it is unknown how many islets survive shortly after transplantation. In the model of islet auto-transplantation performed in patients undergoing total pancreatectomy for untreatable painful pancreatitis, it was shown that the number of islets required to achieve insulin independence is lower than in the setting of allotransplantation. Some minor abnormalities are observed after different insulinogenic stimuli. A normal response is observed during arginine infusion, while first peak insulin secretion after intravenous glucose is missing. Reduced β cell mass, the absence of vascularization/innervation, or the intrahepatic transplantation site can account for the observed impairment in glucose-mediated insulin secretion [24,25]. Furthermore, islet-toxic drugs (ie, FK-506 and sirolimus) are delivered to the liver, exposing the intrahepatic transplanted islets to twofold higher levels of drugs than those that reach the periphery after oral administration of the drugs, the so-called portal immunosuppressive storm [26–32]. These abnormalities were observed also in studies with the clamp technique, where a defect of insulin secretion during the hyperglycemic clamp was observed, when compared with normal subjects or with pancreas-transplanted patients [16,33–35].

In some patients, islet transplantation does not lead to full insulin independence, probably because of a low mass of functioning islets. Nevertheless in these patients, an impressive improvement of metabolic control is observed, with a clear reduction of the rate on hypoglycemic episodes, showing that also in these cases islet transplantation concurs to the maintenance of metabolic control. Furthermore, in these cases, the so-called partial islet function (C peptide greater than 0.5 ng/mL and a 60% reduction in pretransplant insulin requirement), a normalization of postabsorptive and insulin-mediated protein and lipid metabolism, is observed [23]. In contrast, glucose homeostasis remains mildly abnormal [23]. Analysis of studies in which the amino acid and lipid concentrations were measured in patients who had type 1 diabetes receiving conventional or intensive insulin treatment suggests that the metabolic abnormalities of islet-transplanted patients with partial function are comparable to those of type 1 diabetic patients receiving insulin [16]. The positive role played by islet transplantation on the reduction of the rate of hypoglycemic episodes seems the consequence of a correct suppression of endogenous insulin secretion [34–39] and of the inhibition of the sympathoadrenal response during hypoglycemia [34,35,39,40]. On the other hand, glucagon counter-regulation is not corrected completely after islet transplantation [34,35,39]. Whether these effects are also the results of a reduction of the doses of exogenous insulin therapy and/or the consequence of a restoration of a normal counter-regulation, is still matter of debate [41,42].

The first studies on lipid metabolism after islet transplantations were performed in patients submitted to kidney–islet transplantation. These studies showed that, in a cohort of patients who received islet after kidney transplants and submitted to chronic immunosuppression including steroids, islets improved lipid metabolism, with an evident reduction in lipid oxidation, contrary to the impairment in patients whose graft failed [23,43,44]. These results were observed not only in patients who achieved insulin independence, but also in patients showing partial function (C peptide greater than 0.5 ng/mL) [45]. In particular, three groups of patients were compared:

Kidney–pancreas transplanted patients (KP: completely insulin-free)
Islet after kidney transplanted patients (IAK), who experienced insulin independence and after that partial long-term function
Patients with type 1 diabetes who received a kidney transplant (KD) who did not receive, or had previously rejected, a pancreas/islets graft [45]

In these patients, triglyceride levels appeared lower in the KP and IAK groups than in the KD group at 2 and 4 years, whereas at 6 years, only the KP group showed lower triglyceride levels than the KD group. Mean total cholesterol levels were slightly but significantly increased from baseline in the KP and KD groups but not in the IAK group [45]. This was associated with a long-term sustained C peptide secretion in the IAK group. It is interesting to note that these results were better than those observed in patients receiving a kidney–pancreas transplantation, which is considered the benchmark in the treatment of type 1 diabetes. This is probably because the studies performed in kidney–pancreas patients were done in patients who received a pancreas anatomized to the general circulation, which leads to peripheral hyperinsulinemia, a known risk factor toward dyslipidemia.

Studies performed in patients receiving islet transplantation alone did not confirm these data. This is probably because of a confounding factor; this kind of patient generally is treated with rapamycin, an immunosuppressant drug that can induce dyslipidemia [19,46–48].

In conclusion, islet transplantation exerts a positive role on metabolic control in diabetic patients, playing its role at different levels, from glucose metabolism to lipid and protein metabolism.

Islet isolation and transplantation

Isolation technique

Islets are isolated from pancreata obtained from multiple organ donors. The human pancreas is dissected carefully from the duodenum; the main and accessory ducts are identified, clamped, and divided. A cannula is placed in the pancreatic duct to allow for an enzyme blend to distend the organ. Collagenase is injected into the pancreatic duct to separate islets from exocrine tissues and to selectively digest the fibrotic framework of the pancreas.

The pancreas is placed in Ricordi's chamber, and a continuous digestion process disassembles the organ into fragments of decreasing sizes. A heating circuit activates the enzymes in the chamber, allowing the islets to be released and collected at the bottom of the chamber. With the use of dithizone and a transparent chamber, islets can be stained and followed to monitor the progression of the digestion process. At the end of the process, pancreatic cell clusters are collected in separate containers, while the fibrous network of duct and vessels is retained in the chamber.

The small islet fraction is separated from predominantly exocrine tissue and no islet tissue on a discontinuous density gradient using specialized cell processors (COBE 2991 Cell Processor; COBE, Lakewood, Colorado). After this step, the pure islet fraction normally is located in the top layer, while less pure islets and mantled islets (surrounded by exocrine tissue) are located within more dense interfaces. The volume of tissue infused needs to remain within acceptable limits (5 to 7 mL). Satisfactory preparation should meet the following criteria:

- Sterility (assessment for aerobic, anaerobic, fungal, mycoplasmal organisms)
- Number of equivalent islets (EI) greater than 6000/kg of body weight each infusion
- Purity greater than 20% (morphometric determination of islet)

Preoperative management

The immunosuppressive protocol is started then, and islets are infused. Transplantation is performed within 24 hours of islet isolation. Eligible patients receive transplants according to ABO compatibility. HLA matching is not required for humans, and has been shown to be deleterious in mice when the HLA match is too stringent because of accelerated autoimmunity [49].

Postoperative management

Islets are infused into the hepatic portal vein of recipients. A percutaneous transhepatic injection (under local anesthesia) is performed with ultrasound or fluoroscopic guidance. Following the procedure, patients remain hospitalized for few days, according to the schedule of the transplant physicians; ultrasound of the liver is performed every other day along with liver enzyme tests. Stringent glucose metabolic control for several days through the use of an intravenous insulin pump avoids the toxic effect of hyperglycemia on the transplanted islets. Generally, the daily insulin requirement drops by a mean of 30% to 50% in a few days after islet transplantation, but most patients become completely insulin-independent after the second injection. Doppler ultrasound of portal vein and liver enzymes need to be evaluated to monitor the viability of the portal vein and possible hepatic necrosis. To prevent portal vein thrombosis, enoxaparin 30 mg twice daily is started 4 hours after islet infusion for 7 days. Patients are seen in the clinic every week until 3 months after transplantation, then twice a month until 6 months after transplantation, and then monthly unless the physician requests a different schedule.

Complications and adverse events

The most common post-transplant symptoms are transient abdominal pain, nausea, and occasional vomiting [19,50]. In the authors' experience, only three (one hemoperitoneum, one hemothorax, and one partial portal thrombosis) of 58 patients who underwent islet cell transplantation (intrahepatic) experienced symptoms [50]. The rate of acute complications is 2% to 3% for hemorrhage and 3% for partial portal vein thrombosis. Hepatic focal steatosis without functional impairment has been reported in 20% to 30% of cases [51,52]. A different and new spectrum of adverse events was seen in the patients in the Immune Tolerance Network (ITN) Trial of the Edmonton protocol recently published in the *New England Journal of Medicine* [19]. There were no deaths or post-transplant cancer/lymphoproliferative disorders among the study subjects. No major viral infections were evident (ie, cytomegalovirus [CMV] or Epstein-Barr virus [EBV]), but 38 serious events were reported, with at least 23 related to the study therapy. Main portal branch thrombosis was almost absent, and the rate of peripheral branch or partial thrombosis was low (approximately 6%). One recent and potentially harmful adverse event is the worsening of creatinine function [53]. Patients who had microalbuminuria before islet transplantation were most likely to become overtly proteinuric after the introduction of immunosuppressant. A major warning on this topic will be recommended in the following years [19].

Outcomes of islet transplantation

Clinical outcomes for islet transplantation have changed dramatically in the last years with the introduction of safer and less toxic immunosuppressive protocols, even if some historical data and anecdotal reports by the Miami, Minneapolis, and Milan groups previously showed long-term function of more than 4 years [21,22]. The rate of insulin independence increased following the introduction of a steroid-free protocol by the Edmonton group in 2000 [17]. The increase in the rate of insulin independence at 1 year was confirmed in a recent report in the *New England Journal of Medicine* [19]. This success changes the perspective on islet transplantation from that of being considered a procedure for patients with type 1 diabetes with a previous kidney transplant to a procedure applicable to all patients with type 1 diabetes [17,54]. This remarkable accomplishment achieved by Shapiro and colleagues [17], who reported 100% insulin independence in seven patients with type 1 diabetes and life-threatening hypoglycemic unawareness, expedited the growth of the field of islet transplantation.

Although early results were encouraging, the insulin-free survival rate falls dramatically to 15% at 5 years [55]. The data indicate that much progress is necessary to render islet cell transplantation as successful as other solid organ transplantation. Mean glycated hemoglobin generally is normalized in insulin-independent recipients and improved in recipients who remain positive for C peptide. In the authors' experience many patients had C peptide higher than 0.5 ng/mL for many years (Fig. 1). As expected, glycated hemoglobin tends to rise in those patients who lose all graft function. The reason for this decline or complete loss of islet function after transplantation is not clear, but it may involve direct immunosuppressive toxicity, allo- or recurrent autoimmune rejection, or potential islet cell apoptosis reflecting the natural life cycle of islets in the native pancreas [56,57].

Immunosuppression

The IAK group included patients either who lost the pancreatic graft early after simultaneous kidney–pancreas transplantation or who received only a renal a transplant. After induction with antithymoglobulin (125 mg/d for

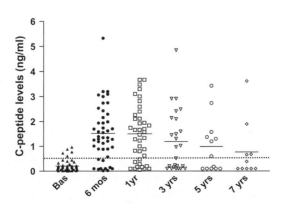

Fig. 1. C-peptide levels (ng/mL) in the authors' group of patients who received islet after kidney transplantation. A long-term sustained C peptide secretion can be achieved in most of the patients.

10 days; Thymoglobulin, SangStat), immunosuppression is maintained with cyclosporine (aiming at trough levels between 100 and 200 ng/mL), mycophenolate mofetil (2 g/d), and metilprednisone (10 mg/d). Steroids are withdrawn 3 to 6 months after islet transplantation.

The ITA group included patients affected by type 1 diabetes with a very poor control of glycemic values or frequent hypoglycemic episodes or emotional or psychological problems associated with insulin therapy. Induction is based on intravenous infusion of anti-IL2r (daclizumab) five times at a dosage of 1 mg/kg over 8 weeks. The maintenance is based on the administration of sirolimus once daily to achieve a target trough therapeutic range of 12 to 15 ng/mL for 3 months after transplantation, after which the target trough range is lowered to 7 to 12 ng/mL. FK-506 (tacrolimus) is administered daily and adjusted to achieve a target trough level of 3 to 6 ng/mL. Steroids are avoided to prevent their deleterious effects on islet cell function and glucose metabolism.

Benefits of islet transplantation

A recent report from our group has analyzed the effect of islet transplantation on patient survival [58]. In a 7-year follow-up study including 34 uremic type 1 diabetic patients who received kidney transplantation, the survival among those patients who received successful islet transplantation with a sustained restoration of β-cell function was significantly higher (90%) than among patients who received unsuccessful islet transplantation (51%). Patients with successful islet transplantation showed a higher C peptide levels and lower insulin requirements, but glycated hemoglobin levels were not significantly different. The rate of cardiovascular deaths (according to the *International Classification of Diseases, Ninth Revision* [ICD-9]) was higher in the group with unsuccessful islet transplants, with a poorer atherosclerotic profile and endothelial function [58,59].

A previous paper reported, for the first time, the course of cardiovascular function over a 3-year follow-up period in 42 kidney transplant recipients with or without a functioning islet transplant [59]. Islet transplantation was associated with an improvement in diastolic function and QT dispersion and a delay in intima media thickening [20,59]. Furthermore, a reduction in atrial/ventricular natriuretic peptide, a marker of atrial and ventricular function, was evident during the follow-up period in patients who received a functioning islet transplantation compared with those who did not [59].

Furthermore, the authors showed that islet transplants, when successful, prevent the worsening of graft survival and vascular function of the kidney graft that may occur in patients with type 1 diabetes with end-stage renal disease receiving kidney transplants [18]. Noninvasive assessments of graft vascular function using the Doppler resistance index and microalbuminuria evaluations showed that the group with type 1 diabetes (24 patients) who received a kidney transplants and also an islet transplant showed better renal vascular function and cumulative kidney graft survival than the group without functioning islets [18,45]. A summary of biological markers that improve after islet transplantation after 4 years of follow-up is provided in Fig. 2.

Restoration of C peptide secretion or improved metabolic control? Explaining the benefits of islet transplantation

In the 1993 the Diabetes Control and Complications Trial (DCCT) [1] established the modern standard of care for the medical management of type 1 diabetes. Two treatments, a classic treatment and an intensive treatment (including multiple daily injections, frequent finger-stick monitoring of glucose, and a dietary approach), randomly were assigned to 1441 patients. Patients in the intensive treatment group showed a dramatic improvement in survival and a lower rate of diabetic complications, initiating a gold standard in diabetes management. For the first time, it was evident that

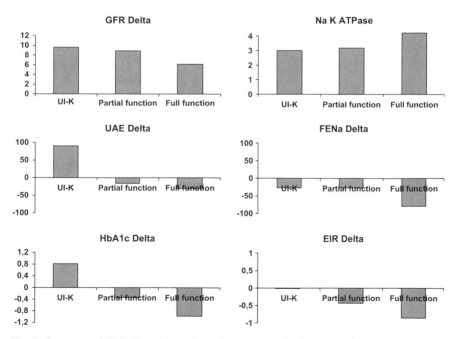

Fig. 2. Summary of clinical parameters in patients who received unsuccessful (UI-K), partial or full-functioning islet transplantation. All parameters are expressed as a delta between 4 years and baseline. Glomerular filtration rate (GFR, mL/min) is unchanged, while for Na-K-ATPase activity in the red blood cells (Na K ATPase, mmol/Na/L cell/h), urinary albumin excretion (mg/dL), urinary fractional sodium excretion (FeNa, µmol/L), glycated hemoglobin (HBA1c, percentage), and exogenous insulin requirement (EIR, unit per day) a clear improvement was evident in patients who had partial and full function of the islets.

better glycometabolic control is associated with a prolongation of life for patients who have type 1 diabetes [1]. The DCCT provided a strong rationale for the use of islet transplantation and for the use of any other approaches to β cell replacement. When islet-transplanted patients experience insulin independence, there is no doubt that the procedure will be helpful and have a positive impact on patients' life expectancy and quality of life [20].

A series of recent studies demonstrated that C peptide exerts several physiological effects [60–63]. In patients who have type 1 diabetes, infusion of exogenous C peptide has ameliorated nerve dysfunction [64], increased forearm blood flow, improved myocardial vasodilatation [65,66], and reduced glomerular hyperfiltration and urinary albumin excretion [61]. C peptide was shown to bind unspecifically to human cell membranes [60,67–73] and to activate intracellular Ca^{2+}-dependent pathways, resulting in stimulation of Na^+-K^+-ATPase [60] and eNOS activities [60]. Indeed, C peptide induces glomerular vasodilatation, contributing to a slowing of the progression of diabetic nephropathy in the transplanted kidney [18,63,67,74].

All these data confirm that C peptide is an outstanding candidate for the beneficial effects of islet transplantation (Fig. 3).

Summary

Many major hurdles must be overcome before successful islet cell transplantation can be accomplished. Most centers currently require islet isolation from more than one pancreata. A limited supply of islets is a major burden because of the shortage of organs. To overcome this problem,

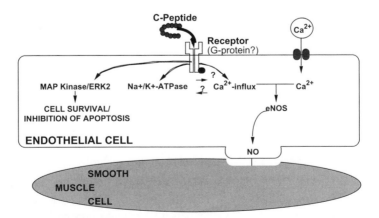

Fig. 3. C peptide can be a candidate for explaining the positive outcomes of islet transplanted patients, particularly those who did not achieve insulin independence. Shown is a potential pathway for C peptide mechanism of action.

investigators seek to improve islet isolation methods, to establish protocols to grow islets from exocrine ducts with the support of gene therapy, and to use xeno-islets. A primary reason for the recent success of clinical islet isolation has been the decrease in the use of immunosuppressants, which are associated with islet toxicity. The use of new immunosuppressive agents, such as the new mTOR-inhibitor everolimus; the IL-2 inhibitor basiliximab; and costimulatory blockade with, for example, humanized anti-CD154, LEA29Y, and hCTLA4Ig, has had promising results [75]. The use of encapsulated islets to protect them from attack by lymphocytes is also an exciting new approach [76]. Tolerance induction that renders the recipient independent of immunosuppressants is the ideal ultimate achievement.

One of the major limiting factors in islet cell transplantation is the lack of adequate knowledge about the fate of the islets following islet cell transplantation in the liver. For instance, it is not known how islets are revascularized or how much ischemic changes or simply nonfunctioning grafts are involved in the unsatisfactory results of islet cell transplantation.

Islet cell transplantation holds great promise as an emerging therapy for patients who have type 1 diabetes [75]. Islet transplantation is a relatively minimally invasive procedure and a promising alternative to pancreas transplantation for restoring endogenous insulin secretion in patients who have type 1 diabetes [5,20,75,77]. Complete insulin independence is presently 70% at 1 year among islet transplant recipients, showing that islet transplantation no longer should be considered an experimental procedure.

Unfortunately, this rate drops dramatically among some patients, although some show very long-term survival, in terms either of insulin independence or of endogenous C peptide secretion [5,20,77]. Recent studies have shown that this partial restoration of insulin and C peptide secretion could improve overall patient survival and cardiovascular outcomes [20,59]. One major advance is the recognition that insulin independence is not the only goal of islet transplantation. Achievement of even partial function dramatically improves quality of life, reduces hypoglycemia, and halts the progression of long-term diabetic complications.

Acknowledgments

The authors thank all the people in their centers who are caring for islet-transplanted patients, isolating islets, and collecting data for research. Paolo Fiorina would like to thank Alessandra Mello for her amazing support.

References

[1] DCCT. The Diabetes Control and Complications Trial Research Group. The effect of intensive. treatment of diabetes on the development and progression of long-term complications in insulin-dependent diabetes mellitus. N Engl J Med 1993;329:977–86.
[2] Bloomgarden ZT. Diabetes complications. Diabetes Care 2004;27(6):1506–14.

[3] Bloomgarden ZT. Glycemic treatment: control of glycemia. Diabetes Care 2004;27(5):
    1227–34.
[4] Bailes BK. Diabetes mellitus and its chronic complications. Aorn J 2002;76(2):266–76,
    278–82 [quiz: 283–6].
[5] Ricordi C. Islet transplantation: a brave new world. Diabetes 2003;52(7):1595–603.
[6] Lacy PE, Kostianovsky M. Method for the isolation of intact islets of Langerhans from the
    rat pancreas. Diabetes 1967;16(1):35–9.
[7] Ballinger WF, Lacy PE. Transplantation of intact pancreatic islets in rats. Surgery 1972;
    72(2):175–86.
[8] Sutherland DE, Matas AJ, Goetz FC, et al. Transplantation of dispersed pancreatic islet
    tissue in humans: autografts and allografts. Diabetes 1980;29(Suppl 1):31–44.
[9] Ricordi C, Lacy PE, Finke EH, et al. Automated method for isolation of human pancreatic
    islets. Diabetes 1988;37(4):413–20.
[10] Lake SP, Bassett PD, Larkins A, et al. Large-scale purification of human islets utilizing
    discontinuous albumin gradient on IBM 2991 cell separator. Diabetes 1989;38(Suppl 1):
    143–5.
[11] Lake SP, Chamberlain J, Bassett PD, et al. Successful reversal of diabetes in nude rats
    by transplantation of isolated adult human islets of Langerhans. Diabetes 1989;38(2):
    244–8.
[12] Tzakis AG, Ricordi C, Alejandro R, et al. Pancreatic islet transplantation after upper
    abdominal exenteration and liver replacement. Lancet 1990;336(8712):402–5.
[13] Ricordi C, Tzakis AG, Carroll PB, et al. Human islet isolation and allotransplantation in 22
    consecutive cases. Transplantation 1992;53(2):407–14.
[14] Hering BJ, Browatzki CC, Schultz AO, et al. Islet Transplant Registry report on adult and
    fetal islet allografts. Transplant Proc 1994;26(2):565–8.
[15] Hering BJ, Browatzki CC, Schultz A, et al. Clinical islet transplantation—registry report,
    accomplishments in the past and future research needs. Cell Transplant 1993;2(4):269–82
    [discussion: 283–305].
[16] Luzi L, Hering BJ, Socci C, et al. Metabolic effects of successful intraportal islet transplan-
    tation in insulin-dependent diabetes mellitus. J Clin Invest 1996;97(11):2611–8.
[17] Shapiro AM, Lakey JR, Ryan EA, et al. Islet transplantation in seven patients with type
    1 diabetes mellitus using a glucocorticoid-free immunosuppressive regimen. N Engl J Med
    2000;343(4):230–8.
[18] Fiorina P, Folli F, Zerbini G, et al. Islet transplantation is associated with improvement of
    renal function among uremic patients with type 1 diabetes mellitus and kidney transplants.
    J Am Soc Nephrol 2003;14(8):2150–8.
[19] Shapiro AM, Ricordi C, Hering BJ, et al. International trial of the Edmonton protocol for
    islet transplantation. N Engl J Med 2006;355(13):1318–30.
[20] Fiorina P, Folli F, Bertuzzi F, et al. Long-term beneficial effect of islet transplantation on
    diabetic macro-/microangiopathy in type 1 diabetic kidney-transplanted patients. Diabetes
    Care 2003;26(4):1129–36.
[21] Davalli AM, Maffi P, Socci C, et al. Insights from a successful case of intrahepatic islet
    transplantation into a type 1 diabetic patient. J Clin Endocrinol Metab 2000;85(10):3847–52.
[22] Alejandro R, Angelico MC, Ricordi C, et al. Long-term function of islet allograft in type 1
    diabetes mellitus. Transplant Proc 1995;27(6):3158.
[23] Luzi L, Perseghin G, Brendel MD, et al. Metabolic effects of restoring partial beta cell func-
    tion after islet allotransplantation in type 1 diabetic patients. Diabetes 2001;50(2):277–82.
[24] Leahy JL, Bonner-Weir S, Weir GC. Abnormal glucose regulation of insulin secretion in
    models of reduced B cell mass. Diabetes 1984;33(7):667–73.
[25] Mattsson G, Jansson L, Nordin A, et al. Evidence of functional impairment of syngenetically
    transplanted mouse pancreatic islets retrieved from the liver. Diabetes 2004;53(4):948–54.
[26] Jindal RM, Sidner RA, Milgrom ML. Post-transplant diabetes mellitus. The role of immu-
    nosuppression. Drug Saf 1997;16(4):242–57.

[27] Filler G, Neuschulz I, Vollmer I, et al. Tacrolimus reversibly reduces insulin secretion in paediatric renal transplant recipients. Nephrol Dial Transplant 2000;15(6):867–71.

[28] Montori VM, Basu A, Erwin PJ, et al. Post-transplantation diabetes: a systematic review of the literature. Diabetes Care 2002;25(3):583–92.

[29] Fabian MC, Lakey JR, Rajotte RV, et al. The efficacy and toxicity of rapamycin in murine islet transplantation. In vitro and in vivo studies. Transplantation 1993;56(5):1137–42.

[30] Bell E, Cao X, Moibi JA, et al. Rapamycin has a deleterious effect on MIN-6 cells and rat and human islets. Diabetes 2003;52(11):2731–9.

[31] Shapiro AM, Gallant H, Hao E, et al. Portal vein immunosuppressant levels and islet graft toxicity. Transplant Proc 1998;30(2):641.

[32] Desai NM, Goss JA, Deng S, et al. Elevated portal vein drug levels of sirolimus and tacrolimus in islet transplant recipients: local immunosuppression or islet toxicity? Transplantation 2003;76(11):1623–5.

[33] Luzi L. Metabolic strategies to predict and improve intrahepatic islet graft function. J Mol Med 1999;77(1):49–56.

[34] Rickels MR, Schutta MH, Markmann JF, et al. β cell function following human islet transplantation for type 1 diabetes. Diabetes 2005;54(1):100–6.

[35] Rickels MR, Schutta MH, Mueller R, et al. Islet cell hormonal responses to hypoglycemia after human islet transplantation for type 1 diabetes. Diabetes 2005;54(11):3205–11.

[36] Gupta V, Wahoff DC, Rooney DP, et al. The defective glucagon response from transplanted intrahepatic pancreatic islets during hypoglycemia is transplantation site-determined. Diabetes 1997;46(1):28–33.

[37] Kendall DM, Rooney DP, Smets YF, et al. Pancreas transplantation restores epinephrine response and symptom recognition during hypoglycemia in patients with long-standing type 1 diabetes and autonomic neuropathy. Diabetes 1997;46(2):249–57.

[38] Kendall DM, Teuscher AU, Robertson RP. Defective glucagon secretion during sustained hypoglycemia following successful islet allo- and autotransplantation in humans. Diabetes 1997;46(1):23–7.

[39] Paty BW, Ryan EA, Shapiro AM, et al. Intrahepatic islet transplantation in type 1 diabetic patients does not restore hypoglycemic hormonal counter-regulation or symptom recognition after insulin independence. Diabetes 2002;51(12):3428–34.

[40] Meyer C, Hering BJ, Grossmann R, et al. Improved glucose counter-regulation and autonomic symptoms after intraportal islet transplants alone in patients with long-standing type 1 diabetes mellitus. Transplantation 1998;66(2):233–40.

[41] Cryer PE, Davis SN, Shamoon H. Hypoglycemia in diabetes. Diabetes Care 2003;26(6):1902–12.

[42] Ryan EA, Shandro T, Green K, et al. Assessment of the severity of hypoglycemia and glycemic lability in type 1 diabetic subjects undergoing islet transplantation. Diabetes 2004;53(4):955–62.

[43] Rickels MR, Naji A, Teff KL. Insulin sensitivity, glucose effectiveness, and free fatty acid dynamics after human islet transplantation for type 1 diabetes. J Clin Endocrinol Metab 2006;91(6):2138–44.

[44] Senior PA, Paty BW, Cockfield SM, et al. Proteinuria developing after clinical islet transplantation resolves with sirolimus withdrawal and increased tacrolimus dosing. Am J Transplant 2005;5(9):2318–23.

[45] Fiorina P, Venturini M, Folli F, et al. Natural history of kidney graft survival, hypertrophy, and vascular function in end-stage renal disease type 1 diabetic kidney-transplanted patients: beneficial impact of pancreas and successful islet cotransplantation. Diabetes Care 2005; 28(6):1303–10.

[46] Digon BJ 3rd, Rother KI, Hirshberg B, et al. Sirolimus-induced interstitial pneumonitis in an islet transplant recipient. Diabetes Care 2003;26(11):3191.

[47] Hirshberg B, Rother KI, Digon BJ 3rd, et al. Benefits and risks of solitary islet transplantation for type 1 diabetes using steroid-sparing immunosuppression: the National Institutes of Health experience. Diabetes Care 2003;26(12):3288–95.

[48] Zhang N, Su D, Qu S, et al. Sirolimus is associated with reduced islet engraftment and impaired beta-cell function. Diabetes 2006;55(9):2429–36.

[49] Makhlouf L, Kishimoto K, Smith RN, et al. The role of autoimmunity in islet allograft destruction: major histocompatibility complex class II matching is necessary for autoimmune destruction of allogeneic islet transplants after T cell costimulatory blockade. Diabetes 2002; 51(11):3202–10.

[50] Venturini M, Angeli E, Maffi P, et al. Technique, complications, and therapeutic efficacy of percutaneous transplantation of human pancreatic islet cells in type 1 diabetes: the role of US. Radiology 2005;234(2):617–24.

[51] Markmann JF, Rosen M, Siegelman ES, et al. Magnetic resonance-defined periportal steatosis following intraportal islet transplantation: a functional footprint of islet graft survival? Diabetes 2003;52(7):1591–4.

[52] Maffi P, Angeli E, Bertuzzi F, et al. Minimal focal steatosis of liver after islet transplantation in humans: a long-term study. Cell Transplant 2005;14(10):727–33.

[53] Maffi P BF, De Taddeo F, Magistretti P, et al. Kidney function after islet transplant alone in type 1 diabetes: impact of immunosuppressive therapy on progression of diabetic nephropathy. Diabetes Care 2007;30(5):1150–5.

[54] Robertson RP. Islet transplantation as a treatment for diabetes—a work in progress. N Engl J Med 2004;350(7):694–705.

[55] Ryan EA, Paty BW, Senior PA, et al. Five-year follow-up after clinical islet transplantation. Diabetes 2005;54(7):2060–9.

[56] Davalli AM, Ogawa Y, Scaglia L, et al. Function, mass, and replication of porcine and rat islets transplanted into diabetic nude mice. Diabetes 1995;44(1):104–11.

[57] Han D, Leith J, Alejandro R, et al. Peripheral blood cytotoxic lymphocyte gene transcript levels differ in patients with long-term type 1 diabetes compared to normal controls. Cell Transplant 2005;14(6):403–9.

[58] Fiorina P, Folli F, Maffi P, et al. Islet transplantation improves vascular diabetic complications in patients with diabetes who underwent kidney transplantation: a comparison between kidney–pancreas and kidney-alone transplantation. Transplantation 2003;75(8):1296–301.

[59] Fiorina P, Gremizzi C, Maffi P, et al. Islet transplantation is associated with an improvement of cardiovascular function in type 1 diabetic kidney transplant patients. Diabetes Care 2005; 28(6):1358–65.

[60] Forst T, De La Tour DD, Kunt T, et al. Effects of proinsulin C peptide on nitric oxide, microvascular blood flow, and erythrocyte Na+,K+-ATPase activity in diabetes mellitus type I. Clin Sci (Lond) 2000;98(3):283–90.

[61] Johansson BL, Borg K, Fernqvist-Forbes E, et al. Beneficial effects of C peptide on incipient nephropathy and neuropathy in patients with type 1 diabetes mellitus. Diabet Med 2000; 17(3):181–9.

[62] Jonasson P, Nygren PA, Jornvall H, et al. Integrated bioprocess for production of human proinsulin C peptide via heat release of an intracellular heptameric fusion protein. J Biotechnol 2000;76(2–3):215–26.

[63] Wahren J, Ekberg K, Johansson J, et al. Role of C peptide in human physiology. Am J Physiol Endocrinol Metab 2000;278(5):E759–68.

[64] Cotter MA, Ekberg K, Wahren J, et al. Effects of proinsulin C peptide in experimental diabetic neuropathy: vascular actions and modulation by nitric oxide synthase inhibition. Diabetes 2003;52(7):1812–7.

[65] Johansson BL, Sundell J, Ekberg K, et al. C peptide improves adenosine-induced myocardial vasodilation in type 1 diabetes patients. Am J Physiol Endocrinol Metab 2004;286(1):E14–9.

[66] Johansson BL, Wahren J, Pernow J. C peptide increases forearm blood flow in patients with type 1 diabetes via a nitric oxide-dependent mechanism. Am J Physiol Endocrinol Metab 2003;285(4):E864–70.

[67] Rigler R, Pramanik A, Jonasson P, et al. Specific binding of proinsulin C peptide to human cell membranes. Proc Natl Acad Sci USA 1999;96(23):13318–23.

[68] Forst T, Kunt T, Pfutzner A, et al. New aspects on biological activity of C peptide in IDDM patients. Exp Clin Endocrinol Diabetes 1998;106(4):270–6.

[69] Forst T, Kunt T, Pohlmann T, et al. Biological activity of C peptide on the skin microcirculation in patients with insulin-dependent diabetes mellitus. J Clin Invest 1998;101(10): 2036–41.

[70] Forst T, Pfutzner A, Kunt T, et al. Skin microcirculation in patients with type 1 diabetes with and without neuropathy after neurovascular stimulation. Clin Sci (Lond) 1998;94(3):255–61.

[71] Kunt T, Schneider S, Pfutzner A, et al. The effect of human proinsulin C peptide on erythrocyte deformability in patients with type 1 diabetes mellitus. Diabetologia 1999;42(4): 465–71.

[72] Kitamura T, Kimura K, Jung BD, et al. Proinsulin C peptide rapidly stimulates mitogen-activated protein kinases in Swiss 3T3 fibroblasts: requirement of protein kinase C, phosphoinositide 3-kinase, and pertussis toxin-sensitive G-protein. Biochem J 2001;355(Pt 1):123–9.

[73] Kitamura T, Kimura K, Jung BD, et al. Proinsulin C-peptide activates cAMP response element-binding proteins through the p38 mitogen-activated protein kinase pathway in mouse lung capillary endothelial cells. Biochem J 2002;366(Pt 3):737–44.

[74] Ido Y, Vindigni A, Chang K, et al. Prevention of vascular and neural dysfunction in diabetic rats by C peptide. Science 1997;277(5325):563–6.

[75] Ricordi C, Strom TB. Clinical islet transplantation: advances and immunological challenges. Nat Rev Immunol 2004;4(4):259–68.

[76] Calafiore R, Basta G, Luca G, et al. Microencapsulated pancreatic islet allografts into nonimmunosuppressed patients with type 1 diabetes: first two cases. Diabetes Care 2006; 29(1):137–8.

[77] Secchi A, Taglietti MV, Socci C, et al. Insulin secretory patterns and blood glucose homeostasis after islet allotransplantation in IDDM patients: comparison with segmental- or whole-pancreas transplanted patients through a long-term longitudinal study. J Mol Med 1999;77(1):133–9.

ELSEVIER
SAUNDERS

Endocrinol Metab Clin N Am
36 (2007) 1015–1038

ENDOCRINOLOGY
AND METABOLISM
CLINICS
OF NORTH AMERICA

Pancreas-Kidney and Pancreas Transplantation for the Treatment of Diabetes Mellitus

Gerald S. Lipshutz, MD, MS, FACS[a,b,*],
Alan H. Wilkinson, MD, FRCP[c]

[a]Kidney and Pancreas Transplant Program, Department of Surgery, 77-120 CHS, David
Geffen School of Medicine at UCLA, Los Angeles, CA 90095, USA
[b]Kidney and Pancreas Transplant Program, Department of Urology, 77-120 CHS, David
Geffen School of Medicine at UCLA, Los Angeles, CA 90095, USA
[c]Kidney and Pancreas Transplant Program, Department of Medicine, 200 Medical Plaza,
Suite 370-12, David Geffen School of Medicine at UCLA, Los Angeles, CA 90095, USA

Diabetes mellitus is a major health problem estimated to affect 100 million people worldwide. It affects 6.3% of the United States population (18.2 million individuals), approximately one half of whom are unaware that they have the disease. It accounts for more than 160,000 deaths per year in the United States, and in 2002, the annual direct and indirect costs of type 1 and 2 diabetes exceeded $130 billion. It is the leading single cause of end-stage renal disease (ESRD), accounting for approximately one third of all new ESRD patients. Retinopathy is the second leading cause of blindness in all persons [1]. Ten percent of diabetics require a major amputation in their lifetime. Life expectancy of diabetics is approximately one third lower than that of nondiabetics; cardiovascular disease is the leading cause of death.

The prevalence of type 1 diabetes in the United States is estimated to be 1 million people with 30,000 new cases diagnosed each year. At the turn of the nineteenth century, a patient diagnosed as having type 1 diabetes had an average life expectancy of 2 years. The isolation and development of insulin as a treatment for diabetes changed the disease from one that is rapidly fatal to a chronic disease with the potential for multiple secondary complications occurring 10 to 20 years after disease diagnosis: blindness, cardiovascular

* Corresponding author. Kidney and Pancreas Transplant Program, Department of Surgery and Department of Urology, 77-120 CHS, David Geffen School of Medicine at UCLA, Los Angeles, CA 90095.
  E-mail address: glipshutz@mednet.ucla.edu (G.S. Lipshutz).

0889-8529/07/$ - see front matter © 2007 Elsevier Inc. All rights reserved.
doi:10.1016/j.ecl.2007.07.010

disease, dyslipidemia, cerebrovascular disease, amputation, and lifespan reduction. Approximately 34% of diabetics develop ESRD as a secondary complication within 15 years of disease onset [2].

The first human pancreas transplantation was pioneered in 1966 by Kelly and colleagues [3]. The major surgical challenge to be overcome was appropriate pancreatic exocrine drainage [4]. They transplanted a duct-ligated segmental pancreatic allograft and a cadaveric kidney into a 28-year-old woman. Posttransplantation immunosuppression was azathioprine and prednisone. Unfortunately, a pancreatic fistula complicated the patient's postoperative course, and both the kidney and pancreas were removed about 2 months later. The patient died from a pulmonary embolus 13 days later. The second patient, a 32-year-old recipient, underwent transplantation 2 weeks after the first recipient. The patient suffered from rejection, and treatment consisted of steroid boluses and graft irradiation. The patient died from sepsis 4.5 months after transplantation. Although the results were poor, these early transplantations did demonstrate that glucose control without exogenous insulin was possible. The procedure established that endogenous secretion of insulin with normal feedback mechanisms could occur with a pancreas transplant.

Although kidney transplantation is the treatment of choice for end-stage diabetic nephropathy, the ultimate treatment today for type 1 diabetes mellitus is the whole vascularized pancreas transplant. By the end of 2004, more than 23,000 pancreas transplantations had been performed worldwide, with more than 17,000 in the United States and approximately 6000 outside the United States [5]. United States 1-year graft survival rates for 2002/2003 were 85% for simultaneous pancreas-kidney (SPK) recipients, 78% for pancreas after kidney (PAK) recipients, and 77% for pancreas transplants alone (PTA) recipients [5].

The benefits of SPK transplantation are improved quality of life, prevention of recurrent diabetic nephropathy, freedom from exogenous insulin with euglycemia and normalization of glycosylated hemoglobin, lack of dietary restrictions and frequent whole blood glucose monitoring, and stabilization or improvement in secondary complications [6–18]. These documented benefits of SPK are the basis for its acceptance as an appropriate therapy for patients who have type 1 diabetes mellitus and renal failure. The trade-off to the patient is the operative risk and the need for chronic immunosuppression. Pancreas transplantation, however, normalizes glucose levels far better than any other strategy available for the treatment of type 1 diabetes mellitus today. (Box 1 lists common abbreviations used in the field of pancreas transplantation.)

Candidacy for pancreas transplantation

Pancreas transplantation usually is performed in combination with kidney transplantation for patients who have renal failure secondary to diabetic

---

Box 1. Abbreviations commonly used in pancreas and kidney transplantation

SPK: simultaneous pancreas and kidney transplantation
PAK: pancreas after kidney transplantation
PTA: pancreas transplantation alone
KTA: kidney transplantation alone

---

nephropathy. Often the patient's decision to undergo pancreas transplantation is not difficult, because he or she already requires lifelong immunosuppression as part of the medical regimen following renal transplantation. The primary significant risk is the operative procedure, and the patient must decide if he or she would like to have both organs transplanted simultaneously (in an SPK) or to undergo two transplantations in sequence with a period of recovery between, as in PAK. Often this decision is affected by whether the patient has a living kidney donor.

Among patients who have insulin-dependent diabetes mellitus and nephropathy, those who have minimal or limited secondary diabetic complications are considered the best candidates for SPK or PAK. These patients tend to be between 20 and 45 years of age. Criteria for a patient considering PTA are based on a significantly impaired quality of life secondary to hypoglycemic unawareness, brittle diabetic control, and with the presence of early diabetic complications [19].

Because diabetes and dialysis dependence are significant risk factors for atherosclerotic disease, candidates for pancreas transplantation require thorough cardiac evaluation. In addition to their long history of diabetes mellitus, these patients often have multiple cardiovascular risk factors including tobacco use, hypertension, hyperlipidemia, family history, and renal failure. Cardiovascular disease is the single greatest cause of mortality in pancreas transplant recipients [20,21]. As many as one third of potential diabetic candidates have significant coronary artery disease, and all patients should undergo appropriate evaluation preoperatively. What constitutes an appropriate evaluation is controversial and often center specific. This controversy probably is related, in part, to the poor predictive value of noninvasive imaging in transplantation candidates [22,23]. Nuclear perfusion imaging is best performed as a screening initial study in all patients. In general, select young patients who have had diabetes mellitus for less than 25 years and who have never smoked tobacco or have other risk factors may be evaluated by stress imaging only. Most other candidates should be evaluated by coronary angiography, and significant coronary artery disease should be treated appropriately before transplantation. In addition, patients should undergo routine reassessment with yearly noninvasive stress imaging until transplantation.

Absolute contraindications to pancreas transplantation are relatively few (Box 2). Exclusion criteria include insufficient cardiac function, active infection, recent malignancy, ongoing substance abuse, ongoing untreated psychiatric illness, recent history of medical noncompliance, lack of social support, inability to provide informed consent, significant irreversible hepatic, gastrointestinal, or pulmonary abnormalities, significant obesity, or untreated significant vascular disease.

Indications for pancreas transplantation

The clinical practice recommendations of the American Diabetes Association state that pancreas transplantation (SPK or PAK) is an acceptable surgical procedure in type 1 diabetic patients also undergoing kidney transplantation [24]. These patients must be medically suitable type 1 diabetic patients also who are candidates for renal transplantation or who have excellent function of a kidney transplant and who are interested in receiving a pancreas transplant. The vast majority of pancreas transplantations are performed as an SPK; the second most common method is a PAK.

Box 2. General patient-selection criteria for kidney/pancreas transplantation

General criteria/indications
- Adults age 18 to 55 (age > 55 on a case-by-case basis)
- Diabetes mellitus type 1 (insulin dependent)
- Chronic renal failure secondary to diabetic nephropathy
- Ability to comply with medical regimen
- Ability to understand risks and benefits of procedure
- Brittle diabetes not controlled by exogenous insulin therapy (PTA)
- Ability to withstand the surgery and immunosuppression
- Absence of contraindications

Contraindications for kidney/pancreas transplantation
- Insufficient cardiac reserve:
  - Noncorrectable coronary artery disease
  - Ejection fraction < 40%
  - Recent myocardial infarction
- Extensive peripheral vascular disease
- Lack of well-defined secondary complications
- Ongoing substance abuse
- Debilitating psychiatric illness
- Significant obesity

Pancreas transplantation can be performed in type 1 diabetics who have preserved native kidney function but suffer from glucose lability and frequent, acute, and severe metabolic complications including repeated episodes of ketoacidosis, who have incapacitating clinical and emotional problems related to insulin therapy, and who have consistent failure of insulin therapy to prevent acute diabetic complications. Significant hypoglycemic unawareness also may be an indication, because achieving an insulin-free state enhances these patients' quality of life. PTA should be performed before secondary complications of diabetes become irreversible and before the need for kidney transplantation. A creatinine clearance above 60 to 70 mL/min usually is required, because calcineurin inhibitors can cause accelerated deterioration of native renal function in patients who have a lower creatinine clearance. This group is the smallest of the three groups receiving pancreas transplantation.

Success in all three groups depends on (1) appropriate patient selection and (2) appropriate donor patient selection, organ procurement, and meticulous backbench preparation of the pancreatic allograft for implantation.

Types of operations

Three groups of patients are considered for pancreas transplantation. For diabetics who are in renal failure, SPK generally is the preferred method of pancreas transplantation, because of its advantages in requiring only one surgical intervention and one source of foreign HLA for the recipient patient.

For diabetic patients who already have a functioning kidney allograft, PAK is the appropriate procedure. Immunosuppressive therapy is not a major concern, because patients already are immunosuppressed for the kidney allograft. The main risk to the patient is the alteration in immunosuppression necessary after pancreas transplantation and the inherent risks of an intra-abdominal surgical procedure. In general, patients who have type 1 diabetes undergoing living or cadaveric renal transplantation should have the kidney placed on the left side in anticipation of a pancreas transplantation in the future.

For the preuremic patient who has no or minimal renal dysfunction but who has brittle diabetic management despite the administration of conventional antidiabetic therapies and hypoglycemic unawareness, PTA is the therapeutic option. The main risks to these patients are the long-term effects of chronic immunosuppression and the surgical procedure itself.

Donor selection and surgical procedures

Donor selection

The ideal organ donor typically is in the age range of 10 to 45 years, has had no trauma to or previous pancreatic surgery, and has no history of diabetes. Organs from older donors have had higher rates of graft thrombosis, intra-abdominal infections, anastomotic or duodenal leaks, re-laparotomy, and decreased graft survival [25]. In general caution should used in using pancreas donors older than 45 years [26]. Weight and body mass are important considerations in a donor organ. The authors often consider 45 kg to be the lower weight limit for a donor, but others require a minimum donor weight of 30 kg [27]. This limitation is set primarily because of concern about size of the pancreatic arterial vasculature for construction of the iliac Y-graft and risk of graft thrombosis. Some, however, have used pancreata from pediatric donor patients successfully [28]. The authors do not consider donor patients who have a body mass index over 30 because of concern about fatty infiltration of the gland and subsequent increased risk of infection, pancreatitis, and allograft thrombosis.

The surgical procedure can be broken down into three parts: organ procurement, backbench pancreas preparation, and pancreas transplantation.

Organ procurement

After opening the lesser sac, the gastrocolic ligament is divided. The pancreas is closely examined and palpated. A Kocher maneuver is performed to the inferior vena cava. The right gastroepiploic and pyloric vessels are ligated and divided. The nasogastric tube is advanced into the second portion of the duodenum and instilled with 200 cm^3 of a solution of 50:50 saline and betadine paint with 100 mg of amphotericin B. The nasogastric tube then is withdrawn to the fundus of the stomach. The short gastrics are divided, allowing the stomach to be separated from the spleen. The transverse colon is mobilized completely by ligating the middle colic vasculature. The stomach then is divided proximal to the pylorus with a gastrointestinal anastomotic (GIA) stapler. The fourth portion of the duodenum is divided similarly just before removal of the pancreas. While the spleen is carefully retracted anteriorly, the splenonephric and renophrenic attachments are divided carefully. The liver is mobilized, and the aorta, vena cava, and inferior mesenteric vein are isolated. The gallbladder is emptied, and the bile duct is flushed. The supraceliac aorta is isolated, and heparin is given intravenously. Cannulas are placed into the aorta and inferior mesenteric vein, and preservation solution is instilled. The surface is cooled by ice slush. The thoracic organs then are procured, and, after division of the gastroduodenal artery, portal vein, and splenic artery, the liver is removed. The pancreas with spleen attached is removed after division of the superior mesenteric artery (SMA) at the aorta. The allograft should be kept ice cold and sterile in preservation solution (Fig. 1) until ready to be prepared on the backbench.

Assessment of the vascular anatomy of the porta hepatis is very important during the procurement. The presence of an accessory or replaced hepatic artery is not a contraindication to using the pancreatic allograft for transplantation. In this situation, however, the right hepatic artery needs

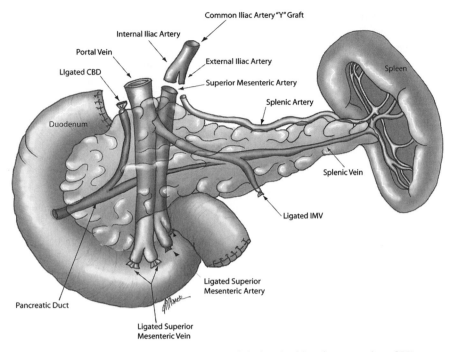

Fig. 1. Anatomy of procured pancreatic allograft before backbench preparation. CBD, common bile duct; IMV, inferior mesenteric vein.

to be dissected to the SMA and the SMA divided distal to the takeoff of the right hepatic artery; a cuff of SMA must remain on the aberrant right hepatic artery for the donor liver. When this dissection is performed, great care must be taken in examining for an inferior pancreaticoduodenal artery, which is critical for vascularization of the head of the pancreas and the duodenal segment. If this vessel must be taken to leave a cuff of SMA on the aberrant right hepatic artery, the pancreatic allograft generally should not be used for whole-organ transplantation.

Backbench pancreas preparation

The backbench preparation of a pancreatic allograft requires very careful preparation and surgical technique. It generally can be divided into four steps. First, the distal and proximal duodenum must be shortened to proper length. This shortening is performed while probing the common bile duct to ensure that the ampulla is in the center of the duodenal segment and is not compromised during duodenal shortening. The ends of the duodenum generally are stapled and then oversewn in a Lembert fashion. The bile duct is ligated. A culture of the excised duodenum should be sent to the laboratory for Gram stain, fungal stain, and bacterial and fungal cultures.

Second, a Y-graft is constructed using the donor common iliac/external iliac/internal iliac artery bifurcation. Typically the internal iliac artery is anastomosed to the splenic artery in an end-to-end fashion; then the external iliac artery is anastomosed to the SMA. The inferior mesenteric vein should be ligated if ligation was not performed during the procurement.

Third, extraneous tissue at the periphery of the gland is ligated and removed. The hilum of the spleen is dissected carefully, and the splenic artery and vein are tied by suture ligature. The stapled mesenteric vasculature is oversewn. The portal vein then is dissected carefully from the surrounding gland, and the coronary vein is tied.

Fourth, the gland should be tested for vascular integrity. Ice-cold preservation solution should be injected carefully into the common iliac artery, using a syringe with a tapered connector attached, and the gland should be examined carefully from all aspects. Evidence of preservation solution extrusion should be addressed with ties or suture ligatures. This precaution will decrease the amount of blood loss and improve hemostasis during implantation.

Surgical implantation techniques

The main issues in pancreatic transplantation surgical techniques involve the method of exocrine drainage and the method of vascular drainage.

Enteric versus bladder drainage

Enteric drainage of the exocrine pancreas (Figs. 2 and 3) is the most physiologic approach for drainage of exocrine secretions. It is associated with fewer urologic problems than exocrine bladder drainage (Fig. 4). There are fewer urinary tract infections or episodes of dehydration and a lower rate of pancreatitis than with bladder drainage, and there are few, if any, significant metabolic derangements [29]. The major specific problem with enteric drainage is the risk of more severe complications from the development of an enteric leak. In addition, when the organ is placed mid-abdomen, there is less access for biopsy (in the case of portal venous drainage).

The main advantage of bladder drainage of exocrine secretions is the ability to monitor urinary amylase for pancreatic allograft rejection. In addition, there tend to be fewer severe complications from duodenal leaks and abscesses, and cystoscopy can be used to perform a biopsy. The anastomosis is nonphysiologic, however, which often results in a number of urologic complications [29,30] and metabolic abnormalities [31].

Systemic versus portal drainage

Most pancreatic allografts have been transplanted like kidneys: heterotopically in the pelvis using the iliac vasculature for inflow and outflow. Advantages of this approach include lower rates of allograft thrombosis, easier

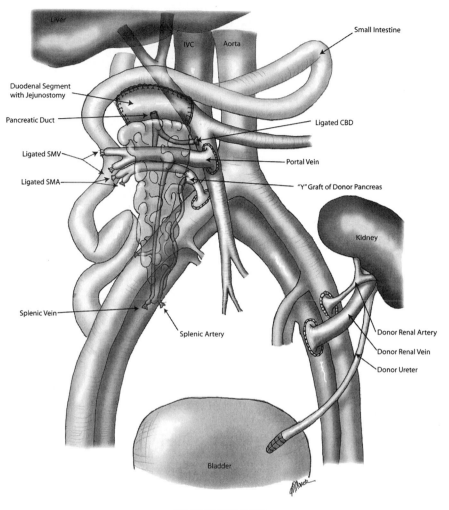

Fig. 2. Portal venous and enterically drained pancreatic allograft with kidney on the left. IVC, inferior vena cava; SMA, superior mesenteric artery; SMV, superior mesenteric vein.

access for percutaneous biopsy, and the ability to use either the bladder or intestine for drainage of exocrine secretions. This approach, however, does result in peripheral hyperinsulinemia with portal hypoinsulinemia [32,33], because the first-pass effect of hepatic degradation is lost. Some report abnormal lipoprotein metabolism [34] with an increased risk of the progression of atherosclerotic cardiovascular disease [35–38] with this approach.

Portal venous drainage results in normal insulin levels, and lipoprotein metabolism is better than with systemic venous drainage. The rate of allograft thrombosis is higher, however, and access is more difficult if

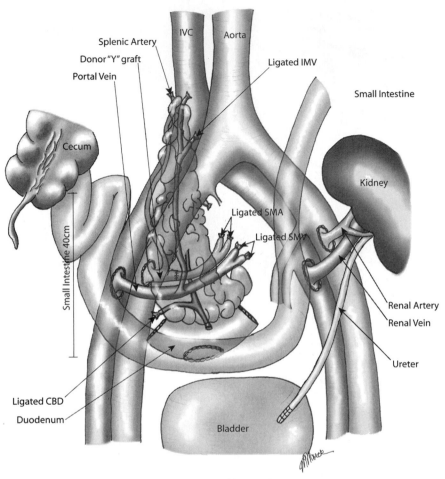

Enteric Drained Systemic Venous

Fig. 3. Systemic venous and enterically drained pancreatic allograft with kidney on the left. CBD, common bile duct; IVC, inferior vena cava; SMA, superior mesenteric artery; SMV, superior mesenteric vein.

percutaneous biopsy is necessary. In addition, drainage must be enteric because of the cephalad placement of the donor duodenum (see Fig. 2).

Complications

Results with pancreas transplantation have improved significantly during the last 25 years, in part because of improvements in antibiotics, surgical techniques, and immunosuppression [39,40]. A number of early postoperative complications still can occur with whole-organ pancreas transplantation, however. These complications include bleeding, infection, rejection, pancreatitis, and allograft thrombosis. The rate of technical complications

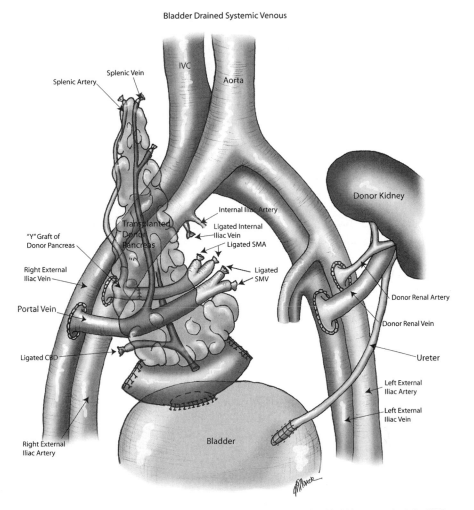

Fig. 4. Systemic venous and bladder-drained pancreatic allograft with kidney on the left. CBD, common bile duct; IVC, inferior vena cava; SMA, superior mesenteric artery; SMV, superior mesenteric vein.

after pancreas transplantation is higher than after most other solid-organ transplantations [41]. Technical failure rates (as opposed to immunologic failure rates) have been reported to be highest in SPK recipients, followed by PAK and PTA recipients [42].

Thrombosis

Graft thrombosis is well recognized and is the most common early cause of loss of a pancreatic allograft. It is a devastating complication that can occur in as many as 10% to 20% of pancreatic transplant recipients. Seventy percent of the time, graft thrombosis occurs in the first week after transplantation. Both recipient and donor factors can lead to graft thrombosis. Recipient factors are ones that decrease blood flow to the allograft and include pancreatitis, hypotension, acute rejection, and reperfusion injury. Donor factors include older age, longer cold ischemia times, and death resulting from cerebrovascular events.

Thrombosis of a pancreatic allograft may occur in either the arterial or the venous system. Arterial thrombosis may occur in the splenic artery (Fig. 5) or in the SMA; it sometimes occurs in both (see Fig. 1 for anatomy). Arterial thrombosis of the SMA leads to nonviability of the duodenal segment. On exploration, the pancreas appears soft and pale. In general, early on the patient feels no abdominal pain, and there typically is an acute rise in serum glucose with a fall in serum amylase. Even if the splenic artery is patent, surgical removal generally is the most appropriate measure.

Venous thrombosis usually presents with graft swelling resulting in symptoms of abdominal pain. Serologically, patients demonstrate a rise in glucose and amylase levels. On abdominal exploration the graft often appears large, dark-blue, and engorged. Doppler ultrasound examination is used routinely to examine vascular flow. In venous thrombosis, there is high resistance in the pancreatic arteries with no flow in the pancreatic veins. Pancreatectomy typically is the next step.

Prevention and postoperative vigilance are the main measures for addressing the risk of allograft thrombosis. Anticoagulation is the main measure to prevent graft thrombosis but increases the risk of postoperative bleeding. Liberal use of Doppler ultrasound imaging should be employed for any indication of early graft dysfunction.

Transplant pancreatitis

Pancreatitis of an allograft, detected postoperatively by a transient rise in serum amylase or lipase levels, tends to occur to some degree in all

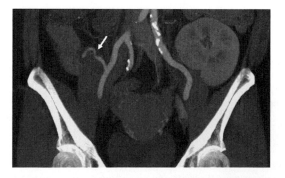

Fig. 5. CT angiogram of pancreatic allograft. Arrow demonstrates thrombosis of splenic artery of allograft with intact and patent superior mesenteric artery. The gland is well perfused because of collateral blood flow.

recipients. These elevations usually are temporary and are without great clinical significance. Pancreatitis typically occurs as a result of cold ischemic storage and reperfusion injury or from handling during organ recovery and implantation and usually is without clinical consequence, is self-limited, and resolves with conservative therapy. In bladder-drained recipients, pancreatitis also may be caused by the irritant effects of urine refluxing into the duodenal segment and pancreatic duct. This situation is more common in recipients of neurogenic and distended bladders and is managed with self-catheterization, double voiding, and alpha-adrenergic–blocking agents. Endocrine function is unaltered, but patients typically present with low-grade fever, elevated serum amylase levels, and graft tenderness. Enteric conversion sometimes is required.

The treatment for transplant pancreatitis mirrors the treatment of pancreatitis in patients who are not transplant recipients. In some patients, peripancreatic fluid collections can occur, and these collections may be high in exocrine enzymes. Patients may require laparotomy, evacuation of collections, and pancreatic débridement if abdominal imaging suggests evidence of necrosis or subsequent infection.

Anastomotic leak

Duodenal segment leaks in the bladder-drained pancreas recipient most often occur in the first 3 months after transplantation and usually present with the acute onset of abdominal pain and elevation of serum amylase levels. Diagnosis can be made by performing a cystogram or by nuclear medicine imaging. Treatment is nonoperative in as many as two thirds of patients [43], usually requiring prolonged Foley urethral drainage. Resistant cases may require exploration and closure of the leakage site or enteric conversion [44].

Enteric exocrine drainage is the most popular method of draining the exocrine pancreas today. The development of an anastomotic leak is the most serious complication of an enterically drained whole-pancreas transplant. Early duodenal segment leaks tend to result from technical complications or ischemia. Late duodenal leaks tend to be caused by rejection, infection, or ischemia of the duodenal staple line. Leaks do not result in alteration of endocrine function, but patients present with elevated white blood cell counts, graft tenderness, and fever, and leaks generally lead to a pancreaticocutaneous fistula or peripancreatic abscess. These developments are particularly serious because of the spillage of succus entericus within the abdomen. CT imaging and percutaneous drainage usually demonstrate a mixed infection of bacteria and often fungus. Broad-spectrum antibiotics are essential, and surgical exploration should be performed without delay. At laparotomy, decisions must be made regarding the extent of the infection, its potential for clearance, and need for removal of the pancreatic allograft. Treatment of the infection, if inadequate, will lead to organ failure, sepsis, and death of the recipient. Some have converted the allograft to a Roux-en-Y limb when there has been evidence of an anastomotic leak, but this conversion has not always been successful in salvaging the allograft.

Abscess and infection

Intra-abdominal infections are much more common after pancreas transplantation than after KTA and represent a significant cause of mortality if inadequately treated. Conservative therapy with percutaneous drains and intravenous antibiotics often is adequate (Fig. 6). Peripancreatic fluid collections can become infected, and persistence or lack of resolution requires consideration of operative exploration and drainage. Pancreatectomy must be considered in these situations. A worrisome and late complication in patients who have peripancreatic abscesses is the development of a mycotic aneurysm and serious and life-threatening bleeding.

Gastrointestinal bleeding

Early gastrointestinal bleeding, typically from the suture line of the duodenal-ileal anastomosis or the duodenal-bladder anastomosis, may occur in both bladder-drained and enterically drained pancreas transplant recipients. This bleeding can be caused by ischemia/reperfusion injury of the duodenal mucosa or by a bleeding vessel at the suture line of the anastomosis. When heparin is used for anticoagulation postoperatively, bleeding can be evident by either a fall in the hematocrit or melenic stool. In addition, in uremic patients who have a delay in graft function of the kidney allograft, platelet

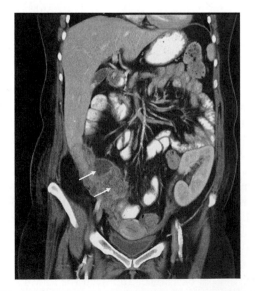

Fig. 6. CT image demonstrates peripancreatic transplant abscess (*arrows*).

dysfunction becomes evident, and bleeding can occur. In both cases, bleeding tends to stop with the cessation of anticoagulation or, in the case of uremia and delayed kidney function, with transfusion of packed red blood cells and platelets. Bleeding in enterically drained patients usually resolves with such therapy. In bladder-drained patients, however, bladder irrigation may be necessary, and cystoscopy may be needed to remove larger clots. Occasionally, open cystotomy may be necessary with fulguration or ligation of a bleeding vessel.

Complications specific to the bladder-drained pancreas

There are specific and unique complications related to the bladder-drained pancreas. Bladder drainage, however, generally is considered safer than enteric drainage because it avoids the concerning complications of enteric leak and formation of an intra-abdominal abscess. Because of the drainage of a large volume of exocrine-rich contents to the bladder, complications can occur, some more serious than others, and some primarily affecting the lifestyle of the recipient. These complications are the primary reasons that this method of drainage has become less popular today and for conversion from a bladder-drained to an enterically drained pancreas in as many as one in four recipients. Complications include urinary tract infections (which are common and may be caused by sutures), urethral stricture with sterile urethritis and balanitis, hematuria (caused by duodenal ulcer or persistent cystitis), ureteral stricture, urethral disruption, ureteral leak, and duodenal segment leak. Metabolic abnormalities can occur because of the loss of large quantities of bicarbonate-rich pancreatic fluid. Hyponatremia, volume loss, and acidemia may occur.

Effect of pancreas transplantation on diabetic complications

The goal of kidney and pancreas transplantation in diabetic recipients is to restore renal function and to normalize carbohydrate metabolism and establish a state of normoglycemia. In general, this process improves the quality of life in diabetic patients who have ESRD and frees patients from exogenous insulin and dietary restrictions. Quality-of-life improvements include greater satisfaction with life, a feeling of control and independence, and improved perceptions of mental and physical health. Although making patients insulin independent is a clear advantage, whether transplantation arrests and sometimes reverses secondary complications of chronic diabetes mellitus is controversial and continues to be studied.

Nephropathy

Renal allografts transplanted into diabetic recipients demonstrate signs of diabetic nephropathy as early as 2 years after transplantation. The first demonstration that diabetic glomerulopathy could be prevented was demonstrated in the 1980s [9,45]. One to 4 years after transplantation, glomerular basement membrane widths in diabetic SPK recipients were compared with those of diabetics who had received KTA. Glomerular basement membrane widths were in the normal range in all SPK recipients but were increased in most diabetic KTA patients. Although these investigations had limitations, they suggest that prolonged normoglycemia prevents the recurrence of diabetic glomerulopathy in kidney allografts.

Studies performed by another group at 5 years [46] and 10 years [47] showed interesting results. At 5 years after PTA, there was no amelioration of established diabetic nephropathy lesions. At 10 years, however, there was reversal of diabetic glomerular lesions in all patients who had functioning pancreatic allografts. Glomerular and tubular basement membrane width, which was unchanged at 5 years, decreased at 10 years, falling into the normal range for some patients and approaching normal in the remaining patients. Kimmelstiel-Wilson nodular lesions disappeared, and glomerular capillaries previously compressed by mesangial expansion were noted to have reopened.

Data also suggest that a successful PAK may halt the progression of diabetic glomerulopathy. In this single study, pancreas transplantation was performed 1 to 7 years after kidney transplantation in diabetic recipients. Kidney transplant biopsies were performed before pancreas transplantation and at 4 years. These biopsies were compared with those in diabetic recipients of a KTA. Microscopic examination demonstrated decreased mesangial fractional volume in PAK recipients as compared with diabetic KTA. In addition, PAK recipients had smaller glomeruli on biopsy, suggesting that glomerular enlargement may be reversible with sustained normoglycemia [48]. These studies demonstrate that diabetic glomerular, tubular, and interstitial lesions can reverse with the prolonged normoglycemia established by successful pancreas transplantation.

Vascular disease

Cardiovascular disease is the most common cause of mortality in patients who have diabetes [20,21]. Whether the risk of cardiovascular disease or cardiovascular disease itself improves or worsens after pancreas transplantation is an important outcome measure. Improvement in glucose levels reduces the risk of microvascular complications in type 1 diabetes mellitus. Few prospective studies with a large number of patients have examined the relationship between the establishment of normoglycemia in long-term diabetic patients and a reduction in cardiovascular morbidity and mortality, however. Some studies that have been performed do suggest benefit.

When radionuclide imaging was used to assess left ventricular diastolic function in kidney/pancreas recipients 4 years after transplantation, peak filling rates as a measure of left ventricular function were higher in kidney/pancreas recipients than in KTA recipients [49]. In addition, the ratio of peak filling rate to peak ejection rate and the endothelial-dependent dilation of the brachial artery were improved when compared with KTA recipients.

In examining atherosclerotic risk factors 3 years after transplantation, kidney/pancreas recipients were found to have decreased levels of von Willebrand's factor, fibrinogen, triglyceride, D-dimers, and homocysteine when compared with KTA recipients. Candidates for pancreas transplantation have greater carotid intima-media thickening (IMT) than age-matched normal control subjects [50]. Ultrasound examination showed that the intimal thickness of the carotid artery was lower in kidney/pancreas recipients than in KTA recipients (0.74 mm versus 0.86 mm; $P = .04$). This study was limited by the small number of patients and by lack of pretransplantation assessment of intimal thickness and atherosclerotic risk factors. In a more recent prospective study that measured carotid IMT before and 2 years after transplantation, however, carotid IMT was improved, and there were no changes in blood pressure, body mass index, smoking, lipid levels, or use of hypolipidemic agents to explain this change [20].

Other investigations have tended to look more closely at pretransplantation studies. In one study, two-dimensional, and M-mode echocardiography before and 1 year after transplantation was performed in both SPK and KTA recipients [14]. This study observed a greater decrease in left ventricular mass and greater normalization of diastolic dysfunction in SPK recipients than in those who underwent KTA. Progression of coronary artery disease, using mean segment diameter loss on coronary angiography, was less in patients who had a functioning graft after SPK than in patients in whom the graft had failed [51]. This observation, and the other improvements in cardiovascular health observed, suggests that future vascular disease events and mortality should be reduced after pancreas transplantation.

Retinopathy

Many studies have examined the impact of pancreas transplantation (in combination with kidney transplantation) on existing diabetic retinopathy. Although limited by including patients who had advanced retinopathy and recent transplantation, most studies have shown transplantation to have little impact on retinopathy [52–55]. Studies of longer duration in patients who had less advanced diabetic retinopathy or those who had macular edema have suggested some improvement with pancreas transplantation. In some patients who had preproliferative retinopathy, stability [56,57] or regression [58] after transplantation was detected, and macular edema was improved [57,59].

Some studies have suggested an unexplained and transient worsening of retinopathy in the first year after transplantation. A trend in these longer-term studies suggests that there is a delayed benefit in euglycemia, because improvement in patients who had less advanced disease occurred 3 years or later after transplantation.

Neuropathy

Diabetic focal or polyneuropathies are common complications of diabetes mellitus and often affect both the autonomic and somatic nervous systems. Polyneuropathy, a diffuse involvement of autonomic, sensory, and motor systems, is disabling, and is the most common neurologic complication of diabetes. It is a contributing factor to foot ulceration [60]. The prevalence of polyneuropathy by clinical symptoms ranges from 26% [61] to 39% [62].

Chronic hyperglycemia generally is considered the most important factor in the development of diabetic neuropathy [63]. It has been suggested that long periods of normoglycemia would be necessary to slow progression of nerve dysfunction [64]; however, such benefits of intensive therapy with insulin generally are associated with increased risks of hypoglycemic episodes [65]. As with other secondary complications of diabetes, extended observation periods as long as 10 years may be necessary to recover from pathologic abnormalities that have developed over the previous 20 or more years since the onset of diabetes mellitus in individual patients [66].

The most comprehensive study with the longest follow-up of patients who had polyneuropathy and who underwent pancreas transplantation was published in 1997 [67]. The study consisted of 115 patients, all of whom were examined before and after transplantation. Comparison was made with a control group of 92 diabetic patients. The control group demonstrated progressive deterioration in neuropathy by neurophysiologic evaluation during the 10-year follow-up period. In patients who underwent successful pancreas transplantation, neurologic evaluation demonstrated a general trend toward improvement in the motor and sensory nerve conduction studies at 1 year and in autonomic function at 5 years. In general, 60% had improvement on motor testing, 50% in sensory testing, and 30% to 45% in autonomic nervous system testing. Patients who had either PTA or a pancreas transplantation in combination with a kidney transplantation (SPK or PAK) showed improvement throughout the 10-year follow-up period, demonstrating that the effect was not related to correction of uremia.

Diabetic autonomic nervous system dysfunction is associated with mortality [68]. Does the improvement in neuropathy after pancreas transplantation result in less mortality? A large group of diabetic patients (n = 545) who had complete autonomic cardiovascular and nerve conduction studies was examined to answer this question [15]. Of these patients, 257 received a pancreas transplant. Of the total cohort, 116 died during the period of observation, and the results of cardiovascular autonomic testing correlated with mortality. Abnormal cardiorespiratory reflexes were present in 417 patients, and there was abnormal nerve conduction in 392. Mortality rates for patients who had abnormal tests were higher than for patients who had normal tests. Patients who had moderate neuropathy (but not those who had severe neuropathy) and who retained a functioning pancreas transplant survived longer than those who lost pancreatic function in the first 3 months.

Impact on survival

There are significant complexities in comparing survival probabilities among patients who have ESRD and who undergo different and subsequent renal replacement therapies [18]. This complexity is reflected in studies regarding the benefit [8,69–71] or detriment [72,73] of SPK over KTA in diabetics. Although both primary and repeat kidney transplantation have been shown to provide greater survival benefit in diabetics than in nondiabetics [74,75], there have been conflicting reports as to whether SPK provides additional survival benefit over KTA [18].

Recently, an evaluation of survival of a cohort of 13,467 uremic type 1 diabetic patients who underwent SPK, cadaveric KTA, living-donor KTA, or who remained on the transplant waiting list was performed [18]. The study analyzed data from the US Scientific Renal Transplant Registry supplemented with data from the US Renal Data System. The data from this study indicate that SPK recipients can expect to live 15 years longer than type 1 diabetics on the wait list who do not receive a transplant. In addition, SPK recipients can expect to live 10 years longer than if they were a type 1 diabetic recipient of a cadaveric KTA. All in all, the projected extra lifetime gained for all SPK recipients is 23.4 years; those in the age cohort of 18 to 29 years are projected to gain as many as 48.8 years, whereas those age 40 to 49 years are expected to gain 18.7 years. The overall adjusted mortality rates for SPK, living-donor kidney recipients, and cadaveric recipients were 40, 41, and 59 deaths per 1000 patient-years, respectively [18]. The results of this analysis suggest that there is a survival advantage for all demographic subgroups except those 50 years old or older at the time of transplantation.

With this increased survival, there is the additional risk of excess initial morbidity and mortality [18]. In SPK recipients the risk of infectious death after transplantation was increased twofold [18]. In addition, their overall risk of mortality was higher after transplantation. When compared with the type 1 diabetic on the dialysis wait list (relative mortality risk of 1), it takes 101 days for SPK recipients to reach the same relative mortality risk (the mortality risk immediately after transplantation is > 1.3). This period is nearly twice as long as that for recipients of cadaveric KTA (43 days) and nearly seven times as long as that for recipients of a living-donor kidney (15 days). The authors conclude that, with the selection criteria in use today and the posttransplantation management of these patients, SPK, despite the early elevated mortality risk, improves longevity more than other existing therapies for type 1 diabetic patients who have renal failure [18].

Survival benefit with PTA is controversial because of the associated morbidity and mortality, the need for immunosuppression, and uncertainty about whether secondary complications are prevented [76]. The recent publication of two large studies has added to the controversy. One study, while confirming the survival benefit of SPK, demonstrated an increase in mortality for at least the first 4 years after transplantation in those receiving PAK or PTA when compared with wait-list patients [76]. The other study demonstrated that the surgical procedure increased the mortality risk in the first 3 months after transplantation when compared with wait-list patients [77]. The overall hazard ratio, however, favored transplantation for the SPK category, was indeterminate for the PAK category, and for the PTA category demonstrated a trend toward a lower mortality for those receiving transplantation ($P = .12$) versus those on the wait-list. The authors concluded that PTA did not give an overall survival advantage versus the waiting list, but there was not a survival disadvantage, and most recipients achieved insulin independence [77].

Summary

Pancreas transplantation currently is the only treatment that restores normoglycemia in patients who have type 1 diabetes. The goal of the procedure is to improve the quality of life of the recipient beyond that obtained with KTA. The tradeoff for the patient's insulin independence is the need for chronic immunosuppression and for undergoing a more extensive surgical procedure. Although controversial, multiple studies demonstrate stabilization or improvement of secondary complications of diabetes and a prolongation of survival in patients who undergo SPK. Recent studies have suggested conflicting results with PTA, but carefully selected patients may have a survival benefit from successful SPK.

Acknowledgment

The authors would like to acknowledge Ms. Michelle Moeck for the original artwork prepared for this article.

References

[1] Deckert T. Insulin-dependent diabetes mellitus and its complications. In: Groth C, editor. Pancreatic transplantation. Philadelphia: WB Saunders & Co; 1988.

[2] American Diabetes Association. American Diabetes Association clinical practice recommendations 2001. Diabetes Care 2001;24(Suppl 1):S1–133.

[3] Kelly WD, Lillehei RC, Merkel FK, et al. Allotransplantation of the pancreas and duodenum along with the kidney in diabetic nephropathy. Surgery 1967;61(6):827–37.

[4] Mai ML, Ahsan N, Gonwa T. The long-term management of pancreas transplantation. Transplantation 2006;82(8):991–1003.

[5] Gruessner AC, Sutherland DE. Pancreas transplant outcomes for United States (US) and non-US cases as reported to the United Network for Organ Sharing (UNOS) and the International Pancreas Transplant Registry (IPTR) as of June 2004. Clin Transplant 2005;19(4): 433–55.

[6] Robertson RP, Davis C, Larsen J, et al. Pancreas and islet transplantation for patients with diabetes. Diabetes Care 2000;23(1):112–6.

[7] American Diabetes Association. American Diabetes Association clinical practice recommendations 2000. Supplement 1. Diabetes Care 2000;23(Suppl 1):S1–116.

[8] Tyden G, Bolinder J, Solders G, et al. Improved survival in patients with insulin-dependent diabetes mellitus and end-stage diabetic nephropathy 10 years after combined pancreas and kidney transplantation. Transplantation 1999;67(5):645–8.

[9] Bohman SO, Tyden G, Wilzcek H, et al. Prevention of kidney graft diabetic nephropathy by pancreas transplantation in man. Diabetes 1985;34(3):306–8.

[10] Tibell A, Linden R, Larsson M, et al. Long-term glucose control after pancreatic transplantation. Transplant Proc 1990;22(2):645–6.

[11] Morel P, Goetz FC, Moudry-Munns K, et al. Long-term glucose control in patients with pancreatic transplants. Ann Intern Med 1991;115(9):694–9.

[12] Solders G, Tyden G, Tibell A, et al. Improvement in nerve conduction 8 years after combined pancreatic and renal transplantation. Transplant Proc 1995;27(6):3091.

[13] Solders G, Tyden G, Persson A, et al. Improvement of nerve conduction in diabetic neuropathy. A follow-up study 4 yr after combined pancreatic and renal transplantation. Diabetes 1992;41(8):946–51.

[14] Gaber AO, el-Gebely S, Sugathan P, et al. Early improvement in cardiac function occurs for pancreas-kidney but not diabetic kidney-alone transplant recipients. Transplantation 1995; 59(8):1105–12.

[15] Navarro X, Kennedey WR, Aeppli D, et al. Neuropathy and mortality in diabetes: influence of pancreas transplantation. Muscle Nerve 1996;19(8):1009–16.

[16] Gross CR, Zehrer CL. Health-related quality of life outcomes of pancreas transplant recipients. Clin Transplant 1992;6(3 part 1):165–71.

[17] Nakache R, Tyden G, Groth CG. Quality of life in diabetic patients after combined pancreas-kidney or kidney transplantation. Diabetes 1989;38(Suppl 1):40–2.

[18] Ojo AO, Meier-Kriesche HU, Hanson JA, et al. The impact of simultaneous pancreas-kidney transplantation on long-term patient survival. Transplantation 2001;71(1):82–90.

[19] Robertson RP. Seminars in medicine of the Beth Israel Hospital, Boston: pancreatic and islet transplantation for diabetes—cures or curiosities? N Engl J Med 1992;327(26):1861–8.

[20] Larsen JL, Colling CW, Ratanasuwan T, et al. Pancreas transplantation improves vascular disease in patients with type 1 diabetes. Diabetes Care 2004;27(7):1706–11.

[21] Larsen JL. Pancreas transplantation: indications and consequences. Endocr Rev 2004;25(6): 919–46.

[22] Bates JR, Sawada SG, Segan DS, et al. Evaluation using dobutamine stress echocardiography in patients with insulin-dependent diabetes mellitus before kidney and/or pancreas transplantation. Am J Cardiol 1996;77(2):175–9.

[23] Vandenberg BF, Rossn JD, Grover-McKay M, et al. Evaluation of diabetic patients for renal and pancreas transplantation: noninvasive screening for coronary artery disease using radionuclide methods. Transplantation 1996;62(9):1230–5.

[24] Robertson P, Davis C, Larsen J, et al. Pancreas transplantation in type 1 diabetes. Diabetes Care 2004;27(Suppl 1):S105.

[25] Gruessner AC, Barrou B, Jones J, et al. Donor impact on outcome of bladder-drained pancreas transplants. Transplant Proc 1993;25(6):3114–5.

[26] Gruessner RW, Sutherland DE, Troppnaum C, et al. The surgical risk of pancreas transplantation in the cyclosporine era: an overview. J Am Coll Surg 1997;185(2):128–44.

[27] Schulz T, Schenke P, Flecken M, et al. Donors with a maximum body weight of 50 kg for simultaneous pancreas-kidney transplantation. Transplant Proc 2005;37(2):1268–70.

[28] Fernandez LA, Turgeon NA, Odorico JS, et al. Superior long-term results of simultaneous pancreas-kidney transplantation from pediatric donors. Am J Transplant 2004;4(12): 2093–101.

[29] Sollinger HW, Messing EM, Eckhoff DE, et al. Urological complications in 210 consecutive simultaneous pancreas-kidney transplants with bladder drainage. Ann Surg 1993;218(4): 561–8, [discussion: 568–70].

[30] Ploeg RJ, Eckhoff DE, D'Alessandro AM, et al. Urological complications and enteric conversion after pancreas transplantation with bladder drainage. Transplant Proc 1994;26(2): 458–9.

[31] Sindhi R, Stratta RJ, Lowell JA, et al. Experience with enteric conversion after pancreatic transplantation with bladder drainage. J Am Coll Surg 1997;184(3):281–9.

[32] Diem P, Abid M, Redmon JB, et al. Systemic venous drainage of pancreas allografts as independent cause of hyperinsulinemia in type I diabetic recipients. Diabetes 1990;39(5):534–40.

[33] Gaber AO, Shokouh-Amiri MH, Hathaway DK, et al. Results of pancreas transplantation with portal venous and enteric drainage. Ann Surg 1995;221(6):613–22, [discussion: 622–4].

[34] Hughes TA, Gaber AO, Armis HS, et al. Kidney-pancreas transplantation. The effect of portal versus systemic venous drainage of the pancreas on the lipoprotein composition. Transplantation 1995;60(12):1406–12.

[35] Stout RW. Insulin and atheroma. 20-yr perspective. Diabetes Care 1990;13(6):631–54.

[36] Goalstone ML, Natarajan R, Standley PR, et al. Insulin potentiates platelet-derived growth factor action in vascular smooth muscle cells. Endocrinology 1998;139(10):4067–72.

[37] Sobel BE. The potential influence of insulin and plasminogen activator inhibitor type 1 on the formation of vulnerable atherosclerotic plaques associated with type 2 diabetes. Proc Assoc Am Physicians 1999;111(4):313–8.

[38] Bagdade JD, Teuscher AH, Ritter MC, et al. Alterations in cholesteryl ester transfer, lipoprotein lipase, and lipoprotein composition after combined pancreas-kidney transplantation. Diabetes 1998;47(1):113–8.

[39] Humar A, Kandaswamy R, Granger D, et al. Decreased surgical risks of pancreas transplantation in the modern era. Ann Surg 2000;231(2):269–75.

[40] Stratta RJ, Lo A, Shokouh-Amiri MD, et al. Improving results in solitary pancreas transplantation with portal-enteric drainage, thymoglobin induction, and tacrolimus/mycophenolate mofetil-based immunosuppression. Transpl Int 2003;16(3):154–60.

[41] Reddy KS, Stratta RJ, Shokouh-Amiri MH, et al. Surgical complications after pancreas transplantation with portal-enteric drainage. J Am Coll Surg 1999;189(3):305–13.

[42] Humar A, Ramcharan T, Kaudaswamy R, et al. Technical failures after pancreas transplants: why grafts fail and the risk factors—a multivariate analysis. Transplantation 2004; 78(8):1188–92.

[43] Nath DS, Greussner A, Kandaswamy R, et al. Late anastomotic leaks in pancreas transplant recipients—clinical characteristics and predisposing factors. Clin Transplant 2005;19(2): 220–4.

[44] West M, Gruessner AC, Metraka P, et al. Conversion from bladder to enteric drainage after pancreaticoduodenal transplantations. Surgery 1998;124(5):883–93.

[45] Bohman SO, Wilczek H, Tyden G, et al. Recurrent diabetic nephropathy in renal allografts placed in diabetic patients and protective effect of simultaneous pancreatic transplantation. Transplant Proc 1987;19(1 Pt 3):2290–3.

[46] Fioretto P, Mauer SM, Bilous RW, et al. Effects of pancreas transplantation on glomerular structure in insulin-dependent diabetic patients with their own kidneys. Lancet 1993; 342(8881):1193–6.

[47] Fioretto P, Steffes MW, Sutherland DE, et al. Reversal of lesions of diabetic nephropathy after pancreas transplantation. N Engl J Med 1998;339(2):69–75.

[48] Bilous RW, Mauer SM, Sutherland DE, et al. The effects of pancreas transplantation on the glomerular structure of renal allografts in patients with insulin-dependent diabetes. N Engl J Med 1989;321(2):80–5.

[49] Fiorina P, LaRorca E, Astorri E, et al. Reversal of left ventricular diastolic dysfunction after kidney-pancreas transplantation in type 1 diabetic uremic patients. Diabetes Care 2000; 23(12):1804–10.

[50] Larsen JL, Lynch T, Al'Halawani M, et al. Carotid intima-media thickness by ultrasound measurement in pancreas transplant candidates. Transplant Proc 1995;27(6):2996.

[51] Jukema JW, Smets YF, van den Pijl JW, et al. Impact of simultaneous pancreas and kidney transplantation on progression of coronary atherosclerosis in patients with end-stage renal failure due to type 1 diabetes. Diabetes Care 2002;25(5):906–11.

[52] Bandello F, Vigano C, Secchi A, et al. Diabetic retinopathy after successful kidney-pancreas allotransplantation: a survey of 18 patients. Graefes Arch Clin Exp Ophthalmol 1991;229(4): 315–8.

[53] Wang Q, Klein R, Moss SE, et al. The influence of combined kidney-pancreas transplantation on the progression of diabetic retinopathy. A case series. Ophthalmology 1994;101(6): 1071–6.

[54] Ramsay RC, Goetz FR, Sutherland DE, et al. Progression of diabetic retinopathy after pancreas transplantation for insulin-dependent diabetes mellitus. N Engl J Med 1988;318(4):208–14.

[55] Petersen MR, Vine AK. Progression of diabetic retinopathy after pancreas transplantation. The University of Michigan Pancreas Transplant Evaluation Committee. Ophthalmology 1990;97(4):496–500, [discussion: 501–2].

[56] Pearce IA, Llango B, Sells RA, et al. Stabilisation of diabetic retinopathy following simultaneous pancreas and kidney transplant. Br J Ophthalmol 2000;84(7):736–40.

[57] Ulbig M, Kampik A, Thurau S, et al. Long-term follow-up of diabetic retinopathy for up to 71 months after combined renal and pancreatic transplantation. Graefes Arch Clin Exp Ophthalmol 1991;229(3):242–5.

[58] Konigsrainer A, Miller K, Steurer W, et al. Does pancreas transplantation influence the course of diabetic retinopathy? Diabetologia 1991;34(Suppl 1):S86–8.

[59] Friberg TR, Tzakis AG, Carroll PB, et al. Visual improvement after long-term success of pancreatic transplantation. Am J Ophthalmol 1990;110(5):564–5.

[60] Boyko EJ, Ahroni JH, Stensel V, et al. A prospective study of risk factors for diabetic foot ulcer. The Seattle Diabetic Foot Study. Diabetes Care 1999;22(7):1036–42.

[61] Franklin GM, et al. Sensory neuropathy in non-insulin-dependent diabetes mellitus. The San Luis Valley Diabetes Study. Am J Epidemiol 1990;131(4):633–43.

[62] The Diabetes Control and Complications Trial Research Group. Factors in development of diabetic neuropathy. Baseline analysis of neuropathy in feasibility phase of Diabetes Control and Complications Trial (DCCT). Diabetes 1988;37(4):476–81.

[63] Bird SJ, Brown MJ. The clinical spectrum of diabetic neuropathy. Semin Neurol 1996;16(2): 115–22.

[64] Ziegler D, Dannahl K, Wietels K, et al. Differential effects of near-normoglycaemia for 4 years on somatic nerve dysfunction and heart rate variation in type 1 diabetic patients. Diabet Med 1992;9(7):622–9.

[65] The Diabetes Control and Complications Trial Research Group. The effect of intensive treatment of diabetes on the development and progression of long-term complications in insulin-dependent diabetes mellitus. N Engl J Med 1993;329(14):977–86.

[66] Pyke D. Pancreas transplantation. Diabetes Metab Rev 1991;7(1):3–14.

[67] Navarro X, Sutherland DE, Kennedy WR. Long-term effects of pancreatic transplantation on diabetic neuropathy. Ann Neurol 1997;42(5):727–36.

[68] Ewing DJ, Campbell IW, Clarke BF. Mortality in diabetic autonomic neuropathy. Lancet 1976;1(7960):601–3.

[69] Rayhill SC, D'Alessandro AM, Odorico JS, et al. Simultaneous pancreas-kidney transplantation and living related donor renal transplantation in patients with diabetes: is there a difference in survival? Ann Surg 2000;231(3):417–23.

[70] Cheung AH, Sutherland DE, Gillingham KJ, et al. Simultaneous pancreas-kidney transplant versus kidney transplant alone in diabetic patients. Kidney Int 1992;41(4):924–9.

[71] Smets YF, Westendorp RG, van den Pijl JW, et al. Effect of simultaneous pancreas-kidney transplantation on mortality of patients with type-1 diabetes mellitus and end-stage renal failure. Lancet 1999;353(9168):1915–9.

[72] Manske CL, Wang Y, Thomas W. Mortality of cadaveric kidney transplantation versus combined kidney-pancreas transplantation in diabetic patients. Lancet 1995; 346(8991–8992):1658–62.

[73] Simultaneous kidney-pancreas transplantation versus kidney transplantation alone: patient survival, kidney graft survival, and post-transplant hospitalization. Am J Kidney Dis 1992; 20(5 Suppl 2):61–7.

[74] Port FK, Wolfe RA, Mauger EA, et al. Comparison of survival probabilities for dialysis patients vs cadaveric renal transplant recipients. JAMA 1993;270(11):1339–43.

[75] Ojo A, Wolfe RA, Agodoa LY, et al. Prognosis after primary renal transplant failure and the beneficial effects of repeat transplantation: multivariate analyses from the United States Renal Data System. Transplantation 1998;66(12):1651–9.

[76] Venstrom JM, McBride MA, Rother KI, et al. Survival after pancreas transplantation in patients with diabetes and preserved kidney function. JAMA 2003;290(21):2817–23.

[77] Gruessner RW, Sutherland DE, Gruessner AC. Mortality assessment for pancreas transplants. Am J Transplant 2004;4(12):2018–26.

ELSEVIER
SAUNDERS

Endocrinol Metab Clin N Am
36 (2007) 1039–1049

ENDOCRINOLOGY
AND METABOLISM
CLINICS
OF NORTH AMERICA

Preemptive Kidney Transplantation in Patients with Diabetes Mellitus

Rajani Dinavahi, MD[a,b], Enver Akalin, MD[a,b,*]

[a]Renal Division, Mount Sinai School of Medicine, New York, NY 10029, USA
[b]Recanati/Miller Transplantation Institute, Mount Sinai School of Medicine,
New York, NY 10029, USA

Twenty-one million patients, approximately 7% of the United States population, are affected by diabetes mellitus. The numbers continue to rise, and by 2025, diabetes will affect 300 million people worldwide [1]. Despite improvements in the management of proteinuric renal diseases and hypertension in the last decade, diabetes remains the most prevalent etiology for end-stage renal disease (ESRD) in the United States. Diabetic nephropathy as an etiology for ESRD accounted for just over 17% of the United States dialysis population in 1980, but now comprises almost 45%, a significant increase within 25 years [2].

Peritoneal dialysis, hemodialysis, and renal transplantation are the three mainstays of renal replacement therapy. Kidney transplantation is the most preferred treatment for ESRD, because it improves not only the patient's survival compared with dialysis, but also the quality of life. Although the mortality rates of dialysis patients have improved over time, 15% to 20% still die each year [2]. With advances in immunosuppressive medications and the care of transplant recipients, 1-year patient and graft survival have increased to over 95% and 90%, respectively, and acute rejection rates have decreased to 10% to 15%. As of December 2006, 74,000 patients were on the waiting list for kidney transplantation in the United States [3]. Only 16,481 patients, however, received kidney transplantation in 2005 (9913 deceased donor and 6568 living donor). Waiting times on the list vary considerably by region of the country, with the median wait time for patients who were listed in 2002 for renal transplantation being 1136 days. Waiting times for deceased donor transplantation more than 5 to 7 years are not

* Corresponding author. Mount Sinai Medical Center, One Gustave L. Levy Place, Box 1104, New York, NY 10029-6574.
E-mail address: enver.akalin@msnyuhealth.org (E. Akalin).

0889-8529/07/$ - see front matter © 2007 Elsevier Inc. All rights reserved.
doi:10.1016/j.ecl.2007.07.005 *endo.theclinics.com*

uncommon in many metropolitan areas. Patients who have ESRD often are started on dialysis during these extended waiting times. Preemptive transplantation is transplantation performed before the initiation of renal dialysis. Preemptive transplantation occurred in 25% of adult living donor recipients and 10% of deceased donor recipients in the United States [4,5]. The rate is slightly higher in pediatric recipients, 34% and 14% of living and deceased donors, respectively, because of preferential allocation of deceased organs to pediatric recipients by the United Network for Organ Sharing (UNOS) point allocation system, and also to the increased availability of living donors to pediatric recipients. Obstacles to the performance of transplantation before the initiation of dialysis were lack of access to health care and timely referral to both nephrologist and transplant center. Preemptive transplantation in deceased donor recipients was performed less often due to prolonged waiting times. Recent observational studies have supported the benefits of preemptive transplantation in ESRD patients. This article summarizes the advantages of kidney transplantation compared with dialysis and the importance of early referral of patients with chronic kidney disease to transplant centers. It also discusses whether preemptive transplantation has any additional benefits to transplant recipients. Diabetic patients who have ESRD are also candidates for pancreas transplantation, either in the form of simultaneous pancreas and kidney transplantation (SPK) or pancreas after kidney transplantation (PAK), and the article discusses preemptive SPK in diabetic patients.

Renal replacement treatment: dialysis versus transplantation

Mortality rates across all age groups are 10- to 20-fold higher in the dialysis population compared with the general population, with greater than 50% of that mortality being attributed to cardiovascular disease [2,6]. Cardiovascular disease risk increases across the spectrum of severity in chronic kidney disease, peaking in the ESRD population. There is an increased incidence of acute myocardial infarction, congestive heart failure, and sudden cardiac death in dialysis patients [2]. Twenty-seven percent of all causes of mortality in ESRD patients may be attributed to arrhythmias and sudden cardiac death. Hypertension and left ventricular hypertrophy are very common in patients who have ESRD. Risk of acute myocardial infarction, congestive heart failure, or sudden cardiac death appear to be greater in diabetics across all stages of chronic kidney disease and all modalities of renal replacement therapy, and these risks appear to increase exponentially in relation to the overall duration of dialysis. Overall, 5-year survival is only 27.2% in hemodialysis and 23.3% in peritoneal dialysis diabetic patients [2]. Cerebrovascular disease in ESRD patients is also significantly higher, with the overall incidence of stroke being 15%, almost four times the general population.

The association between cardiovascular disease and renal failure is explained in part by traditional risk factors shared by the both diseases, such as diabetes, hypertension, hyperlipidemia, smoking, and older age. Renal failure and ESRD, however, carry additional nontraditional cardiac risk factors that contribute to accelerated atherosclerosis, such as calcium phosphate deposition, secondary hyperparathyroidism, hyperhomocysteine-mia, increased advanced glycation end products, volume overload, electro-lyte abnormalities, and altered nitric oxide/endothelin levels [7]. Poor nutritional status, a chronic inflammatory state, thrombogenic factors, and altered immunologic function also may place these patients at addi-tional risk.

Another important factor for the increased morbidity and mortality in ESRD patients is dialysis-related vascular access procedures and infection, totaling almost 1.5 million access procedures in the United States for ESRD patients in 2004. Over 50% of dialysis-related hospital admissions are secondary to dialysis access-associated infections [2].

Renal transplantation was shown to confer a survival benefit to the patient by Wolfe and colleagues [8] in a landmark 1999 article. The benefit was sustained across all races, ages, and primary causes of renal disease, establishing it as the standard of care for patients who had ESRD. This was a longitudinal study examining mortality in 228,552 dialysis patients. Of these, 46,164 patients were placed on a waiting list for deceased donor renal transplantation; 23,275 received a deceased donor transplant between 1991 and 1997. The annual death rate per 100 patient years was 2.8 in trans-plant recipients, compared with 6.3 in patients on the waiting list and 16.1 in dialysis patients not listed for transplantation. The projected increase in life expectancy by transplantation was 10 years overall (range 3 to 17 years, according to patient groups by age). Thirty-three percent of patients on the waiting list and 31% of transplant recipients were diabetic. Among the diabetic patients on the waiting list, the annual mortality rate was 11%, and transplant reduced the risk of death by 73%. The greatest increase in life expectancy in terms of the etiology of the ESRD was observed in dia-betics (11 years, compared with 7 years among the patients with glomerulo-nephritis, and 8 years among those with other causes of ESRD). Further studies demonstrated an improved survival benefit in patients receiving mar-ginal deceased donor organs and in obese recipients, as well as in patients outside the United States [9–12].

Cardiac disease progression appears to halt after successful renal trans-plantation and maintenance of graft function. Meier-Kriesche and col-leagues [13] analyzed 60,141 primary renal transplant patients registered in the United States Renal Data System (USRDS) registry between 1995 and 2000 for cardiac mortality, and compared them with 66,813 adult dial-ysis patients on the waiting list. Although cardiovascular risk increases in the immediate postoperative period, this risk diminishes with time as long as renal function is preserved. This even held true in diabetic patients, where the cardiovascular death rates were about twice as high compared with non-diabetic patients. In contrast, the cardiovascular disease rates on the transplant waiting list increased progressively over time.

In addition to the morbidity and mortality benefits received by renal transplantation, the major economic advantage of renal transplantation makes it a significant medical and societal concern. Inpatient Medicare expenses for dialysis during 2004 reached $5.6 billion, with outpatient costs reaching an astronomical $6.7 billion [2]. ESRD patients with diabetes incur 33% overall higher costs than their nondiabetic counterparts, almost $72,000 per patient per year in 2004, the largest percentage of any single group. Although the cost of transplantation per patient per year is higher than dialysis during the first year after transplantation, it significantly reverses after the first year, and becomes cost-effective compared with dialysis [2]. Additionally, USRDS data showed 0.79 days of admission per patient-year for renal transplant recipients, versus almost 2 days of admission for patients receiving either hemodialysis or peritoneal dialysis.

Referral to transplantation

Because the risk of cardiovascular disease and mortality in dialysis patients is increased, prompt referral to renal transplant centers is a critical and life-saving step. The average waiting time for deceased donor transplantation is almost 3 years from listing, exceeding 5 to 7 years in some regions, so early listing is important to achieve prompt transplantation and decrease the time on dialysis. A prospective study at the University of Pennsylvania evaluated the factors affecting transplantation referral practices, where 129 patients had preemptive and 161 patients had nonpreemptive renal transplant evaluations [14]. Seventy-six percent of patients undergoing preemptive evaluation and 53% of patients undergoing nonpreemptive renal transplant evaluation stated that the person most influential in their decision to undergo transplantation was their nephrologist. Preemptive group members saw their nephrologists an average of 71 months before transplant evaluation; nonpreemptive group members saw their nephrologists an average of 25 months before the initiation of dialysis. This study suggested the importance of early referral to nephrologists leading to early referral for transplant evaluation. Many patients, however, are not being seen by nephrologists until late into their course, thereby delaying the recognition of severe renal disease. Arora and colleagues [15] reported that late referral to the nephrologist was common at New England Medical Center and associated with poor pre-ESRD care.

A retrospective analysis using USRDS data of 38,836 primary kidney transplant recipients between 1995 and 1998 demonstrated that the factors associated with preemptive renal transplantation included Caucasian race, higher education, and coverage by private insurance versus Medicare [16].

Although the accepted UNOS guideline for placement onto renal transplant waiting lists in the United States is 20 mL/min, the average glomerular filtration rate (GFR) in the United States at the time of listing, is 9.9 mL/min, suggesting that patients are being referred later than necessary for a life-saving procedure. Referral to renal transplant centers should occur when GFR is under 30 mL/min, or if it is predictable that a patient's renal function will decline steadily.

Preemptive kidney transplantation

Although most transplants in the United States are performed after the initiation of dialysis, there has been much interest in the advantage of preemptive renal transplantation. Living transplantation more often occurs preemptively as there is no waiting time, and it has superior outcomes compared with deceased donor transplantation in terms of the allograft and patient survival. Lack of published evidence until the last decade regarding the survival benefit of preemptive renal transplantation may have resulted in later referrals of patients to transplant centers until the initiation of renal replacement therapy. The authors have summarized the published studies about preemptive transplantation in Table 1 and will discuss each study briefly. These studies did not focus mainly on diabetic patients and used USRDS or UNOS databases.

Earlier retrospective and single-center studies involving small numbers of patients transplanted between 1970s and 1980s showed conflicting results regarding the beneficial effects of preemptive transplantation on allograft outcome [17–19]. The impact of pretransplant dialysis on patient and graft survival first was studied in a large single-center study by Cosio and colleagues [20] involving 523 kidney transplant recipients. Only 7% of preemptively transplanted recipients died during follow-up compared with 23% of patients dialyzed for less than 3 years and 44% dialyzed for more than 3 years. The authors also reported that increasing time on dialysis increases the prevalence of left ventricular hypertrophy and cardiomegaly. The type of dialysis did not impact patient outcome. Another single-center study, analyzing 385 preemptive and 1464 nonpreemptive adult primary kidney transplant recipients, demonstrated a significant difference in the 5-year patient survival: 92.6% versus 76.6% in deceased donor and 93.3% versus 89.5% in living donor transplants, respectively [21]. Graft survival was increased in preemptive living donor recipients but not in deceased donor recipients.

Meier-Kriesche and colleagues [22] analyzed 73,103 primary adult renal transplant registered in the United States Renal Data System (USRDS) registry between 1988 and 1997 to investigate the effect of waiting time on renal transplant outcome. The authors showed that relative to preemptive transplants, waiting times on dialysis of 6 to 12, 12 to 24, 24 to 36, 36 to 48, and

Table 1
Preemptive kidney transplantation

Author	Database	Patient number	Outcome
Cosio [20]	Ohio State University 1984–1991	523	↑ mortality and ↑ LVH with duration of pretransplant dialysis
Mange [24,25]	USRDS 1994–1997	9130	↑ GS and ↓ AR with preemptive KTx
Papalois [21]	University of Minnesota 1984–1998	1849	↑ PS in preemptive KTx and ↑ GS in preemptive living donor KTx
Vats [30]	NAPRTCS 1992–1996	2495	↑ GS in preemptive pediatric living donor KTx
Meier-Kreische [22]	USRDS 1988–1997	73,103	↑ mortality and ↓ GS with increased duration on dialysis
Meier-Kreische [23]	USRDS 1988–1998	2405 (paired donors)	↑ mortality and ↓ GS with increased duration on dialysis
Kasiske [16]	UNOS and USRDS 1995–1998	38,836	↓ mortality and ↑ GS with preemptive KTx
Ishani [27]	USRDS 1994–2000	4,046	No benefit of residual renal function on post-transplant GFR
Gill [28]	USRDS 1987–1996	40,063	No benefit of residual renal function on post-transplant GFR
Innocenti [29]	Mayo Clinics 2000–2002	438	Similar mortality and GS in preemptive and nonpreemptive KTx

Abbreviations: AR, acute rejection; GFR, glomerular filtration rate; GS, graft survival; HD, hemodialysis; KTx, kidney transplantation; LVH, left ventricular hypertrophy; NAPRTCS, North American Pediatric Renal Transplantation Cooperative Study; PS, patient survival; UNOS, United Network for Organ Sharing; USRDS, United States Renal Data System.

over 48 months conferred a 21%, 28%, 41%, 53%, and 72% increase in mortality risk after transplantation, respectively. This study found a time-dependent detrimental effect of dialysis on patient survival, but also the graft survival, where patients on dialysis more than 2 years had a 68% increased risk of death-censored graft loss. The authors subsequently published a paired kidney donor analysis model, where one kidney of the pair went to a patient who had been on dialysis for less than 6 months, and the other kidney went to a patient who had been on dialysis for longer than 2 years, to avoid potential donor-related confounding factors [23]. This study excluded patients who had an HLA-identical or zero-antigen mismatched kidney transplant. The data analysis of 2405 kidney pairs harvested from the same donor between 1988 and 1998 revealed that recipients who had less than 6 months of dialysis before transplant had much better 5- and 10-year unadjusted allograft survival rates than those who had greater than 2 years on dialysis (78% and 63% versus 58% and 29%, respectively). Ten-year graft survival in deceased donor recipients was shown to be 69% for preemptive transplants and 39% for patients after 24 months of hemodialysis. In living transplants, preemptive transplantation resulted in 75% 10-year allograft survival, which decreased to 49% for those on pretransplant hemodialysis for more than 24 months. The authors concluded that waiting time on dialysis is the strongest independent modifiable risk factor for renal transplant outcomes. This effect is so significant that even deceased donor recipients who were on dialysis for less than 6 months had graft survival equivalent to living donor recipients who were on dialysis for more than 2 years.

Kasiske and colleagues [16] reviewed the data of 38,836 first kidney-only transplants between 1995 and 1998. In adjusted Cox proportional hazard analysis, the relative risk of graft failure for preemptive transplantation was 0.75 (0.67 to 0.84) among 25,758 deceased donor transplants and 0.73 (0.64 to 0.83) among 13,708 living donor transplants, compared with patients who received a transplant after initiating dialysis. Preemptive transplantation also was associated with a reduced risk of death: 0.84 (0.72 to 0.99) for deceased donor transplants and 0.69 (0.56 to 0.85) for living donor transplants.

How does preemptive transplantation improve patient and graft survival after transplantation? The most plausible explanation is the avoidance of dialysis-associated morbidities with preemptive transplantation. The other explanation could be selection bias, where healthier, younger, more educated, and more compliant patients are more likely to receive preemptive transplantation. Other factors that have been investigated included acute rejection episodes and residual renal function. Mange and colleagues [24] analyzed the outcomes of 8481 first living donor kidney transplant recipients between January 1994 and June 1997 and reported that preemptive transplantation was associated with 52%, 82%, and 86% reductions in the risk of allograft failure during the first, second, and subsequent years after transplantation, respectively. Interestingly, increasing duration of dialysis was associated with increasing odds of rejection within 6 months of transplantation. Renal biopsy-confirmed acute rejection rates during the first month were 2.5-fold higher among recipients of nonpreemptive living renal transplants compared with preemptive patients, even when accounting for high panel reactive antibody titers and delayed graft function [25]. These results suggest a stimulatory effect of the immune system by dialysis exposure before transplantation. T cell activity has been shown to be suppressed in patients who have chronic kidney disease, and the initiation of dialysis may improve the T cell proliferation and responsiveness to alloantigen. Increased levels of T cell activation markers and complement cascade caused by exposure to dialysis membranes also have been suggested [26].

Residual renal function improves outcome in hemodialysis and peritoneal dialysis patients and is thought to play role in better outcomes with preemptive transplantation. Two studies, however, failed to confirm that higher levels of pretransplant GFR are associated with improved outcomes. Ishani and colleagues [27] retrospectively reviewed the USRDS data of living donor transplant recipients between 1994 and 2000. There were no differences in allograft survival and 6-month post-transplant estimated GFR, when patients with pretransplant GFR greater than or equal to15 mL/min were compared with patients with GFR levels less than 15 mL/min. Gill and colleagues [28] compared 6-month GFR levels after transplantation in 5966 preemptive transplant recipients with 34,997 nonpreemptive transplant recipients, and found no difference (49.5 versus 49.2 mL/min, respectively). Both groups had a similar rate of decline in kidney function after transplantation.

The Minnesota Mayo Clinic group reported a high preemptive living donor transplant rate (44%) in patients transplanted between 2000 and 2002 [29]. This study excluded highly sensitized patients with positive cross-matches and ABO-incompatible transplants. There was no difference in patient survival at 3 years in diabetic preemptive and nonpreemptive patients (88% versus 89%, respectively). Preemptive transplant recipients had higher 3-year graft survival compared with nonpreemptive recipients (97% versus 90%, respectively) but the difference was not statistically significant by multivariate analysis, probably because of the small number of patients. The beneficial effect of preemptive kidney transplantation in graft survival was shown in pediatric primary living kidney transplant recipients between 1992 and 1996 [30].

Preemptive kidney/pancreas transplantation

Diabetic kidney transplant recipients have lower patient survival compared with kidney transplant recipients without diabetes. The SPK has been advocated to improve survival in diabetic patients. A study by Ojo and colleagues [31] evaluating 13,467 diabetic patients showed 67% 10-year patient survival in SPK recipients, compared with 46% in recipients of deceased donor kidneys alone. Reddy and colleagues [32] reviewed the UNOS database of 18,459 type 1 diabetic patients transplanted between 1987 and 1996, and reported increased 8-year patient survival in SPK recipients (72%) compared with patients receiving only deceased donor kidney transplantation (55%). SPK has been hypothesized to improve kidney allograft survival by better glycemic control and shorter cold ischemia time, leading to decreased delayed graft function. There are only three studies that investigated the effects of preemptive SPK on allograft outcome (Table 2) [33–35].

Israni and colleagues [33] examined UNOS data for 8323 diabetic patients waitlisted for SPK and received either SPK or kidney transplantation alone to avoid the selection bias of healthier patients listed for SPK compared with diabetic patients listed for only kidney transplantation. SPK recipients had adjusted risk ratio (RR) for kidney allograft loss of 0.63 (0.51 to 0.77, $P < .001$) compared with kidney transplant recipients without pancreas

Table 2
Preemptive simultaneous pancreas and kidney transplantation

Israni [33]	SRTR 1990–2002	8323	↑ GS in preemptive SPK
Becker [34]	SRTR 1997–2002	23,328	↑ GS in SPK, ↓ mortality risk in DM I and DM II with preemptive KTx
Pruijm [35]	Leiden University 1986–2004	180	↑ PS in preemptive SPK, no change in GS

Abbreviations: GS, graft survival; KTx, kidney transplantation; PS, patient survival; SPK, simultaneous pancreas kidney transplantation; SRTR, Scientific Registry for Transplant Recipients.

allograft. Preemptive SPK recipients demonstrated a lower rate of allograft loss compared with SPK recipients transplanted after initiation of dialysis [RR = 0.83 (0.69 to 0.99, P = .042)], even though the duration of pretransplant dialysis was less than 2 years in 70% of the nonpreemptive recipients.

Becker and colleagues [34] investigated the impact of preemptive kidney transplantation on patient and graft survival in 23,238 adult type 1 and 2 diabetic patients receiving a first kidney transplantation alone or SPK, analyzing data from the Scientific Registry of Transplant Recipients between 1997 and 2002. Preemptive kidney transplantation was provided to 14.4% type 1 and 6.7% type 2 diabetic patients. Preemptive SPK and preemptive living kidney alone transplantation conferred significantly lower adjusted mortality risks for type 1 diabetic patients (RR, 0.50 and 0.57, respectively). The mortality benefit of preemptive kidney transplantation was also evident for type 2 diabetic patients (RR, 0.65). Preemptive SPK was associated with lower risk for allograft loss (RR = 0.79). Preemptive kidney transplantation, however, did not affect graft survival in type 2 diabetic patients, although there was a trend toward lower risk for type 2 living donor recipients (RR, 0.081; P = .09). This somewhat differed from the analysis by Meier-Kriesche examining an earlier cohort of patients (1988 to 1997). The reasons for this discrepancy could be attributed to different immunosuppressive regimens, decreasing acute rejection rates over time, and different comorbid conditions of the patients receiving transplantation.

A recent single-center study from the Netherlands comparing preemptive versus nonpreemptive SPK showed a survival benefit and decreased cardiovascular deaths in preemptive patients [35]. This study involved 180 patients who received SPK between 1986 and 2004. Sixty-five patients (36%) were transplanted preemptively. Ten- and 15-year patient survivals were 71.3% and 64.8% in the preemptive group, compared with 63.8% and 45% in the nonpreemptive group, leading to an RR for mortality of 0.50 (P = .07). The difference was not statistically significant, probably because of the number of patients studied. There was no difference in kidney and pancreas allograft survival between the two groups. The mean GFR at the time of transplantation was 21.4 mL/min, which is higher than expected, where patients start on dialysis when the GFR is less than 15 mL/min in diabetics.

Patients on the waiting list for kidney transplantation start to recruit time when the GFT is less than 20 mL/min in the United States.

Summary

Kidney transplantation is the best treatment for ESRD. It improves not only patient life expectancy, but also the quality of life. Preemptive transplantation further improves patient and graft survival by avoiding dialysis-related morbidities, including the increased risks of cardiovascular disease and infection. Transplantation also brings economic advantages to health care system. The most important factor is the early referral of patients with chronic kidney disease to nephrologists and transplant centers to discuss the options for renal replacement therapy. Patients should start work up for transplantation when the GFR reaches 30 mL/min or if there is inevitable and predictable decline in renal function, so that they may receive kidney transplantation before initiation of dialysis.

Acknowledgment

The authors thank Dr. Jonathan S. Bromberg for critical review of the manuscript.

References

[1] King H, Aubert R, Herman WH. Global burden of diabetes, 1995–2025. Diabetes Care 1998;21:1414–31.

[2] Annual report. USRDS 2006.

[3] United Network for Organ Sharing Web site. Available at: www.unos.org.

[4] Mange KC, Weir M. Preemptive renal transplantation: why not? Am J Transplant 2003;3: 1336–40.

[5] Meier-Kriesche H, Schold JD. The impact of pretransplant dialysis on outcomes in renal transplantation. Semin Dial 2005;18(6):499–504.

[6] Muntner P, He J, Hamm L, et al. Renal insufficiency and subsequent death resulting from cardiovascular disease in the United States. J Am Soc Nephrol 2002;13:745–53.

[7] Sarnak MJ, Levey AS. Cardiovascular disease and chronic renal disease: a new paradigm. Am J Kidney Dis 2000;35(4 Suppl 1):S117–31.

[8] Wolfe R, Ashby VB, Milford EL. Comparison of mortality in all patients on dialysis, patients on dialysis awaiting transplantation, and recipients of a first cadaveric transplant. N Engl J Med 1999;341(23):1725–30.

[9] Ojo AO, Hanson JA, Meier-Kreische HU, et al. Survival in recipients of marginal cadaveric donor kidneys compared with other recipients and wait-listed transplant candidates. J Am Soc Nephrol 2001;12:589–97.

[10] Glanton CW, Kao TC, Cruess D, et al. Impact of renal transplantation on survival in end-stage renal disease patients with elevated body mass index. Kidney Int 2003;63:647–53.

[11] McDonald SP, Russ GR. Survival of recipients of cadaveric kidney transplants compared with those receiving dialysis treatment in Australia and New Zealand, 1991–2001. Nephrol Dial Transplant 2002;17:2212–9.

[12] Schnuelle P, Lorenz D, Trede M, et al. Impact of renal cadaveric transplantation on survival in end-stage renal failure: evidence for reduced mortality risk compared with hemodialysis during long-term follow-up. J Am Soc Nephrol 1998;9:2135–41.

[13] Meier-Kriesche H, Schold J, Srinivas TR, et al. Kidney transplantation halts cardiovascular disease progression in patients with end-stage renal disease. Am J Transplant 2004;4:1662–8.

[14] Weng FL, Mange KC. A comparison of persons who present for preemptive and nonpreemptive kidney transplantation. Am J Kidney Dis 2003;42(5):1050–7.

[15] Arora P, Obrador G, Ruthazer R. Prevalence, predictors, and consequences of late nephrology referral at a tertiary care center. J Am Soc Nephrol 1999;10:1281–6.

[16] Kasiske BL, Snyder JJ, Matas AJ, et al. Preemptive kidney transplantation: the advantage and the advantaged. J Am Soc Nephrol 2002;13:1358–64.

[17] Migliori RJ, Simmons RL, Payne WD, et al. Renal transplantation done safely without prior chronic dialysis therapy. Transplantation 1987;43(1):51–5.

[18] Katz SM, Kerman RH, Golden D, et al. Preemptive transplantation—an analysis of benefits and hazards in 85 cases. Transplantation 1991;51(2):351–5.

[19] Roake JA, Cahill AP, Gray CM, et al. Preemptive cadaveric renal transplantation—clinical outcome. Transplantation 1996;62(10):1411–6.

[20] Cosio FG, Alamir A, Yim S, et al. Patient survival after renal transplantation: the impact of dialysis pretransplant. Kidney Int 1998;53:767–72.

[21] Papalois VE, Moss A, Gillingham KJ, et al. Preemptive transplants for patients with renal failure. Transplantation 2000;70(4):625–31.

[22] Meier-Kriesche H, Port FK, Ojo AO, et al. Effect of waiting time on renal transplantation outcome. Kidney Int 2000;58:1311–7.

[23] Meier-Kriesche H, Kaplan B. Waiting time on dialysis as the strongest modifiable risk factor for renal transplantation outcomes: a paired donor kidney analysis. Transplantation 2002; 74(10):1377–81.

[24] Mange K, Joffe M, Feldman HL. Effect of the use or nonuse of long-term dialysis on the subsequent survival of renal transplants from living donors. N Engl J Med 2001;344(10):726–31.

[25] Mange KC, Joffe MM, Feldman HI. Dialysis prior to living donor kidney transplantation and rates of acute rejection. Nephrol Dial Transplant 2003;18:172–7.

[26] Kaul GM, Sester U, Sester M, et al. Initiation of hemodialysis treatment leads to improvement of T cell activation in patients with end-stage renal disease. Am J Kidney Dis 2000;35: 611–6.

[27] Ishani A, Ibrahim H, Gilbertson D, et al. The impact of residual renal function on graft survival and patient survival rates in recipients of preemptive renal transplants. Am J Kidney Dis 2003;42(6):1275–82.

[28] Gill JS, Tonelli M, Johnson N, et al. Why do preemptive kidney transplant recipients have an allograft survival advantage? Transplantation 2004;78(6):873–9.

[29] Innocenti GR, Wadei HM, Prieto M, et al. Preemptive living donor kidney transplantation. Transplantation 2007;83(2):144–9.

[30] Vats A, Donaldson L, Fine R, et al. Pretransplant dialysis status and outcome of renal transplantation in North American children: an NAPRTCS study. Transplantation 2000;69: 1414–9.

[31] Ojo AO, Meier-Kriesche H, Hanson J, et al. The impact of simultaneous pancreas–kidney transplantation on long-term patient survival. Transplantation 2001;71:82–90.

[32] Reddy SK, Stablein D, Taranto S, et al. Long-term survival following simultaneous kidney–pancreas transplantation alone versus kidney transplantation alone in patients with type 1 diabetes mellitus and renal failure. Am J Kidney Dis 2003;41(2):464–70.

[33] Israni AK, Feldman HI, Propert KJ, et al. Impact of simultaneous kidney–pancreas transplant and timing of transplant on kidney allograft survival. Am J Transplant 2005;5:374–82.

[34] Becker B, Rush SH, Dykstra D, et al. Preemptive transplantation for patients with diabetes-related kidney disease. Arch Intern Med 2006;166:44–8.

[35] Pruijm MT, de Fijter HJW, Doxiadis II, et al. Preemptive versus nonpreemptive simultaneous pancreas–kidney transplantation: a single-center, long-term, follow-up study. Transplantation 2006;81(8):1119–24.

ENDOCRINOLOGY
AND METABOLISM
CLINICS
OF NORTH AMERICA

ELSEVIER
SAUNDERS

Endocrinol Metab Clin N Am
36 (2007) 1051–1066

Interferon Alpha Treatment and Thyroid Dysfunction

Yaron Tomer, MD[a,b,*], Jason T. Blackard, PhD[c], Nagako Akeno, PhD[b]

[a]Division of Endocrinology, Cincinnati VA Medical Center
[b]Division of Endocrinology, University of Cincinnati College of Medicine, 3125 Eden Avenue, Cincinnati, OH 45267, USA
[c]Division of Digestive Diseases, University of Cincinnati College of Medicine, Cincinnati, 3125 Eden Ave, Cincinnati, OH 45267, USA

Interferon alpha (IFNα) is a type I IFN that has been used widely as a therapeutic agent [1]. IFNα binds to IFN receptors, which are transmembrane glycoproteins containing cytoplasmic domains that activate various signaling pathways, including the janus kinas signal transducer and activation of transcription (JAK-STAT) pathway, the Crk-pathway, the insulin receptor substrate (IRS) signaling pathway, and the mitogen-activated protein (MAP) kinase pathway [2,3]. More than 24 IFNα-induced proteins have been identified [4]. In the past several decades IFNα has emerged as a major therapeutic modality for several malignant and nonmalignant diseases [4]. By far the most common indication for IFNα treatment is hepatitis C virus (HCV) infection. In two pivotal randomized trials, approximately 50% of patients with chronic hepatitis C, who were treated with peginterferon alpha-2a plus ribavirin, achieved a sustained virologic response [5,6]. Despite its success, IFNα has a well-known adverse effect profile, ranging from influenza-like symptoms to hematologic effects, neuropsychiatric symptoms, and thyroid disease, which cumulatively can lead to dose reductions in up to 40% of patients and drug discontinuation in up to 14% of patients [7]. One of the most common adverse effects of IFNα therapy is thyroiditis. The association between IFNα and thyroid disease was recognized as early as 1985 in patients being treated with IFNα for carcinoid tumors and breast

This work was supported in part by: DK61659 and DK067555 from NIDDK (to YT) and DA022148 (to JTB).

* Corresponding author. Division of Endocrinology, University of Cincinnati College of Medicine, 3125 Eden Avenue, ML 0547, Cincinnati, OH 45267.

E-mail address: yaron.tomer@uc.edu (Y. Tomer).

cancer [8,9]. Since then, numerous studies have reported a high incidence of thyroid disease in patients treated with IFNα [10,11]. Some of these complications of IFNα therapy, especially thyrotoxicosis, can be severe and may interfere with adequate IFNα therapy in patients who have hepatitis C [12–15]. Moreover, because the symptoms of hypothyroidism such as fatigue, and weight gain might be attributable to hepatitis C or IFNα therapy [7], the diagnosis of hypothyroidism in these patients might be delayed, leading to development of further complications. Thus, IFNα-induced thyroiditis (IIT) is a major clinical problem for patients receiving IFNα therapy. This article focuses on the mechanisms leading to IIT and the role of HCV in the pathogenesis of IIT.

The epidemiology of interferon-induced thyroiditis

The authors recently proposed a new classification of IIT into autoimmune IIT and nonautoimmune IIT [16]. Autoimmune IIT includes Graves' disease (GD), Hashimoto's thyroiditis (HT), and the production of thyroid autoantibodies (TAbs) without clinical disease, while nonautoimmune IIT includes destructive thyroiditis and nonautoimmune hypothyroidism.

Autoimmune interferon-induced thyroiditis

The most common clinical manifestation of IIT is HT [17–20]. Most studies have shown that the presence of TAbs before the initiation of IFNα therapy is a significant risk factor for developing IIT manifesting as Hashimoto's thyroiditis [11,17,21,22]. The development of HT in a Tab-positive patient who receives IFNα often is accompanied by a significant increase in the levels of the antibodies [21]. Roti and colleagues [12] calculated that having positive thyroid peroxidase (TPO) antibodies before IFNα therapy had a positive predictive value of 67% for the development of thyroid dysfunction. Therefore, screening for TAbs should be performed before the initiation of IFNα therapy to assess the risk of developing HT [16]. Less commonly, treatment with IFNα can result in the development of GD [12,23]. A retrospective review of 321 patients with hepatitis B or C treated with IFNα found 10 patients who developed thyrotoxicosis characterized by a completely suppressed thyrotropin (TSH) [23]. Six of these patients developed GD based on diffusely increased uptake on thyroid scintigraphy and positive thyroid-stimulating antibodies. All GD patients had symptomatic thyrotoxicosis, and in all cases, the thyrotoxicosis failed to resolve after cessation of IFNα [23]. In another large multicenter study, 3 of 237 patients receiving IFNα developed GD requiring definitive treatment [24]. In most reported cases of GD developing secondary to IFNα therapy, the disease did not go into remission when IFNα therapy was completed or stopped [17,23,24]. There is one case report of Graves' ophthalmopathy that developed following IFNα treatment for hepatitis C [14], underscoring the fact that IIT can result in more severe complications [15]. The most common form of thyroid autoimmunity is the presence of thyroid antibodies (including thyroid peroxidase antibodies [TPO-Ab], and thyroglobulin antibodies [Tg-Ab]), without clinical disease [25]. The presence of TAbs, is usually a preclinical phase of autoimmune thyroid disease AITD [26]. TAbs without clinical disease also have been shown to develop during or following IFNα therapy. The TAbs can develop de novo during IFNα, or IFNα can cause a significant increase in Tab levels in individuals who were positive for TAb before IFN therapy. Thus, it seems that IFNα can induce thyroid autoimmunity de novo, and exacerbate pre-existing thyroid autoimmunity [17,22,27]. The incidence of de novo development of TAbs secondary to IFNα therapy varied widely in different studies, from 1.9% to 40.0%, most likely because of the different assays used to test for thyroid antibodies [16]. The newer immunoassays have up to a tenfold higher sensitivity to detect TAbs than the older assays [28,29]. Indeed, recent studies are more consistent and report an incidence of TAbs in IFN-treated HCV patients of around 10% [12,17,21,22,30]. Marazuela and colleagues [27] found that development of antithyroid antibodies was significantly higher in women compared with men, 14.8% versus 1% ($P < .01$), and was also related directly to increasing age. Most individuals who develop de novo TAbs on IFNα therapy remain Tab-positive after the end of treatment. In one long-term study in which patients were followed for a median of 6.2 years (5.5 to 8.4 years) after completion of IFNα therapy, 72.2% of patients who became TAb-positive during IFNα therapy continued to have TAbs at the end of the study [20].

Nonautoimmune interferon-induced thyroiditis

Nonautoimmune thyroiditis is seen in up to 50% of patients who develop IIT, suggesting that thyroid dysfunction may be mediated by a direct effect of IFNα on thyroid cell function and not only by immune-mediated effects [12,23,31]. Nonautoimmune IIT usually manifests as destructive thyroiditis. Destructive thyroiditis is a self-limited inflammatory disorder of the thyroid gland. The disease is characterized by three phases—a sudden onset of hyperthyroidism, followed by a hypothyroid phase, and eventually resolution and normalization of thyroid functions—usually within several weeks to months [32]. In less than 5% of the cases, permanent hypothyroidism develops [33]. More than 50% of patients who have IIT with thyrotoxicosis have destructive thyroiditis, while the remainder have GD [11,12,21,23,24,31]. The diagnosis of destructive thyroiditis in patients receiving IFNα therapy is based on negative TSH-receptor antibodies (TRAb) and low thyroid radioactive iodine uptake [12,23]. Because many cases of destructive thyroiditis secondary to IFNα are mild or subclinical, it is possible that subacute thyroiditis occurs more frequently than reported. On retreatment with IFNα, patients may develop recurrent thyroiditis, and therefore, thyroid functions should be monitored carefully upon rechallenge with IFNα [34]. Destructive thyroiditis caused by IFNα therapy of hepatitis C infection is usually benign. However, in the authors' experience, some of these patients may develop complications, such as rapid atrial fibrillation, requiring thyroid ablation before retreatment with IFNα. In addition, a subset of these patients may progress to permanent hypothyroidism, usually accompanied by the development of thyroid antibodies [13]. Clinical and subclinical hypothyroidism without thyroid antibodies also have been described secondary to IFNα therapy [22,24,35]. In many of these cases, the hypothyroidism is transient, and permanent hypothyroidism usually is seen when patients develop thyroid antibodies [12,17,19,20].

The role of hepatitis C virus in the development of interferon-induced thyroiditis

Although IIT has been reported in patients receiving IFNα for various medical conditions [36], most cases of IIT have been reported in patients with chronic HCV infection. Thus, it is plausible that HCV infection plays an important role in the etiology of thyroiditis in patients treated with IFN. Infectious agents long have been suspected to trigger thyroid autoimmunity [37], and among the possible infectious triggers of thyroid autoimmunity, HCV has shown the strongest association with AITD [38].

Epidemiological observations

Earlier studies of patients with hepatitis C who never received IFNα showed no significant correlation between hepatitis C infection and the presence of thyroid antibodies [39–41]. For example, in one large community-based study in Sardinia, where infection with hepatitis viruses is endemic, 1310 were surveyed, and no association was found between the presence of hepatitis C antibodies and thyroid antibodies [39]. On the other hand, other studies have shown a significant correlation between hepatitis C infection and thyroid disorders [21,42–45]. In two studies from France of patients with hepatitis C infection who had not received IFNα therapy, the incidence of thyroid antibodies and/or dysfunction was significantly higher in the patients than in the controls [42,43]. Another study from France in hepatitis C patients who had not received IFNα revealed that 13.6% had positive TAbs [46]. Although this study lacked a control group, this incidence is greater than expected by age and gender [46,47]. Moreover, in most studies examining the frequency of thyroid disorders in IFNα-treated hepatitis C patients, approximately 10% of the patients had positive TAbs before initiation of IFNα therapy [12,17,27,30,48].

Some of the problems of earlier studies included the use of less sensitive TAb assays and the lack of control for factors, which may affect the development of thyroid autoimmunity, mainly iodine intake. Moreover, the definition of HCV infection was not standard across different studies. Some studies defined HCV infection as the presence of positive HCV antibodies (indicative of past and/or present infection), while other studies measured HCV RNA (indicative of current HCV infection only) [49]. Thus, one could speculate that past versus current HCV infection could influence the development of thyroiditis. One recent very large study demonstrated that both hypothyroidism and thyroid autoimmunity were significantly more common in patients with hepatitis C compared with controls [45]. Patients were considered having chronic HCV based on positive HCV antibodies and elevated transaminase levels for more than 6 months. The authors studied four groups: 630 IFNα-naïve patients who had hepatitis C, 389 gender- and age-matched subjects from an iodine-sufficient region, 268 people from an iodine-deficient region, and 86 patients who had hepatitis B virus infection. They found that the presence of thyroid antibodies (both Tg-Ab and TPO-Ab) was significantly higher in patients who had hepatitis C infection than in the other three groups. Clinical hypothyroidism was also significantly more frequent in patients who had hepatitis C compared with the three control groups [45]. This study controlled for both intake of iodine and treatment with IFNα. In summary, while earlier studies did not show an association between HCV infection and AITD consistently, more recent data support such an association. Moreover, pooling of data from all studies on HCV infection (as measured by either HCV antibodies or RNA) and thyroid autoimmunity demonstrated a significant increase in the risk of thyroiditis in patients who have HCV [49].

Pathogenesis of hepatitis C virus

Globally, hepatitis C virus infects more than 170 million people, while over 4.1 million people have been exposed to HCV in the United States alone [50]. Although some individuals may resolve acute HCV infection spontaneously, most infected individuals will develop chronic HCV infection characterized by HCV antibody seropositivity and persistent viremia. Importantly, chronic HCV infection may result in significant hepatic fibrosis, cirrhosis, and hepatocellular carcinoma, and is the major reason for liver transplantation in the United States. The genome of this enveloped, single-stranded, positive-sense RNA virus is organized as a single polyprotein that encodes for multiple structural and nonstructural proteins and is flanked by untranslated regulatory (UTRs). A comprehensive review of the HCV life cycle has been presented elsewhere [51]. Viral replication is extremely robust. This, coupled with the error-prone nature of the viral RNA polymerase (NS5B), results in production of a heterogenous viral population, termed the viral quasispecies, within an infected individual. These viral variants may display divergent phenotypic properties, such as altered replication capacity or fitness, cell tropism, immunologic escape, and antiviral drug resistance [52]. At the population level, HCV also consists of multiple genotypes, an important determinant of the virologic response to HCV therapy [53].

Interestingly, there is also some suggestion that a portion of the HCV genome could share partial sequence homology with thyroid tissue antigens [54]. Thus, persons with chronic HCV infection might be more susceptible to autoimmune thyroid diseases.

Innate immunity to hepatitis C virus

Viral infection triggers activation of several antiviral effectors, including IFN, that represent an early host defense mechanism that occurs before the development of adaptive immune responses. Nonetheless, it is rare that these innate antiviral responses completely eliminate virus production. Several HCV proteins, including core, E2, NS3/4A, and NS5A have been implicated in inhibition of IFNα-inducible genes and/or key components of IFNα signaling pathways [55]. Furthermore, host immune selection pressures may drive the outgrowth and selection of viral variants capable of persisting despite the presence of an antiviral response directed against HCV or antiviral treatment. Thus, HCV can trigger and control the response to infection, and HCV's ability to antagonize these antiviral responses is crucial to its persistence in a host. Among the structural proteins, the two envelope glycoproteins (E1 and E2) interact with components of the adaptive immune response and are essential for host cell entry. Several cell surface molecules have been proposed to play a role in mediating HCV attachment and entry, including CD81, scavenger receptor class B type I (SR-BI), heparin sulfate, dendritic cell-specific intercellular adhesion molecule-3–grabbing nonintegrin (DC-SIGN)/L-SIGN, and the low-density lipoprotein (LDL) receptor [56]. Importantly, a recent study has demonstrated that hepatic binding of envelope glycoproteins—without productive HCV infection—results in a cascade of intracellular signals that modulate cellular gene expression, in particular genes critical to innate immune responses and lipid metabolism [57]. Furthermore, cross-linking of CD81 by HCV E2 protein blocks NK cell activation, cytokine production, cytotoxic granule release, and proliferation and results in costimulatory signals for T cells [58,59]. Similarly, engagement of CD81 on B cells by E2 protein and anti-CD81 antibody triggers the jun N-terminal kinas (JNK) pathway and leads to proliferation of naïve B lymphocytes. Thus, any cell type that expresses potential HCV receptors and/or entry cofactors, including thyrocytes, potentially could engage HCV glycoproteins, even in the absence of productive HCV infection. This engagement then can activate intracellular signaling pathways, triggering a tissue inflammatory response. Indeed, the authors recently have shown (N. Akeno and Y. Tomer, unpublished data, 2007) expression of CD81 in thyroid cells. Thus, it is possible that CD81 engagement by HCV E2 proteins in thyrocytes can trigger intracellular signaling cascades that ultimately induce thyroiditis and may contribute to the etiology of ITT.

Extrahepatic replication of hepatitis C virus

Although hepatocytes are the major site of HCV replication, numerous extrahepatic complications of HCV infection also exist, including autoimmune diseases, rheumatic diseases, and lymphoproliferative disorders [60]. HCV is also lymphotropic; thus, extrahepatic reservoirs of viral replication are relevant to the maintenance of viral persistence. Accurately demonstrating extrahepatic HCV replication, however, has been challenging because of the lack of robust models of HCV replication in vitro. Thus, to date, such studies have been performed almost exclusively using cells and tissues collected from HCV-infected patients. Because hepatitis C virions themselves contain positive-sense RNA genomes, the detection of positive-strand HCV RNA is not sufficient to demonstrate HCV replication. Rather, detection of actively replicating viral genomes, as indicated by negative-strand HCV RNA (so-called replicative intermediates) is necessary. Using highly sensitive, strand-specific polymerase chain reaction, negative-strand HCV RNA has been amplified in the peripheral blood, granulocytes, monocytes/macrophages, dendritic cells, and lymphocytes [60]. Negative-strand HCV RNA also has been demonstrated in the thyroid. For instance, Laskus and colleagues [61] investigated extrahepatic replication of HCV in various tissues from HCV-infected patients who died of AIDS-related complications and detected negative-strand HCV RNA in the thyroid of two individuals. The immunologic, virologic, and genetic factors that regulate HCV replication in extrahepatic sites, such as the thyroid, have not been explored, however, nor have the precise cell types supporting replication been identified.

Is the thyroid exposed to hepatitis C virus?

While intact, infectious hepatitis C virions are responsible for productive infection; viral proteins that are shed for virions or that are part of noninfectious virions also may have important physiological consequences. For instance, it has been demonstrated that HCV E2 proteins induce apoptosis through STAT1 induction and up-regulation of Fas ligand and the proapoptotic molecule Bid [62–64]. The proinflammatory cytokine interleukin 8 (IL-8) also is up-regulated by HCV E2 protein [65]. These data suggest that HCV proteins themselves could impact the thyroid environment significantly and contribute to thyroid dysfunction. Hence, it is possible that HCV infection of thyrocytes and/or exposure of thyrocytes to HCV proteins could trigger a thyroidal innate immune response to HCV, which, together with exogenous IFNα therapy, may activate IFNα-stimulated genes, resulting in thyroidal inflammation. Similarly, it is unknown if thyroid-tropic variants of HCV exist and what role if any these may have on thyroid dysfunction.

Genetic predisposition to interferon-induced thyroiditis

Autoimmune thyroid diseases (AITD) are influenced strongly by genetic factors [66]. Therefore genetic factors are likely to influence the etiology of IIT. In fact, the combination of HCV infection and IFNα therapy might trigger thyroiditis in genetically predisposed individuals [16]. Epidemiological data support a genetic predisposition for IIT. IIT is more common in females than in males [11,17,27,30,67]. In a compilation of data from different studies, females were shown to have a 4.4 times higher risk of developing thyroid dysfunction secondary to IFNα therapy compared with males [10]. Although the female preponderance of IIT potentially may be explained by the effects of estrogenic sex steroids in promoting autoimmunity [68], it also could be secondary to X chromosome susceptibility genes, as has been suggested for AITD [66]. How can a susceptibility gene on the X chromosome explain the increased frequency of IIT in females? Because females have two X chromosomes, and males have only one, females are more likely to inherit an X chromosome susceptibility gene [69]. Variations in the prevalence of a disease among ethnic groups could be another indication that genetic factors influence its etiology. Indeed, one study found that Asian origin was an independent predictor of thyroid dysfunction in patients receiving IFNα [67]. The influence of ethnicity on the incidence of IIT could be caused by genetic factors. No other studies, however, have shown that ethnicity influenced the incidence of IIT. Additional evidence for a genetic predisposition to IIT comes from data showing that the presence of baseline TAbs is a strong risk factor for the development of IIT [11,12,17]. The presence of TAbs is a preclinical stage of AITD, and may represent a marker for genetic predisposition to AITD [26]. Data from pooled studies showed that the risk of developing thyroid dysfunction in patients with baseline positive thyroid autoantibodies was 46.1% compared with only 5.4% in patients with baseline-negative thyroid auto-antibodies [11]. Specifically, the presence of TPO-Ab before treatment was a statistically significant risk factor for developing thyroid disease in patients treated with IFNα [12,17]. Thus IFNα may trigger AITD in genetically predisposed individuals, as manifested by the presence of baseline TAbs. Additional evidence for genetic predisposition to IIT comes from the authors' studies, which have suggested that IFNα accelerates thyroiditis in a thyroiditis-prone mouse model, the NOD-H2h4 mouse [70]. The authors treated NOD-H2h4 mice with IFNα for 8 weeks and examined for the development of thyroiditis. In the IFNα-injected group 6 of 13 (46.2%) developed thyroiditis and/or thyroid antibodies, while in the saline-injected group, only four of 13 (30.8%) developed thyroiditis and/or thyroid antibodies; however, this difference was not statistically significant, and more studies are needed to examine the effects of IFNα on thyroiditis in NOD-H2h4 mice [70]. In recent years, several genes have been found to be associated with thyroid autoimmunity [71]. The AITD genes include genes involved in immune regulation such as HLA-DR [72,73], CTLA-4 [74–76], and PTPN22 [77,78], and thyroid-specific genes, including thyroglobulin [79] and TSHR [80]. It is likely that some of these genes also contribute to the genetic susceptibility to IIT. Two studies examined the HLA gene locus for association with IIT [18,81]. In one study from Japan, an association was found between HLA-A2 and IFNα-induced autoimmune thyroid disorders [81], and another small study in a Caucasian population reported an association with DRB1*11, an allele that is not known to [17] be associated with AITD [15]. We recently tested several candidate genes for association with IIT, and our preliminary data showed evidence for association of IIT with polymorphisms in the CTLA-4 and CD40 genes [82]. Taken together, this preliminary evidence supports a genetic role in the etiology of IIT.

The etiology of interferon-induced thyroiditis

The mechanisms by which IFNα induces thyroid autoimmunity remain unknown. Recent data from several groups, including our group, however, have suggested that both immune-mediated and direct thyroid-toxic effects of IFNα play a role in the etiology of IIT.

Immune-mediated effects of interferon alpha

IFNα exerts various effects on the immune system, many of which might be implicated in the development of autoimmunity. IFNα receptor activation results in activation of the JAK-STAT pathway [83], leading to activation of numerous INF-stimulated genes (ISGs), including cytokine and adhesion molecule genes [84,85]. These combined effects can induce thyroid autoimmunity. One of the cardinal effects of IFNα is to increase major histocompatibility complex (MHC) class 1 antigen expression on cells. Indeed, IFNα was shown to increase the expression of MHC class 1 antigens on thyroid epithelial cells [12]. Overexpression of class 1 antigens is associated with activation of cytotoxic T cells, and thus can lead to tissue damage and inflammatory response [84]. Another potential mechanism of IIT is that IFNα shifts the immune response to a Th1-mediated pattern [86], resulting in the production of IFNγ and IL-2, two potent proinflammatory cytokines [87]. Indeed, it was reported recently that hepatitis C patients who developed IIT showed Th1 polarization of their innate immune response [88]. In some patients who have IIT, however, the clinical picture is that of GD, which generally is believed to be a Th2-mediated disease [89,90]. Because INFα has been shown to drive Th1 lymphocyte switching, it is unclear how IFNα can induce GD in some patients. One clue to this puzzle comes from recent studies by Rapoport and colleagues, suggesting that the initiation of GD is likely to be Th1-mediated [91]. Other potential mechanisms of IIT exist, as IFNα exerts many effects on the immune system. IFNα enhances the activity of lymphocytes, macrophages, and NK cells [1,84,92,93]. In addition, IFNα stimulates neutrophil and monocyte activation [84]. IFNα can induce the release of other cytokines, such as IL-6 [84], a cytokine that has been associated with autoimmune thyroiditis [94]. Thyroid cells have been shown to have specific binding sites for IL-6 [84], which decreases TSH-mediated iodine uptake, TSH-mediated expression of thyroid peroxidase mRNA, and TSH-mediated thyroid hormone release in vitro [84,95]. In addition, IFNα can alter immunoglobulin production and decrease T regulatory cell function, thereby promoting an autoimmune inflammatory response [96,97].

Direct effects of interferon alpha on the thyroid

Because up to 50% of patients who have IIT have nonautoimmune thyroiditis, it is likely that IFNα exerts direct effects on the thyroid. When type 1 IFNs were cultured with human thyroid follicular cells, they were found to inhibit TSH-induced gene expression of thyroglobulin (Tg), TPO, and sodium iodide symporter (NIS) [98]. The authors recently tested the expression levels of the TSHR, Tg, and TPO genes in rat thyroid cell line. Their results were consistent with the results of Caraccio and colleagues, showing an early increase but a late decrease in the levels of Tg and TPO. In addition, the authors have shown up-regulation of the TSHR gene upon exposure of thyroid cells to IFNα, and increased thyroid cell death induced by IFNα [99]. Combined, these results demonstrate that IFNα has direct toxic effects on the thyroid. Such effects may be responsible for the nonautoimmune thyroiditis induced by IFNα.

Diagnosis and management of interferon-induced thyroiditis

Recently, the authors suggested an algorithm for diagnosing and treating IIT [16]. It is important that hepatologists and endocrinologists work together in the care of these patients.

Diagnosis of interferon-induced thyroiditis

Previous studies have shown that IIT can result in serious complications from hyper-or hypothyroidism [12–15,27,100]; therefore, careful screening of all HCV patients before, during, and after IFNα treatment is recommended. Because many symptoms of thyroid dysfunction could be attributed to HCV infection or IFNα therapy, clinicians should look for signs of thyroid dysfunction such as tachycardia or bradycardia, sweating, heat or cold intolerance, unexpected weight loss or weight gain, and extreme fatigue and weakness routinely. Regardless of symptoms, the authors recommend that all hepatitis C patients be screened for thyroid disease before starting IFNα therapy. The authors recommend testing TSH levels to screen for abnormal thyroid functions, and thyroid antibody (TPO-Ab, Tg-Ab) levels, because positive TAbs are associated with significantly higher frequency of IIT [11]. If the TSH is normal and TAbs negative, TSH levels should be followed every 3 months until IFNα therapy is completed. If TSH levels are normal, but TAbs are positive (either TPO-Ab and/or Tg-Ab), the patient is at a higher risk of developing clinical thyroid dysfunction [12,17]. Therefore, in these cases, the authors recommend that TSH levels be followed every 2 months to monitor for the development thyroid dysfunction, either hypothyroidism or hyperthyroidism. If the patient develops hypo- or hyperthyroidism, a full workup needs to be completed. If serum TSH is low, fT4 and fT3 levels should be measured. Workup also should include checking TSH receptor antibody (TRAb), TPO-Ab, and Tg-Ab levels. If the etiology of hyperthyroidism cannot be revealed by these tests, a thyroid I-123 uptake and scan may be performed also. If serum TSH is high, fT4 and fT3 levels should be measured to confirm the diagnosis of primary hypothyroidism.

Treatment of interferon-induced thyroiditis

Hyperthyroidism

If the workup is consistent with destructive thyroiditis (ie, negative TAbs and low radio-iodine uptake on I-123 scan), the patient should be treated with a beta-blocker, if symptomatic. Patients with destructive thyroiditis should be monitored for the development of hypothyroidism, which usually follows the hyperthyroid phase within a few weeks. Corticosteroids, while helpful in subacute thyroiditis, generally are contraindicated in patients who have chronic hepatitis C infection. In cases of symptomatic thyrotoxicosis, withholding IFNα therapy should be considered in consultation with an endocrinologist [23]. It is should be remembered that rechallenge with IFNα may result in a recurrence of destructive thyroiditis and hyperthyroidism (sometimes severe) [34]; therefore, patients need close monitoring of thyroid if they are re-treated with IFNα. If the workup is consistent with GD, treatment with radioactive iodine and/or surgery should be considered [101]. The authors do not recommend treating patients who have IFNα-induced GD with antithyroid medications, because they worsen the liver dysfunction.

Hypothyroidism

Treatment usually consists of thyroid hormone replacement, with no need to stop IFNα therapy. Patients need to be monitored with thyroid functions every 2 months, because the disease may progress, leading to increased T4 requirements. In addition, T4 replacement requirements may increase if patients are treated with a second course of IFN, or may decrease or end altogether after cessation of IFNα treatment [19,27].

Summary

IIT is common among HCV patients treated with IFNα [10,11]. Preliminary studies suggest at least two different models by which IFNα may induce thyroid dysfunction, immune-mediated effects and direct thyroid-toxic effects of IFNα. Chronic HCV infection most likely plays a significant role in the triggering of thyroiditis among IFNα-treated patients. Given the high prevalence of this disease, it is essential that physicians treating patients who have IFNα are aware of the clinical spectrum of IIT, and screen their patients for IIT.

References

[1] Pfeffer LM, Dinarello CA, Herberman RB, et al. Biological properties of recombinant alpha interferons: 40th anniversary of the discovery of interferons. Cancer Res 1998; 58(12):2489–99.

[2] Parmar S, Platanias LC. Interferons: mechanisms of action and clinical applications. Curr Opin Oncol 2003;15(6):431–9.

[3] Jonasch E, Haluska FG. Interferon in oncological practice: review of interferon biology, clinical applications, and toxicities. Oncologist 2001;6(1):34–55.

[4] Baron S, Tyring SK, Fleischmann WR Jr, et al. The interferons. Mechanisms of action and clinical applications. JAMA 1991;266(10):1375–83.

[5] Manns MP, McHutchison JG, Gordon SC, et al. Peginterferon alpha-2b plus ribavirin compared with interferon alpha-2b plus ribavirin for initial treatment of chronic hepatitis C: a randomised trial. Lancet 2001;358(9286):958–65.

[6] Fried MW, Shiffman ML, Reddy KR, et al. Peginterferon alpha-2a plus ribavirin for chronic hepatitis C virus infection. N Engl J Med 2002;347(13):975–82.

[7] Russo MW, Fried MW. Side effects of therapy for chronic hepatitis C. Gastroenterology 2003;124(6):1711–9.

[8] Burman P, Totterman TH, Oberg K, et al. Thyroid autoimmunity in patients on long-term therapy with leukocyte-derived interferon. J Clin Endocrinol Metab 1986;63(5):1086–90.

[9] Fentiman IS, Thomas BS, Balkwill FR, et al. Primary hypothyroidism associated with interferon therapy of breast cancer. Lancet 1985;1(8438):1166.

[10] Prummel MF, Laurberg P. Interferon alpha and autoimmune thyroid disease. Thyroid 2003;13(6):547–51.

[11] Koh LK, Greenspan FS, Yeo PP. Interferon alpha-induced thyroid dysfunction: three clinical presentations and a review of the literature. Thyroid 1997;7(6):891–6.

[12] Roti E, Minelli R, Giuberti T, et al. Multiple changes in thyroid function in patients with chronic active HCV hepatitis treated with recombinant interferon alpha. Am J Med 1996;101(5):482–7.

[13] Mazziotti G, Sorvillo F, Stornaiuolo G, et al. Temporal relationship between the appearance of thyroid autoantibodies and development of destructive thyroiditis in patients undergoing treatment with two different type 1 interferons for HCV-related chronic hepatitis: a prospective study. J Endocrinol Invest 2002;25(7):624–30.

[14] Villanueva RB, Brau N. Graves' ophthalmopathy associated with interferon alpha treatment for hepatitis C. Thyroid 2002;12(8):737–8.

[15] Kryczka W, Brojer E, Kowalska A, et al. Thyroid gland dysfunctions during antiviral therapy of chronic hepatitis C. Med Sci Monit 2001;7(Suppl 1):221–5.

[16] Mandac JC, Chaudhry S, Sherman KE, et al. The clinical and physiological spectrum of interferon alpha-induced thyroiditis: toward a new classification. Hepatology 2006;43(4): 661–72.

[17] Watanabe U, Hashimoto E, Hisamitsu T, et al. The risk factor for development of thyroid disease during interferon alpha therapy for chronic hepatitis C. Am J Gastroenterol 1994; 89(3):399–403.

[18] Martocchia A, Labbadia G, Paoletti V, et al. Hashimoto's disease during interferon alpha therapy in a patient with pretreatment-negative antithyroid autoantibodies and with the specific genetic susceptibility to the thyroid disease. Neuro Endocrinol Lett 2001;22(1): 49–52.

[19] Baudin E, Marcellin P, Pouteau M, et al. Reversibility of thyroid dysfunction induced by recombinant alpha interferon in chronic hepatitis C. Clin Endocrinol (Oxf) 1993;39(6): 657–61.

[20] Carella C, Mazziotti G, Morisco F, et al. Long-term outcome of interferon alpha-induced thyroid autoimmunity and prognostic influence of thyroid autoantibody pattern at the end of treatment. J Clin Endocrinol Metab 2001;86(5):1925–9.

[21] Preziati D, La Rosa L, Covini G, et al. Autoimmunity and thyroid function in patients with chronic active hepatitis treated with recombinant interferon alpha-2a. Eur J Endocrinol 1995;132(5):587–93.

[22] Imagawa A, Itoh N, Hanafusa T, et al. Autoimmune endocrine disease induced by recombinant interferon alpha therapy for chronic active type C hepatitis. J Clin Endocrinol Metab 1995;80(3):922–6.

[23] Wong V, Fu AX, George J, et al. Thyrotoxicosis induced by alpha interferon therapy in chronic viral hepatitis. Clin Endocrinol (Oxf) 2002;56(6):793–8.

[24] Lisker-Melman M, Di Bisceglie AM, Usala SJ, et al. Development of thyroid disease during therapy of chronic viral hepatitis with interferon alpha. Gastroenterology 1992;102(6): 2155–60.

[25] Hollowell JG, Staehling NW, Flanders WD, et al. Serum TSH, T(4), and thyroid antibodies in the United States population (1988 to 1994): National Health and Nutrition Examination Survey (NHANES III). J Clin Endocrinol Metab 2002;87(2):489–99.

[26] Vanderpump MPJ, Tunbridge WMG, French JM, et al. The incidence of thyroid disorders in the community: a twenty-year follow-up of the Whickham survey. Clin Endocrinol (Oxf) 1995;43:55–68.

[27] Marazuela M, Garcia-Buey L, Gonzalez-Fernandez B, et al. Thyroid autoimmune disorders in patients with chronic hepatitis C before and during interferon alpha therapy. Clin Endocrinol (Oxf) 1996;44(6):635–42.

[28] Kohno T, Tsunetoshi Y, Ishikawa E. Existence of antithyroglobulin IgG in healthy subjects. Biochem Biophys Res Commun 1988;155:224–9.

[29] Ericsson UB, Christensen SB, Thorell J. A high prevalence of thyroglobulin autoantibodies in adults with and without thyroid disease as measured with a sensitive solid-phase immunosorbent radioassay. Clin Immunol Immunopathol 1985;37:154–62.

[30] Carella C, Amato G, Biondi B, et al. Longitudinal study of antibodies against thyroid in patients undergoing interferon alpha therapy for HCV chronic hepatitis. Horm Res 1995;44(3):110–4.

[31] Monzani F, Caraccio N, Dardano A, et al. Thyroid autoimmunity and dysfunction associated with type I interferon therapy. Clin Exp Med 2004;3(4):199–210.

[32] Volpe R. Etiology, pathogenesis, and clinical aspects of thyroiditis. Pathol Annu 1978;13: 399–413.

[33] Weetman AP, Smallridge RC, Nutman TB, et al. Persistent thyroid autoimmunity after subacute thyroiditis. J Clin Lab Immunol 1987;23:1–6.

[34] Parana R, Cruz M, Lyra L, et al. Subacute thyroiditis during treatment with combination therapy (interferon plus ribavirin) for hepatitis C virus. J Viral Hepat 2000;7(5):393–5.

[35] Okanoue T, Sakamoto S, Itoh Y, et al. Side effects of high-dose interferon therapy for chronic hepatitis C. J Hepatol 1996;25(3):283–91.

[36] Oppenheim Y, Ban Y, Tomer Y. Interferon-induced autoimmune thyroid disease (AITD): a model for human autoimmunity. Autoimmun Rev 2004;3(5):388–93.

[37] Tomer Y, Davies TF. Infection. Thyroid disease and autoimmunity. Endocr Rev 1993;14: 107–20.

[38] Tomer Y, Villanueva R. Hepatitis C and thyroid autoimmunity: is there a link? Am J Med 2004;117(1):60–1.

[39] Loviselli A, Oppo A, Velluzzi F, et al. Independent expression of serological markers of thyroid autoimmunity and hepatitis virus C infection in the general population: results of a community-based study in northwestern Sardinia. J Endocrinol Invest 1999;22(9):660–5.

[40] Metcalfe RA, Ball G, Kudesia G, et al. Failure to find an association between hepatitis C virus and thyroid autoimmunity. Thyroid 1997;7(3):421–4.

[41] Boadas J, Rodriguez-Espinosa J, Enriquez J, et al. Prevalence of thyroid autoantibodies is not increased in blood donors with hepatitis C virus infection. J Hepatol 1995;22(6):611–5.

[42] Tran A, Quaranta JF, Benzaken S, et al. High prevalence of thyroid autoantibodies in a prospective series of patients with chronic hepatitis C before interferon therapy. Hepatology 1993;18(2):253–7.

[43] Ganne-Carrie N, Medini A, Coderc E, et al. Latent autoimmune thyroiditis in untreated patients with HCV chronic hepatitis: a case–control study. J Autoimmun 2000;14(2): 189–93.

[44] Fernandez-Soto L, Gonzalez A, Escobar-Jimenez F, et al. Increased risk of autoimmune thyroid disease in hepatitis C vs hepatitis B before, during, and after discontinuing interferon therapy. Arch Intern Med 1998;158(13):1445–8.

[45] Antonelli A, Ferri C, Pampana A, et al. Thyroid disorders in chronic hepatitis C. Am J Med 2004;117(1):10–3.

[46] Pateron D, Hartmann DJ, Duclos-Vallee JC, et al. Latent autoimmune thyroid disease in patients with chronic HCV hepatitis. J Hepatol 1993;17(3):417–9.

[47] Tunbridge WMG, Evered DC, Hall R, et al. The spectrum of thyroid disease in a community: the Whickham survey. Clin Endocrinol Oxf 1977;7:481–93.

[48] Carella C, Mazziotti G, Morisco F, et al. The addition of ribavirin to interferon alpha therapy in patients with hepatitis C virus-related chronic hepatitis does not modify the thyroid autoantibody pattern but increases the risk of developing hypothyroidism. Eur J Endocrinol 2002;146(6):743–9.

[49] Antonelli A, Ferri C, Fallahi P, et al. Thyroid disorders in chronic hepatitis C virus infection. Thyroid 2006;16(6):563–72.

[50] Armstrong GL, Wasley A, Simard EP, et al. The prevalence of hepatitis C virus infection in the United States, 1999 through 2002. Ann Intern Med 2006;144(10):705–14.

[51] Bartenschlager R, Lohmann V. Replication of hepatitis C virus. J Gen Virol 2000;81(Pt 7): 1631–48.

[52] Simmonds P. Genetic diversity and evolution of hepatitis C virus—15 years on. J Gen Virol 2004;85(Pt 11):3173–88.

[53] Hnatyszyn HJ. Chronic hepatitis C and genotyping: the clinical significance of determining HCV genotypes. Antivir Ther 2005;10(1):1–11.

[54] Hsieh MC, Yu ML, Chuang WL, et al. Virologic factors related to interferon alpha-induced thyroid dysfunction in patients with chronic hepatitis C. Eur J Endocrinol 2000;142:431–7.

[55] Gale M Jr, Foy EM. Evasion of intracellular host defense by hepatitis C virus. Nature 2005; 436(7053):939–45.

[56] Barth H, Liang TJ, Baumert TF. Hepatitis C virus entry: molecular biology and clinical implications. Hepatology 2006;44(3):527–35.

[57] Fang X, Zeisel MB, Wilpert J, et al. Host cell responses induced by hepatitis C virus binding. Hepatology 2006;43(6):1326–36.

[58] Crotta S, Stilla A, Wack A, et al. Inhibition of natural killer cells through engagement of CD81 by the major hepatitis C virus envelope protein. J Exp Med 2002;195(1):35–41.

[59] Wack A, Soldaini E, Tseng C, et al. Binding of the hepatitis C virus envelope protein E2 to CD81 provides a costimulatory signal for human T cells. Eur J Immunol 2001;31(1): 166–75.

[60] Blackard JT, Kemmer N, Sherman KE. Extrahepatic replication of HCV: insights into clinical manifestations and biological consequences. Hepatology 2006;44(1):15–22.

[61] Laskus T, Radkowski M, Wang LF, et al. Search for hepatitis C virus extrahepatic replication sites in patients with acquired immunodeficiency syndrome: specific detection of negative-strand viral RNA in various tissues. Hepatology 1998;28(5):1398–401.

[62] Munshi N, Balasubramanian A, Koziel M, et al. Hepatitis C and human immunodeficiency virus envelope proteins cooperatively induce hepatocytic apoptosis via an innocent bystander mechanism. J Infect Dis 2003;188(8):1192–204.

[63] Balasubramanian A, Ganju RK, Groopman JE. Signal transducer and activator of transcription factor 1 mediates apoptosis induced by hepatitis C virus and HIV envelope proteins in hepatocytes. J Infect Dis 2006;194(5):670–81.

[64] Balasubramanian A, Koziel M, Groopman JE, et al. Molecular mechanism of hepatic injury in coinfection with hepatitis C virus and HIV. Clin Infect Dis 2005;41(Suppl 1): S32–7.

[65] Balasubramanian A, Ganju RK, Groopman JE. Hepatitis C virus and HIV envelope proteins collaboratively mediate interleukin-8 secretion through activation of p38 MAP kinase and SHP2 in hepatocytes. J Biol Chem 2003;278(37):35755–66.

[66] Tomer Y, Davies TF. Searching for the autoimmune thyroid disease susceptibility genes: from gene mapping to gene function. Endocr Rev 2003;24:694–717.

[67] Dalgard O, Bjoro K, Hellum K, et al. Thyroid dysfunction during treatment of chronic hepatitis C with interferon alpha: no association with either interferon dosage or efficacy of therapy. J Intern Med 2002;251(5):400–6.

[68] Grossman CJ, Roselle GA, Mendenhall CL. Sex steroid regulation of autoimmunity. J Steroid Biochem Mol Biol 1991;40(4-6):649–59.

[69] Barbesino G, Tomer Y, Concepcion ES, et al. Linkage analysis of candidate genes in autoimmune thyroid disease: 2. Selected gender-related genes and the X chromosome. J Clin Endocrinol Metab 1998;83:3290–5.

[70] Oppenheim Y, Kim G, Ban Y, et al. The effects of alpha interferon on the development of autoimmune thyroiditis in the NOD H2h4 mouse. Clin Dev Immunol 2003;10(2–4):161–5.

[71] Jacobson EM, Tomer Y. The CD40, CTLA-4, thyroglobulin, TSH receptor, and PTPN22 gene quintet and its contribution to thyroid autoimmunity: back to the future. J Autoimmun 2007;28:85–98.

[72] Stenszky V, Kozma L, Balazs C, et al. The genetics of Graves' disease: HLA and disease susceptibility. J Clin Endocrinol Metab 1985;61:735–40.

[73] Ban Y, Davies TF, Greenberg DA, et al. Arginine at position 74 of the HLA-DRb1 chain is associated with Graves' disease. Genes Immun 2004;5:203–8.

[74] Yanagawa T, Hidaka Y, Guimaraes V, et al. CTLA-4 gene polymorphism associated with Graves' disease in a Caucasian population. J Clin Endocrinol Metab 1995;80:41–5.

[75] Vaidya B, Imrie H, Perros P, et al. The cytotoxic T lymphocyte antigen-4 is a major Graves' disease locus. Hum Mol Genet 1999;8(7):1195–9.

[76] Tomer Y, Greenberg DA, Barbesino G, et al. CTLA-4 and not CD28 is a susceptibility gene for thyroid autoantibody production. J Clin Endocrinol Metab 2001;86:1687–93.

[77] Smyth D, Cooper JD, Collins JE, et al. Replication of an association between the lymphoid tyrosine phosphatase locus (LYP/PTPN22) with type 1 diabetes and evidence for its role as a general autoimmunity locus. Diabetes 2004;53(11):3020–3.

[78] Velaga MR, Wilson V, Jennings CE, et al. The codon 620 tryptophan allele of the lymphoid tyrosine phosphatase (LYP) gene is a major determinant of Graves' disease. J Clin Endocrinol Metab 2004;89(11):5862–5.

[79] Ban Y, Greenberg DA, Concepcion E, et al. Amino acid substitutions in the thyroglobulin gene are associated with susceptibility to human and murine autoimmune thyroid disease. Proc Natl Acad Sci USA 2003;100:15119–24.

[80] Hiratani H, Bowden DW, Ikegami S, et al. Multiple SNPs in intron 7 of thyrotropin receptor are associated with Graves' disease. J Clin Endocrinol Metab 2005;90(5):2898–903.

[81] Kakizaki S, Takagi H, Murakami M, et al. HLA antigens in patients with interferon alpha-induced autoimmune thyroid disorders in chronic hepatitis C. J Hepatol 1999;30(5): 794–800.

[82] Jacobson EM, Chaudhry S, Mandac JC, et al. Immune-regulatory gene involvement in the etiology of interferon-induced thyroiditis (IIT). Thyroid 2006;16:926.

[83] Nguyen KB, Watford WT, Salomon R, et al. Critical role for STAT4 activation by type 1 interferons in the interferon gamma response to viral infection. Science 2002;297(5589): 2063–6.

[84] Corssmit EP, de Metz J, Sauerwein HP, et al. Biologic responses to IFN-alpha administration in humans. J Interferon Cytokine Res 2000;20(12):1039–47.

[85] You X, Teng W, Shan Z. Expression of ICAM-1, B7.1 and TPO on human thyrocytes induced by IFN-alpha. Chin Med J (Engl) 1999;112(1):61–6.

[86] Farrar JD, Murphy KM. Type I interferons and T helper development. Immunol Today 2000;21(10):484–9.

[87] Tilg H. New insights into the mechanisms of interferon alpha: an immunoregulatory and anti-inflammatory cytokine. Gastroenterology 1997;112(3):1017–21.

[88] Mazziotti G, Sorvillo F, Piscopo M, et al. Innate and acquired immune system in patients developing interferon alpha-related autoimmune thyroiditis: a prospective study. J Clin Endocrinol Metab 2005;90(7):4138–44.

[89] Land KJ, Moll JS, Kaplan MH, et al. Signal transducer and activator of transcription (Stat)-6-dependent, but not Stat4-dependent, immunity is required for the development of autoimmunity in Graves' hyperthyroidism. Endocrinology 2004;145(8):3724–30.

[90] Mazziotti G, Sorvillo F, Carbone A, et al. Is the IFN-alpha-related thyroid autoimmunity an immunologically heterogeneous disease? J Intern Med 2002;252(4):377–8.

[91] Nagayama Y, Mizuguchi H, Hayakawa T, et al. Prevention of autoantibody-mediated Graves'-like hyperthyroidism in mice with IL-4, a Th2 cytokine. J Immunol 2003;170(7): 3522–7.

[92] Corssmit EP, Heijligenberg R, Hack CE, et al. Effects of interferon alpha (IFN-alpha) administration on leucocytes in healthy humans. Clin Exp Immunol 1997;107(2):359–63.

[93] Aulitzky WE, Tilg H, Vogel W, et al. Acute hematologic effects of interferon alpha, interferon gamma, tumor necrosis factor alpha, and interleukin 2. Ann Hematol 1991;62(1): 25–31.

[94] Ajjan RA, Watson PF, McIntosh RS, et al. Intrathyroidal cytokine gene expression in Hashimoto's thyroiditis. Clin Exp Immunol 1996;105(3):523–8.

[95] Sato K, Satoh T, Shizume K, et al. Inhibition of 125I organification and thyroid hormone release by interleukin-1, tumor necrosis factor alpha, and interferon gamma in human thyrocytes in suspension culture. J Clin Endocrinol Metab 1990;70(6):1735–43.

[96] Krause I, Valesini G, Scrivo R, et al. Autoimmune aspects of cytokine and anticytokine therapies. Am J Med 2003;115(5):390–7.

[97] Lindahl P, Leary P, Gresser I. Enhancement by interferon of the expression of surface antigens on murine leukemia L 1210 cells. Proc Natl Acad Sci USA 1973;70(10):2785–8.

[98] Caraccio N, Giannini R, Cuccato S, et al. Type I interferons modulate the expression of thyroid peroxidase, sodium/iodide symporter, and thyroglobulin genes in primary human thyrocyte cultures. J Clin Endocrinol Metab 2005;90(2):1156–62.

[99] Akeno N, Tomer Y. Dissecting the mechanisms of interferon-induced thyroiditis (IIT): direct effects of interferon alpha on thyroid epithelial cells. Presented at the 89th Meeting of the Endocrine Society, Toronto (Canada), June 2, 2007.

[100] Deutsch M, Koskinas J, Tzannos K, et al. Hashimoto encephalopathy with pegylated interferon alpha-2b and ribavirin. Ann Pharmacother 2005;39(10):1745–7.

[101] Weetman AP. Graves' disease. N Engl J Med 2000;343(17):1236–48.

ELSEVIER
SAUNDERS

Endocrinol Metab Clin N Am
36 (2007) 1067–1087

ENDOCRINOLOGY
AND METABOLISM
CLINICS
OF NORTH AMERICA

Use of Insulin Sensitizers in NASH

Mouen Khashab, MD, Naga Chalasani, MD*

*Division of Gastroenterology and Hepatology, Indiana University School of Medicine,
WD OPW 2005, 1001 West 10th Street, Indianapolis, IN 46202, USA*

Nonalcoholic fatty liver disease (NAFLD) is a common chronic liver disease that histologically resembles alcoholic liver disease but occurs in individuals without excessive alcohol consumption. Obesity and type 2 diabetes are the two most common risk factors for developing NAFLD. NAFLD can be categorized broadly into simple steatosis (nonalcoholic fatty liver [NAFL]) and nonalcoholic steatohepatitis (NASH). NASH is characterized histologically by the presence of steatosis, cytologic ballooning, Mallory's hyaline, scattered inflammation, and pericellular fibrosis [1]. Simple steatosis is largely benign with very minimal risk of cirrhosis, whereas NASH is a progressive liver disorder that can lead to cirrhosis and liver failure. Cryptogenic cirrhosis, a frequent indication for liver transplantation in the United States, likely is caused by NASH in more than 80% of patients [1]. It is believed that over next 20 years, NAFLD and NASH will surpass hepatitis C as the leading cause for liver transplantation in the United States. This article briefly discusses NAFLD and its association with the metabolic syndrome, its pathogenesis and natural history, and then presents a detailed discussion on the efficacy and safety of different insulin sensitizers in patients who have NAFLD.

Insulin resistance and metabolic syndrome in nonalcoholic fatty liver disease

The close association between metabolic syndrome and NAFLD is described well in the literature. The metabolic syndrome's core cluster includes diabetes, hypertension, dyslipidemia, and obesity. During the last decade, it

Supported in part by K24 DK 069,290 (NC). Authors have no relevant financial conflicts to declare.

* Corresponding author.

E-mail address: nchalasa@iupui.edu (N. Chalasani).

has become clear that NAFLD is frequently present in patients who have the metabolic syndrome. Depending on the method of detection, up to 40% of patients who have metabolic syndrome have evidence for ongoing NAFLD [2].

Insulin resistance is very common in patients who have NAFLD, and it is thought play an important role in its pathogenesis. Several studies have assessed the prevalence of insulin resistance in patients who have NASH (Table 1). Willner and colleagues [3] reported their experience with 90 patients with NASH. Studies of glucose tolerance demonstrated unsuspected diabetes in six patients and insulin resistance in 85% of those tested. The authors proposed that patients who have NASH and not known to be diabetic should undergo oral glucose tolerance testing with concomitant insulin levels. Chitturi and colleagues [4] tested the hypothesis that insulin resistance is an essential requirement for the development of NASH and that a high association between insulin resistance and liver disease is specific for NASH. The principal findings of this study were that virtually all patients (98%) who had NASH were insulin resistant and that most patients (87%) had the metabolic syndrome. The relative specificity of insulin resistance for NASH was confirmed by the finding that insulin resistance was present more often and appeared to be more profound in patients who had milder cases of NASH than in patients who had chronic hepatitis C virus (HCV) infection of similar severity. This study also established that hyperinsulinemia was attributable to increased insulin secretion and was not the consequence of reduced hepatic extraction of insulin as occurs in all forms of chronic liver diseases at the stage of advanced fibrosis or cirrhosis. Another study by Pagano and colleagues [5] also assessed the association between insulin resistance and NASH. Compared with controls, the NASH group had significantly lower insulin sensitivity and higher total insulin secretion. Hepatic insulin extraction was similar in both groups.

The authors published a study to characterize the metabolic response to a standard mixed meal and to identify anthropometric determinants of insulin resistance in nondiabetic patients who had NASH [6]. Eighteen nondiabetic patients who had biopsy-proven NASH and 18 age-, gender-, body mass index (BMI)-, and body fat-matched controls without liver disease were included in this metabolic study. Subjects in the NASH group had

Table 1
Selected studies of insulin resistance in nonalcoholic steatohepatitis

Author (reference number)	Number of patients	Study design	Year of publication	Prevalence of insulin resistance	Prevalence of metabolic syndrome
Willner et al [3]	90	Retrospective	2001	85%	Not reported
Chitturi et al [4]	66	Case–control	2002	98%	87%
Pagano et al [5]	38	Case–control	2002	Not reported	47%
Chalasani et al [6]	36	Case–control	2003	83%	Not reported

significantly higher levels of insulin and C peptide at fasting and after the meal; however, glucose levels were similar between the groups at baseline and after the meal, suggesting preservation of glucose homeostasis. The homeostatic model assessment (HOMA) values were significantly higher in the NASH group. A statistically significant association existed between HOMA and BMI, percent visceral fat and visceral fat area. One important observation noted in this study was that the subjects who had NASH had a significantly higher visceral fat when compared with BMI- and body fat-matched controls. Because visceral fat is an important determinant of insulin resistance, this finding supports the notion that insulin resistance is the cause rather than the consequence of NASH.

Pathogenesis

The prevailing hypothesis is the two-hit model, with insulin resistance at the core of the pathogenesis. Obesity and diabetes mellitus are associated with increased tissue resistance to insulin; hyperinsulinemia develops and impairs mitochondrial β-oxidation of free fatty acids. Because of this block in fatty acid catabolism, fat accumulates in zone 3 hepatocytes, and thus the development of NAFL. The progression to NASH entails a second hit that is believed to be caused by oxidative stress. This might result from peroxisomal fatty acid metabolism (when mitochondrial pathways are saturated) and cytochrome P450 CYP-2E1 induction, which produces oxygen free radicals. These reactive oxygen species activate liver stellate cells to produce collagen and attract neutrophils that generate an inflammatory reaction. Sanyal and colleagues [7] tested the two-hit hypothesis, insulin resistance accounting for the first hit, and a specific intrahepatic mitochondrial defect that would render the hepatocytes more susceptible to oxidative injury accounting for the second hit. The hypothesis was tested partly by evaluation of insulin resistance by a two-step hyperinsulinemic euglycemic clamp and of the frequency and severity of structural defects in hepatocyte mitochondria in vivo by using transmission electron microscopy. Subjects who had NASH (n = 6 to 10 for different studies) were compared with those who had NAFL (n = 6) or normal controls (n = 6). There was a significant step-wise increase in mean baseline fasting plasma insulin concentrations from normal individuals to those with fatty liver and subjects with NASH. The sensitivity to insulin was reduced both in subjects who had fatty liver and in those who had NASH. The findings were most pronounced, however, in those who had NASH. Insulin infusion produced a decrease in the plasma concentrations of both free fatty acids and glycerol, with the least suppression noted in NASH patients and the greatest suppression in normal individuals. This suggested the presence of insulin resistance at the level of the adipose tissue. Using electron microscopy, NASH patients, in sharp contrast to NAFL patients, had highly abnormal subcellar morphology. The mitochondria were swollen, rounded, and often multila-mellar with loss of cristae. Within the mitochondria, there were stacks of paracrystalline inclusion bodies. The authors hypothesized that such mito-chondrial abnormalities are present in a certain percentage of the general population, and that when such individuals develop insulin resistance, they are at higher risk for developing NAFLD and NASH. Loria and col-leagues [8] suggested that a single hit, insulin resistance, could be enough to explain the whole spectrum of NAFLD. Other authors proposed a four-step model [9]:

Steatosis facilitated by insulin
Necrosis induced by intracellular lipid toxicity or lipid peroxidation
Release of bulk lipid from hepatocytes into the interstitium, leading to direct and inflammatory injury to hepatic veins
Venous obstruction with secondary collapse and, ultimately, fibrous septation and cirrhosis

Thus, all these hypotheses propose that insulin resistance is the central pathophysiological problem in patients who have NAFLD.

There has been recent interest in studying the association between specific derangements of various hormones and NAFLD. Hormonal derangements can be primarily responsible for the development of NAFLD by means of anthropometric changes and/or alterations in the homeostasis of energy and metabolism of glucose and lipids [10]. Studies have shown higher prev-alence of NAFLD in patients who have hypothyroidism [11], panhypopitui-tarism [12], and other endocrine disorders [10].

Epidemiology

More than half of the United States population are either overweight (BMI greater than 25 but less than 29 kg/m^2) or obese (BMI greater than 29 kg/m^2) [13]. It is also estimated that 47 million individuals in the United States have the metabolic syndrome [14]. Thus, a high proportion of the United States population is at risk for NAFLD. NAFLD occurs in 9% of overweight patients and 21% to 33% of those with morbid obesity. Ultra-sonography surveys of the general population indicate the presence of fatty liver in 16% to 25% of adults in the United States. It is the most common cause of increased serum level of alanine aminotransferase (ALT) in blood donors [15,16]. NAFLD is more common than chronic hepatitis C in the United States, and its prevalence is expected to rise with the epidemic of obesity, especially in the pediatric and adolescent populations [17].

One population-based study evaluated the prevalence and the indepen-dent risk factors of primary NAFLD in Israel [18]. The prevalence of NAFLD among the 326 patients included in this study was 30%; it was more prevalent in men than women (38% versus 21%, $P = .001$). Risk factors independently associated with NAFLD included male gender, abdominal obesity, homeostasis model assessment, hyperinsulinemia, and hypertriglyceridemia. Another cross-sectional community study from Taiwan examined the prevalence and risk factors of NAFLD in 3245 adults [19]. The prevalence of NAFLD was 11.5%. The risk factors for NAFLD were male sex, obesity, fasting plasma glucose of at least 126 mg/dL, total cholesterol of at least 240 mg/dL, triglycerides of at least 150 mg/dL, and hyperuricemia. Among the metabolic disorders, only hypertriglyceridemia was related to NAFLD in nonobese subjects.

Multiple other studies have confirmed the association of NAFLD with central obesity, type 2 diabetes, high triglycerides, low high-density lipoprotein (HDL) cholesterol and insulin resistance, and globally with the presence of the metabolic syndrome [20]. The relative importance of each of these risk factors is difficult to determine, because they often coexist in many patients [20].

Few studies have examined the prevalence of NAFLD among different United States ethnic groups. Caldwell and colleagues [21] reported that African Americans were represented infrequently among patients with NASH in a tertiary referral liver transplant center. The authors, however, were unable to determine whether this observation represents differing rates of NASH or simply under-referral, underdiagnosis, or underuse of medical resources by African Americans. One study assessed the demographic characteristics of 41 patients with cryptogenic cirrhosis at a United States county hospital with a racially and ethnically diverse patient population [22]; 74% of the patients had one or more features of NASH on liver biopsies. Although Hispanics comprised less than 26% and African Americans greater than 40% of adult medicine patients, 68% of patients with cryptogenic cirrhosis were Hispanic, while only 7% were African American. Prevalence of cryptogenic cirrhosis among African American and Hispanic patients was 3.9-fold lower and 3.1-fold higher, respectively, than among European American patients despite similar prevalence of diabetes among both ethnic groups. This study supported the belief that NASH is responsible for most cryptogenic cirrhosis cases and indicated that this form of cirrhosis is rare among African Americans.

Prognosis and natural history

Prognosis of patients who have NAFLD depends on hepatic histology and coexisting comorbidities. Patients with underlying metabolic syndrome are especially at risk for cardiovascular morbidity and mortality. A recent study of 420 patients with NAFLD in the community setting found both liver-related and overall mortality higher than the general population [23]. Studies that included mainly patients who had bland steatosis described a benign long-term prognosis, whereas those that included mainly patients who had NASH suggested a more aggressive disorder. Cirrhosis occurs in 15% to 20% of patients who have NASH [24]. NASH and liver fibrosis have been associated with an 11% mortality rate after 10 years. The 5- and 10-year survival rates for patients who have NASH may be as low as 67% and 59%, respectively, if deaths caused by comorbid conditions are included.

Therapy

Improvement of insulin resistance, or insulin sensitivity, has therapeutic potential in preventing the progression of NASH, because the accumulation of triglycerides in hepatocytes is believed to be the first step in the current two-hit hypothesis of the pathophysiological development of NAFLD. The goals of therapy include risk factor modification, avoidance of factors that promote progression of liver disease, and specific treatment of NASH. The ultimate goal is to prevent end-organ damage associated with insulin resistance and metabolic syndrome including end-stage liver disease and ischemic heart disease. The authors focus on the two most promising types of insulin sensitizers in NAFLD, the PPAR-γ agonists known as thiazolidinediones (TZDs), and the only available biguanide agent, metformin, and then briefly discuss the incretins and their potential role in improving insulin sensitivity in patients who have NAFLD.

Thiazolidinediones

Mechanism of action

Thiazolidinediones, more commonly known as glitazones, are a new class of oral antidiabetic drugs that improve insulin sensitivity by acting as selective agonists of the nuclear peroxisome proliferators-activated receptor (PPAR)-γ. Three PPARs, designated PPAR-α, PPAR-δ (also known as PPAR-β), and PPAR-γ, have been identified. PPAR-α is expressed predominantly in muscle, liver, vascular wall, and heart [25]. PPAR-δ is expressed mostly in adipose tissue, skin, brain and hepatic stellate cells, and PPAR-γ is expressed mostly in adipose tissue, pancreatic β-cells, vascular endothelium, macrophages and hepatic stellate cells [26,27].

The first TZD, troglitazone, was approved in the United States in 1997 as a glucose-lowering therapy for patients with type 2 diabetes. Troglitazone was withdrawn from the market in March 2000 because of hepatotoxicity. The two currently available PPAR-γ agonists, rosiglitazone and pioglitazone, were approved in the United States in 1999. TZDs exert insulin-sensitizing actions directly on adipocytes and indirectly by means of altered adipokine release (Fig. 1). According to the first or direct mechanism, TZDs promote fatty acid uptake and storage in adipose tissue and thus

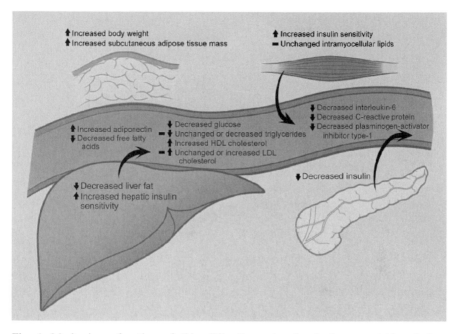

Fig. 1. Mechanism of action of thiazolidinediones in vivo in humans. (*Adapted from* Yki-Jarvinen H. Thiazolidinediones. N Engl J Med 2004;351(11):1106–18; with permission. Copyright © 2004, Massachusetts Medical Society.)

increase adipose tissue mass and spare other insulin-sensitive tissues such as skeletal muscles and the liver, the harmful metabolic effects of high concentrations of free fatty acids [28]. In other words, TZDs promote the distribution of fat from the liver and muscle cells to adipocytes [29]. Consequently, TZDs lower circulating free fatty acid concentrations in the liver and thus restore insulin sensitivity, because fatty acid metabolism is an important determinant of insulin sensitivity [30].

The indirect effects of TZDs on adipose tissue and improvement in insulin sensitivity also are believed to be mediated through adiponectin. Adiponectin, an adipokine produced exclusively by adipose tissue, has insulin-sensitizing properties in mice [31]. Treatment of type 2 diabetic patients with pioglitazone resulted in a significant increase in plasma adiponectin concentration, which was associated with the improvement of insulin resistance and decrease in hepatic fat content [32]. The importance of this study is that plasma adiponectin concentrations correlated with the liver fat content both before and after treatment with pioglitazone. Lutchman and colleagues [33] conducted an open-label study to assess changes in serum adiponectin level and proinflammatory cytokines, and to relate these changes to the improved liver histology resulting from pioglitazone therapy in 18 patients with NASH. Serum levels of adiponectin increased significantly at week 48, but the levels of other inflammatory cytokines, tumor necrosis factor α (TNF- α), interleukin (IL)-1a, and IL-6, did not. Pioglitazone therapy was associated with significant improvement in aminotransferases, steatosis, hepatic fat content as measured by MRI, NASH activity index, and fibrosis ($P < .001$ for all). There was no correlation between changes in NASH activity index score or the individual features of the score and serum TNF-α, IL-1a, or IL-6 levels. In contrast, there was a marked inverse correlation between improvements in the NASH activity index score and adiponectin levels ($P = .01$). Of the individual histological features scored, the correlation was the strongest for hepatic steatosis ($P = .03$). The authors concluded that improvements in liver histology during TZD treatment may be modulated by an adiponectin-mediated effect on insulin sensitivity and hepatic fatty acid metabolism rather than by changes in proinflammatory cytokines.

Clinical studies of thiazolidinediones in nonalcoholic steatohepatitis

Several studies with various study endpoints evaluated the role of TZDs in patients with NAFLD (Table 2) [34,35]. The initial drug in this class, troglitazone, was studied by Caldwell and colleagues [36] in 10 patients with biopsy-proven NASH before its removal from the market secondary to reports of significant hepatotoxicity [37,38]. This suggested that troglitazone may lead to biochemical and possibly histological improvements in patients who have NASH.

Neuschwander-Tetri [39,40] evaluated the use of rosiglitazone in 30 patients who had biopsy-proven NASH. All patients received rosiglitazone, 4 mg twice per day for 48 weeks. The main end points were liver fat content by CT, insulin sensitivity, and a global score of histologic injury. Repeat liver biopsies were obtained in 26 patients. Insulin sensitivity and ALT levels significantly improved over the course of therapy. More importantly, however, necroinflammatory activity and zone-3 perisinusoidal fibrosis improved significantly, with 45% of patients not meeting histologic criteria for NASH at the end of treatment.

Another study by Promrat and colleagues [41] examined 18 patients with biopsy-proven NASH who were treated with pioglitazone 30 mg daily for 48 weeks. The primary outcome was an improvement in hepatic histology. Secondary outcome measures were improvement in serum aminotransferase levels and measures of insulin sensitivity. ALT normalized in 72% of patients at the end of therapy. The ALT decreases were gradual, beginning after 4 weeks of treatment, and reaching lowest levels between 40 and 48 weeks. Repeat liver biopsies were available on all 18 patients. Fibrosis was reduced in 61% of patients; it remained stable in 22% and worsened in 17%. Nine patients had bridging fibrosis at study entry. Among these nine patients, three had stable fibrosis, and six had improvement of fibrosis. Lobular inflammation, hepatocellular injury, Mallory bodies and NASH activity index improved significantly. The changes were associated with improved indices of insulin sensitivity.

Table 2
Selected human studies of thiazolidinediones in nonalcoholic steatohepatitis

Author (reference number)	N	Study design	Year	Agent	Daily dose	Treatment duration	Aminotransferases	Histology
Caldwell et al [36]	10	Open-label	2001	Tro	400 mg	3–6 months	Improved	Improved inflammation
Neuschwander-Tetri et al [40]	30	Open-label	2003	Rosi	8 mg	48 weeks	Improved	Improved steatosis, inflammation and fibrosis
Promrat et al [41]	18	Open-label	2004	Pio	30 mg	48 weeks	Improved	Improved steatosis, inflammation and fibrosis
Shadid and Jensen [34]	5	Open-label	2003	Pio	30 mg	4–5 months	Improved	Not evaluated
Sanyal et al [35]	21	Randomized clinical trial	2002	Pio	30 mg	6 months	Not reported	Improved steatosis and inflammation
Belfort et al [43]	55	Randomized, placebo controlled, double blind clinical trial	2006	Pio	45 mg	6 months	Improved	Improved steatosis and inflammation
Ratziu et al [45] (abstract)	63	Randomized, placebo controlled, double-blind clinical trial	2006	Rosi	8 mg	12 months	Improved	Improved steatosis and delayed disease progression

Abbreviations: Pio, pioglitazone; Rosi, rosiglitazone; Tro, troglitazone.

The same group studied the effects of discontinuing pioglitazone in the same cohort of patients with NASH who demonstrated significant benefit from pioglitazone during the 48-week treatment period [42]. Of the patients who completed the 48-week therapy with pioglitazone, 13 completed a further 48 weeks of follow-up after stopping therapy. Nine of these 13 patients underwent a repeat liver biopsy approximately 48 weeks after stopping the initial course of therapy. ALT values were significantly higher at 48 weeks off pioglitazone compared with end-of-treatment values and were similar to pretreatment levels. Repeat liver biopsy in nine patients showed a significant worsening in inflammation, steatosis, and overall NASH activity index (compared with end of treatment). Also, stopping pioglitazone was associated with a decrease in adiponectin, worsening insulin sensitivity, and increase in total hepatic fat as assessed by MRI. Therefore, this study suggested that long-term therapy with pioglitazone may be necessary for a sustained biochemical and histological improvement in patients who have NASH.

Belfort and colleagues [43] recently reported the first randomized and placebo-controlled trial of pioglitazone in 55 patients who had biopsy-proven NASH. Diet plus pioglitazone, as compared with diet plus placebo, improved glycemic control and glucose tolerance ($P<.001$), normalized liver aminotransferase levels as it decreased plasma aspartate aminotransferase levels (by 40% versus 21%, $P = .04$), decreased alanine aminotransferase levels (by 58% versus 34%, $P<.001$), decreased hepatic fat content as measured by magnetic resonance spectroscopy (by 54% versus 0%, $P<.001$), and increased hepatic insulin sensitivity (by 48% versus 14%, $P = .008$) (Fig. 2). At 6 months, the TNF-α level decreased by 11% ($P = .002$), and the transforming growth factor β (TGF-β) level decreased by 18% ($P = .03$), whereas neither value changed significantly in the placebo group. In the placebo group, the only histologic improvement from baseline to 6 months was a reduction in inflammation ($P = .03$). The combined necroinflammation score improved in 85% of subjects who received pioglitazone, as compared with 38% of those who received placebo ($P = .001$). The fibrosis scores improved in the pioglitazone group ($P = .002$ for the comparison of scores before and after treatment), but the change from baseline did not differ significantly between the treatment group and the placebo group ($P = .08$) (Fig. 3). This study suggested that pioglitazone not only may improve insulin resistance, but also may have direct anti-inflammatory effects on the liver. Pioglitazone lowered TNF-α, TGF-β, and intracellular adhesion molecule and vascular-cell adhesion molecule concentrations [44].

Another randomized, placebo-controlled trial of rosiglitazone in NASH recently was published in abstract form [45]. Patients who had a biopsy-proven NASH were randomized to a 1-year treatment with rosiglitazone (n = 32), 8 mg/d, or placebo (n = 31). The primary endpoint was reduction in steatosis by greater than 30% and secondary end points were normalization of ALT and improvement in necroinflammation and fibrosis. Histologic response was significantly higher in the rosiglitazone group as compared

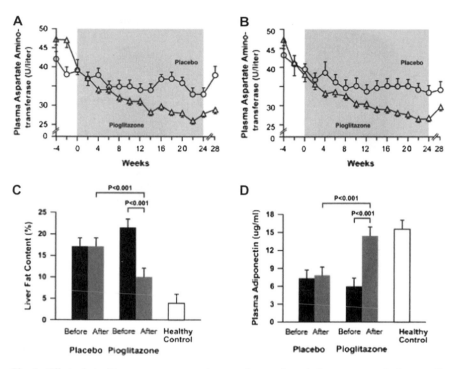

Fig. 2. Effect of pioglitazone on serum aminotransferases, hepatic fat content, and plasma adiponectin levels in patients with nonalcoholic steatohepatitis. Compared with placebo, patients receiving pioglitazone had significant improvement in serum aminotransferases, hepatic fat content, and plasma adiponectin concentration. (*A, B*) Open circles denote placebo, and open triangles denote pioglitazone. (*C, D*) Black bars indicate pre-treatment, and grey bars indicate post-treatment. (*From* Belfort R, Harrison SA, Brown K, et al. A placebo-controlled trial of pioglitazone in subjects with nonalcoholic steatohepatitis. N Engl J Med 2006;355(22): 2297–307; with permission. Copyright © 2006, Massachusetts Medical Society.)

with the placebo group (47% versus 16%, $P < .015$). The mean reduction in steatosis was 20% in the treatment group and 5% in the placebo group ($P = .02$). Biochemical response occurred in 38% of the treatment group and 7% of the placebo group ($P = .005$). Histologic response was correlated with improvement in ALT and serum insulin. There was also a significant delay in disease progression in rosiglitazone patients compared with placebo patients for hepatocyte ballooning, inflammation, and fibrosis. Independent predictors of histologic response were rosigliazone treatment, absence of diabetes, and a high steatosis grade. Although this study showed that rosiglitazone significantly improved liver injury in NASH, more than half of the treated patients were nonresponders. Thus, alternative treatments and large-scale trials with longer treatment durations were suggested by authors.

In summary, several studies have tested the hypothesis that TZDs, by improving insulin resistance, may be beneficial in treating patients who have NAFLD. Aminotransferases improved or normalized in all of these studies.

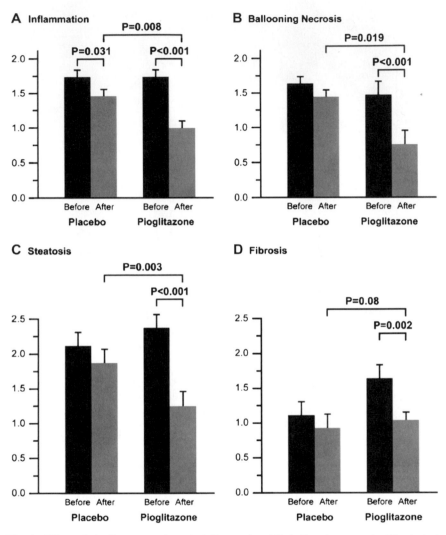

Fig. 3. Effect of pioglitazone on hepatic inflammation (*A*), ballooning necrosis (*B*), steatosis (*C*), and fibrosis (*D*) in patients with nonalcoholic steatohepatitis. Compared with placebo, patients receiving pioglitazone had significant improvement in hepatic steatosis, lobular inflammation, balloon degeneration of hepatocytes, and fibrosis. (*From* Belfort R, Harrison SA, Brown K, et al. A placebo-controlled trial of pioglitazone in subjects with non-alcoholic steatohepatitis. N Engl J Med 2006;355(22):2297–307; with permission. Copyright © 2006, Massachusetts Medical Society.)

Also, there is a suggestion of improved histology. Interpretation of these studies without a placebo group is difficult, however, as ALT levels, hepatic steatosis, and inflammation tend to improve over time as fibrosis progresses in NAFLD [46,47]. The results from two randomized and placebo-controlled trials are encouraging, but larger-scale randomized clinical trials of at least 1 or 2 years' duration are needed to identify the exact role of TZDs in NASH patients. The National Institutes of Health (NIH)-funded NASH Clinical Research Network is conducting a large multicenter randomized study of pioglitazone versus vitamin E versus placebo in nondiabetic patients with NASH (PIVENS), and the results from this 2-year treatment study should be available within next 2 to 3 years.

Safety of thiazolidinediones in nonalcoholic fatty liver disease patients

Pioglitazone and rosiglitazone generally are considered to be very safe from a hepatotoxic stand point [48–50]. Isolated case reports of severe liver damage following their use, however, have appeared in the literature [51–56]. It is recommended by the manufacturers that liver enzymes should be checked in all patients before prescribing these agents, and they should be not used in those with increased liver enzymes (ALT greater than 2.5 times the upper limit of normal) [57]. It is further recommended that the initiation of therapy in patients with mild elevations in liver enzymes should be undertaken with caution [57]. One study by the authors' group examined the effect of rosiglitazone on serum liver biochemistries in diabetic patients with normal and elevated baseline liver enzymes [58]. In this study, the authors showed that diabetic patients who have elevated baseline liver enzymes do not have a higher risk of hepatotoxicity from rosiglitazone than those who have normal baseline liver enzymes (Table 3). Because elevated liver enzymes in patients who have diabetes are likely to represent an underlying NAFLD, this study suggested the safety of rosiglitazone in these patients, although it might have not been powered enough to demonstrate a difference in the incidence of severe hepatotoxicity.

Table 3
Lack of hepatotoxicity from rosiglitazone in diabetic patients with elevated baseline liver tests

	Cohort 1[a] (n = 210)	Cohort 2[a] (n = 628)
Mean aspartate aminotransferase during follow-up (IU/L)	38 ± 35	29 ± 28
Mean alanine aminotransferase during follow-up (IU/L)	36 ± 30	26 ± 23
Mean bilirubin during follow-up (mg/dL)	0.4 ± 0.4	0.5 ± 0.6
Discontinuation of rosiglitazone[c]	18 (8.6%)	51 (8.1%)[b]
Mild–moderate elevations in liver tests[c]	21 (10%)	42 (6.6%)[b]
Severe elevations in liver tests[c]	2 (0.9%)	4 (0.6%)[b]
Hy's rule[c]	0	2 (0.3%)[b]

[a] Cohort 1: Type 2 diabetics with elevated baseline liver tests who received rosiglitazone. Cohort 2: Type 2 diabetics with normal baseline liver tests who received rosiglitazone.

[b] *p* = ns versus variable in the next column.

[c] An article by Chalasani and colleagues contains more detailed definitions [58].

Modified from Chalasani N, Teal E, Hall SD. Effect of rosiglitazone on serum liver biochemistries in diabetic patients with normal and elevated baseline liver enzymes. Am J Gastroenterol 2005;100(6):1317–21; with permission.

Weight gain of 2 to 6 kg is the most common adverse effect noted in the existing studies of TZDs for NASH, and this occurs in 67% to 72% of subjects. The causal relationship between TZD and congestive heart failure is debated [59]. Furthermore, the recently raised concerns of bone fractures from TZDs and increased cardiovascular mortality from rosiglitazone demand caution in defining the role of TZDs to treat NASH [60,61].

Metformin

Mechanism of action

Metformin first was described in the scientific literature in 1957 [62,63], but it did not receive approval by the US Food and Drug administration (FDA) for type 2 diabetes until 1994. The exact mechanism of action of metformin is uncertain despite its known therapeutic benefits. Its mode of action appears to be reduction of hepatic gluconeogenesis, decreased absorption of glucose from the gastrointestinal (GI) tract, and increased insulin sensitivity. The improvement in insulin sensitivity is by increasing glucose uptake and use. It also was shown that metformin stimulates the hepatic enzyme AMP-activated protein kinase, which plays an important role in metabolism of fats and glucose [62]; it reduces plasma lipids and fatty acid oxidation in the liver [64].

Lin and colleagues [65] tested the use of metformin in ob/ob mice. These mice, which are leptin-deficient because of ob gene mutation, have been studied extensively as a naturally occurring model of hepatic steatosis. Treatment with metformin improved fatty liver disease and reversed hepatomegaly, steatosis, and aminotransferase abnormalities in these morbidly obese mice. Also metformin reduced hepatic TNF-α expression in these insulin-resistant mice. The authors of this study concluded that the therapeutic mechanism of metformin likely involved inhibited hepatic expression of TNF-α and TNF-inducible factors that promote hepatic lipid accumulation.

Clinical studies of metformin in nonalcoholic fatty liver disease

Several studies evaluated the role of metformin in patients who had NAFLD (Table 4). Marchesini and colleagues [66] demonstrated improved liver enzymes and reduction in hepatomegaly as measured by ultrasound in 14 patients who had NAFLD treated with metformin (1500 mg/d) for 4 months. Unfortunately, follow-up histopathology was not obtained.

Nair and colleagues [67] reported another trial of 15 patients treated with 20 mg/kg/d of metformin for 48 weeks. Fifteen patients completed 1 year of treatment, and 10 underwent a post-treatment biopsy. Although there was a significant decrease in transaminases by the third month of treatment, there was a gradual rise to pretreatment levels thereafter. In the initial 3 months of treatment, there was a significant increase in insulin sensitivity

Table 4
Selected human studies of metformin in nonalcoholic steatohepatitis

Author	N	Study design	Year	Daily dose	Treatment duration	Aminotransferases	Histology
Marchesini et al [66]	14	Open-label	2001	1.5 g	4 months	Improved	Not evaluated
Nair et al [67]	15	Open-label	2004	20 mg/kg	12 months	Improved	Improved inflammation
Uygun et al [68]	36	Open-label	2004	1.5 g	6 months	Improved	Improved inflammation
Bugianesi et al [69]	55	Randomized clinical trial	2005	2 g	12 months	Improved	Improved steatosis, inflammation and fibrosis
Schwimmer et al [70]	10	Open-label	2005	1 g	6 months	Improved	Not evaluated
Loomba et al [71]	14	Open-label	2006	2 g	48 weeks	Improved	Improved steatosis and inflammation

that corresponded to the fall in the aminotransferases. In the subsequent months, however, there was no further improvement in insulin sensitivity, and this paralleled the rebound in the aminotransferase levels. Among the 10 patients who had post-treatment liver biopsy, three patients (33%) showed improvement in steatosis; two (20%) showed improvement in inflammation, and one (10%) showed improvement in fibrosis.

In a controlled trial, Uygun and colleagues [68] randomized 36 patients who had NASH to receive either dietary modification or dietary modification plus metformin for 6 months. As compared with the former, the latter group had a significant decrease in aminotransferases, insulin, and C peptide. Both groups showed improvements in necroinflammation following therapy without a significant advantage to metformin, although steatosis, as measured by ultrasound, showed improvement with the addition of metformin. Another study from Italy [69] randomized NAFLD patients to 2 g/d of metformin (n = 55), diet (n = 27), or 800 IU/d of vitamin E (n = 28). Significantly more patients taking metformin had normalization of their ALT levels compared with those taking vitamin E or diet treatment. Follow-up liver biopsy was performed in 17 of the 55 subjects in the metformin group; significant improvements were seen in steatosis, inflammation, and fibrosis compared with baseline.

Schwimmer and colleagues [70] studied metformin as a treatment for 10 pediatric patients who had NASH. Aminotransferase levels improved significantly or normalized in 40% to 50% of patients. Patients demonstrated significant improvements in liver fat measured by magnetic resonance spectroscopy.

More recently, Loomba and colleagues [71] conducted an open-label study to evaluate the effects of a 48-week course of metformin on biochemical and histological features of NASH. Twenty four patients started metformin in daily doses of 500 mg for 2 weeks, 1000 mg for 2 weeks, followed by 2000 mg for the remaining 44 weeks. Fourteen patients completed 48 weeks of treatment and had repeat liver biopsies. Five patients (36%) had a histological response, with three of them no longer meeting criteria for NASH. Three patients had a 2-point decrease in NASH activity index, which comprises scores for parenchymal inflammation, cellular injury, and steatosis. The remaining six patients showed no histological response. The responders had a statistically significant change in their BMI, transaminases, and NASH activity as compared with the nonresponders (Table 5). It was concluded that metformin therapy may cause biochemical and histological improvement in NASH by improving insulin sensitivity and inducing weight loss.

In summary, many small trials have shown encouraging results for metformin in patients who have NAFLD, but these results should be reproduced in larger clinical trials with valid end points before one is able to define the role of metformin for treating NASH, especially in those without type2 diabetes.

Table 5
Effects of metformin on weight, alanine aminotransferase and nonalcoholic steatohepatitis activity index

Variable	Responders [5]	Nonresponders [9]	P value
Change in body mass index (kg/m^2)	−5.6 ± 1.4	+0.38 ± 0.23	0.0006
Normalization of alanine aminotransferase	4/5	1/9	0.02
Change in nonalcoholic steatohepatitis activity index	5.2 ± 1.48	0.77 ± 1.39	0.0001

Data from Loomba R, Lutchman G, Kleiner D, et al. Pilot study of metformin in patients with nonalcoholic steatohepatitis [abstract]. Hepatology 2006;44(Suppl 1):260A.

Safety of metformin in nonalcoholic fatty liver disease patients

Metformin seems to be very well tolerated in NAFLD patients. There is one case report of possible hepatitis from metformin in a diabetic patient, with aminotransferases rising to the 500 range [72]. Metformin should be avoided in patients who have renal insufficiency or congestive heart failure because of increased risk of lactic acidosis in these patients. In NAFLD patients, minor elevations of lactate levels are infrequently reported, but no cases of lactic acidosis have been noted [73]. In contrast to TZDs, many patients treated with metformin lose weight. GI intolerance is the most frequent adverse effect.

Other insulin sensitizers

Exendin-4, a naturally occurring peptide that has 50% identity with the amino acid sequence of glucagon-like peptide 1 (GLP-1), binds to GLP-1 receptor and acts similarly to GLP-1 [74]. Both exendin-4 and GLP-1 augment pancreatic β cell function by enhancing glucose-stimulated insulin secretion, restoring first-phase insulin secretion, and stimulating β cell growth and neogenesis under conditions of increased insulin demand. Also, these compounds promote satiety [75–78]. Ding and colleagues [79] conducted a study to determine whether administration of exendin-4 would reverse hepatic steatosis in ob/ob mice. Exendin-4 improved insulin sensitivity in ob/ob mice; serum glucose and hepatic steatosis also were reduced significantly. Future work should be undertaken to confirm and expand these potentially important therapeutic and novel biologic findings.

Summary

NAFLD is very common in the Western world and it can be divided broadly into simple steatosis, which is benign, and NASH, which can progress to cirrhosis and liver failure. Insulin resistance is essential for developing

NAFLD, and thus insulin sensitizers are emerging as promising agents to treat NASH. Many preliminary studies have suggested that second generations are effective in improving hepatic histology in patients who have NASH, but many important safety and practical issues need to be addressed before they can be accepted as first-line agents. The relevance of weight gain caused by TZDs in this patient population is not known. Furthermore, the recently raised concerns of bone fractures from TZDs and increased cardiovascular mortality from rosiglitazone demand caution in defining the role of TZDs to treat NASH. The efficacy of metformin to treat NASH does not appear to be as robust as TZDs, but its safety profile is possibly more desirable.

References

[1] Contos MJ, Sanyal AJ. The clinicopathologic spectrum and management of nonalcoholic fatty liver disease. Adv Anat Pathol 2002;9:37–51.

[2] Hamaguchi M, Kojima T, Takeda N, et al. The metabolic syndrome as a predictor of nonalcoholic fatty liver disease. Ann Intern Med 2005;143(10):722–8.

[3] Willner IR, Waters B, Patil SR, et al. Ninety patients with nonalcoholic steatohepatitis: insulin resistance, familial tendency, and severity of disease. Am J Gastroenterol 2001; 96(10):2957–61.

[4] Chitturi S, Abeygunasekera S, Farrell GC, et al. NASH and insulin resistance: insulin hypersecretion and specific association with the insulin resistance syndrome. Hepatology 2002; 35(2):373–9.

[5] Pagano G, Pacini G, Musso G, et al. Nonalcoholic steatohepatitis, insulin resistance, and metabolic syndrome: further evidence for an etiologic association. Hepatology 2002;35(2): 367–72.

[6] Chalasani N, Deeg MA, Persohn S, et al. Metabolic and anthropometric evaluation of insulin resistance in nondiabetic patients with nonalcoholic steatohepatitis. Am J Gastroenterol 2003;98(8):1849–55.

[7] Sanyal AJ, Campbell-Sargent C, Mirshahi F, et al. Nonalcoholic steatohepatitis: association of insulin resistance and mitochondrial abnormalities. Gastroenterology 2001;120(5):1183–92.

[8] Loria P, Lonardo A, Carulli N. Relative contribution of iron burden, HFE mutations, and insulin resistance to fibrosis in nonalcoholic fatty liver. Hepatology 2004;39:1748.

[9] Wanless IR, Shiota K. The pathogenesis of nonalcoholic steatohepatitis and other fatty liver diseases: a four-step model including the role of lipid release and hepatic venular obstruction in the progression to cirrhosis. Semin Liver Dis 2004;24:99–106.

[10] Lonardo A, Carani C, Carulli N, et al. Endocrine NAFLD, a hormonocentric perspective of nonalcoholic fatty liver disease pathogenesis. J Hepatol 2006;44(6):1196–207.

[11] Liangpunsakul S, Chalasani N. Is hypothyroidism a risk factor for nonalcoholic steatohepatitis? J Clin Gastroenterol 2003;37(4):340–3.

[12] Adams LA, Feldstein A, Lindor KD, et al. Nonalcoholic fatty liver disease among patients with hypothalamic and pituitary dysfunction. Hepatology 2004;39(4):909–14.

[13] Flegal KM, Carroll MD, Ogden CL, et al. Prevalence and trends in obesity among US adults, 1999–2000. JAMA 2002;288:1723–7.

[14] Ford ES, Giles WH, Dietz WH. Prevalence of the metabolic syndrome among US adults: findings from the third National Health and Nutrition Examination Survey. JAMA 2002; 287:356–9.

[15] Pourshams A, Malekzadeh R, Monavvari A, et al. Prevalence and etiology of persistently elevated alanine aminotransferase levels in healthy Iranian blood donors. J Gastroenterol Hepatol 2005;20(2):229–33.

[16] Sampliner RE, Beluk D, Harrow EJ, et al. The persistence and significance of elevated alanine aminotransferase levels in blood donors. Transfusion 1985;25(2):102–4.

[17] Schwimmer JB, Deutsch R, Kahen T, et al. Prevalence of fatty liver in children and adolescents. Pediatrics 2006;118(4):1388–93.

[18] Zelber-Sagi S, Nitzan-Kaluski D, Halpern Z, et al. Prevalence of primary nonalcoholic fatty liver disease in a population-based study and its association with biochemical and anthropometric measures. Liver Int 2006;26(7):856–63.

[19] Chen CH, Huang MH, Yang JC, et al. Prevalence and risk factors of nonalcoholic fatty liver disease in an adult population of Taiwan: metabolic significance of nonalcoholic fatty liver disease in nonobese adults. J Clin Gastroenterol 2006;40(8):745–52.

[20] Clark JM. The epidemiology of nonalcoholic fatty liver disease in adults. J Clin Gastroenterol 2006;40(3 Suppl 1):S5–10.

[21] Caldwell SH, Harris DM, Patrie JT, et al. Is NASH underdiagnosed among African Americans? Am J Gastroenterol 2002;97(6):1496–500.

[22] Browning JD, Kumar KS, Saboorian MH, et al. Ethnic differences in the prevalence of cryptogenic cirrhosis. Am J Gastroenterol 2004;99(2):292–8.

[23] Adams LA, Lymp JF, St Sauver J, et al. The natural history of nonalcoholic fatty liver disease: a population-based cohort study. Gastroenterology 2005;129:113–21.

[24] Powell EE, Cooksley WG, Hanson R, et al. The natural history of nonalcoholic steatohepatitis: a follow-up study of forty-two patients for up to 21 years. Hepatology 1990;11: 74–80.

[25] Barbier O, Torra IP, Duguay Y, et al. Pleiotropic actions of peroxisome proliferator-activated receptors in lipid metabolism and atherosclerosis. Arterioscler Thromb Vasc Biol 2002;22:717–26.

[26] Willson TM, Lambert MH, Kliewer SA. Peroxisome proliferator-activated receptor gamma and metabolic disease. Annu Rev Biochem 2001;70:341–67.

[27] Dubois M, Pattou F, Kerr-Conte J, et al. Expression of peroxisome proliferator-activated receptor gamma (PPARgamma) in normal human pancreatic islet cells. Diabetologia 2000;43:1165–9.

[28] Yki-Jarvinen H. Thiazolidinediones. N Engl J Med 2004;351(11):1106–18.

[29] Shulman GI. Cellular mechanisms of insulin resistance. J Clin Invest 2000;106:171–6.

[30] Taylor R. Causation of type 2 diabetes: the Gordian knot unravels. N Engl J Med 2004;350: 639–41.

[31] Maeda N, Shimomura I, Kishida K, et al. Diet-induced insulin resistance in mice lacking adiponectin/ACRP30. Nat Med 2002;8:731–7.

[32] Bajaj M, Suraamornkul S, Piper P, et al. Decreased plasma adiponectin concentrations are closely related to hepatic fat content and hepatic insulin resistance in pioglitazone-treated type 2 diabetic patients. J Clin Endocrinol Metab 2004;89:200–6.

[33] Lutchman G, Promrat K, Kleiner DE, et al. Changes in serum adipokine levels during pioglitazone treatment for nonalcoholic steatohepatitis: relationship to histological improvement. Clin Gastroenterol Hepatol 2006;4(8):1048–52.

[34] Shadid S, Jensen MD. Effect of pioglitazone on biochemical indices of nonalcoholic fatty liver disease in upper body obesity. Clin Gastroenterol Hepatol 2003;1(5):384–7.

[35] Sanyal AJ, Mofrad PS, Contos MJ, et al. A pilot study of vitamin E versus vitamin E and pioglitazone for the treatment of nonalcoholic steatohepatitis. Clin Gastroenterol Hepatol 2004;2:1107–15.

[36] Caldwell SH, Hespenheide EE, Redick JA, et al. A pilot study of a thiazolidinedione, troglitazone, in nonalcoholic steatohepatitis. Am J Gastroenterol 2001;96(2):519–25.

[37] Menon KVN, Angulo P, Lindor KD. Severe cholestatic hepatitis from troglitazone in a patient with nonalcoholic steatohepatitis and diabetes mellitus. Am J Gastroenterol 2001;96(5): 1631–4.

[38] Neuschwander-Tetri BA, Isley WL, Oki JC, et al. Troglitazone-induced hepatic failure leading to liver transplantation. A case report. Ann Intern Med 1998;129(1):38–41.

[39] Neuschwander-Tetri BA, Brunt EM, Wehmeier KR, et al. Interim results of a pilot study demonstrating the early effects of the PPAR-[gamma] ligand rosiglitazone on insulin sensitivity, aminotransferases, hepatic steatosis, and body weight in patients with nonalcoholic steatohepatitis. J Hepatol 2003;38:434–40.

[40] Neuschwander-Tetri BA, Brunt EM, Wehmeier KR, et al. Improved nonalcoholic steatohepatitis after 48 weeks of treatment with the PPAR-[gamma] ligand rosiglitazone. Hepatology 2003;38:1008–17.

[41] Promrat K, Lutchman G, Uwaifo GI, et al. A pilot study of pioglitazone treatment for nonalcoholic steatohepatitis. Hepatology 2004;39:188–96.

[42] Lutchman G, Modi A, Kleiner DE, et al. The effects of discontinuing pioglitazone in patients with nonalcoholic steatohepatitis. Hepatology 2007;46:424–9.

[43] Belfort R, Harrison SA, Brown K, et al. A placebo-controlled trial of pioglitazone in subjects with nonalcoholic steatohepatitis. N Engl J Med 2006;355(22):2297–307.

[44] Harrison SA, Schenker S, Cusi K. Pioglitazone in nonalcoholic steatohepatitis. N Engl J Med 2007;356:1067–9, Correspondence.

[45] Ratziu V, Charlotte F, Jacqueminet S, et al. One year randomized placebo-controlled double-blind trial of rosigletazone in nonalcoholic steatohepatitis: results of the Pilot trial. Hepatology 2006;44(Suppl 1): [Abstract Form].

[46] Fassio E, Alvarez E, Dominguez N, et al. Natural history of nonalcoholic steatohepatitis: a longitudinal study of repeat liver biopsies. Hepatology 2004;40:820–6.

[47] Adams LA, Sanderson S, Lindor KD, et al. The histological course of nonalcoholic fatty liver disease: a longitudinal study of 103 patients with sequential liver biopsies. J Hepatol 2005;42:132–8.

[48] Isley WL. Hepatotoxicity of thiazolidinediones. Expert Opin Drug Saf 2003;2:581–6.

[49] Scheen AJ. Hepatotoxicity with thiazolidinediones: is it a class effect? Drug Saf 2001;24: 873–88.

[50] Tolman KG, Chandramouli J. Hepatotoxicity of the thiazolidinediones. Clin Liver Dis 2003; 7:369–79.

[51] Bonkovsky HL, Azar R, Bird S, et al. Severe cholestatic hepatitis caused by thiazolidinediones: risks associated with substituting rosiglitazone for troglitazone. Dig Dis Sci 2002; 47:1632–7.

[52] Forman LM, Simmons DA, Diamond RH. Hepatic failure in a patient taking rosiglitazone. Ann Intern Med 2000;132:118–21.

[53] Al-Salman J, Heider A, Kemp D, et al. Hepatocellular injury in a patient receiving rosiglitazone: a case report. Ann Intern Med 2000;132:121–4.

[54] May LD, Lefkowitch JH, Kram MT, et al. Mixed hepatocellular–cholestatic liver injury after pioglitazone therapy. Ann Intern Med 2002;136:449–52.

[55] Pinto AG, Cummings OW, Chalasani N. Severe but reversible cholestatic liver injury after pioglitazone therapy. Ann Intern Med 2002;137:857.

[56] Maeda K. Hepatocellular injury in a patient receiving pioglitazone. Ann Intern Med 2001; 135:306.

[57] Physician Desk Reference (PDR). 58th edition. Montvale (NJ): Thompson Healthcare; 2004.

[58] Chalasani N, Teal E, Hall SD. Effect of rosiglitazone on serum liver biochemistries in diabetic patients with normal and elevated baseline liver enzymes. Am J Gastroenterol 2005; 100(6):1317–21.

[59] Kennedy FP. Do thiazolidinediones cause congestive heart failure? Mayo Clin Proc 2003;78: 1076–7.

[60] Schwartz AV, Sellmeyer DE. Thiazolidinediones: new evidence of bone loss. J Clin Endocrinol Metab 2007;92:1232–4.

[61] Nissen SE, Wolshik K. Effect of rosiglitazone on the risk for myocardial infarction and death from cardiovascular causes. N Engl J Med 2007;356:2457–71.

[62] Ungar G, Freedman L, Shapiro S. Pharmacological studies of a new oral hypoglycemic drug. Proc Soc Exp Biol Med 1957;95(1):190–2.

[63] Zhou G, Myers R, Li Y, et al. Role of AMP-activated protein kinase in mechanism of metformin action. J Clin Invest 2001;108(8):1167–74.

[64] Perriello G, Misericordia P, Volpi E, et al. Acute antihyperglycemic mechanisms of metformin in NIDDM: evidence for suppression of lipid oxidation and glucose production. Diabetes 1994;43:920–8.

[65] Lin HZ, Yang SQ, Chuckaree C, et al. Metformin reverses fatty liver disease in obese, leptin-deficient mice. Nat Med 2000;6(9):998–1003.

[66] Marchesini G, Brizi M, Bianchi G, et al. Metformin in nonalcoholic steatohepatitis. Lancet 2001;358:893–4.

[67] Nair S, Diehl AM, Wiseman M, et al. Metformin in the treatment of nonalcoholic steatohepatitis. Aliment Pharmacol Ther 2004;20:23–38.

[68] Uygun A, Kadayifci A, Isik AT, et al. Metformin in the treatment of patients with nonalcoholic steatohepatitis. Aliment Pharmacol Ther 2004;19:537–44.

[69] Bugianesi E, Gentilcore E, Manini R, et al. A randomized controlled trial of Metformin versus vitamin E or prescriptive diet in nonalcoholic fatty liver disease. Am J Gastroenterol 2005;100:1082–90.

[70] Schwimmer JB, Middleton MS, Deutsch R, et al. A phase 2 clinical trial of metformin as a treatment for nondiabetic paediatric nonalcoholic steatohepatitis. Aliment Pharmacol Ther 2005;21(7):871–9.

[71] Loomba R, Lutchman G, Kleiner D, et al. Pilot study of metformin in patients with nonalcoholic steatohepatitis [abstract]. Hepatology 2006;44:260.

[72] Babich MM, Pike I, Shiffman ML. Metformin-induced acute hepatitis. Am J Med 1998;104:490–2.

[73] Misbin RI, Green L, Stadel LG, et al. Lactic acidosis in patients with diabetes treated with metformin. N Engl J Med 1998;338:265–6.

[74] Doyle M, Egan J. Glucagon-like peptide 1. Recent Prog Horm Res 2001;56:377–99.

[75] Doyle M, Egan J. Pharmacological agents that directly modulate insulin secretion. Pharmacol Rev 2003;55:105–31.

[76] Drucker D. Minireview: the glucagon-like peptides. Endocrinology 2001;142:521–7.

[77] Drucker D. Biological actions and therapeutic potential of the glucagon-like peptides. Gastroenterology 2002;122:531–44.

[78] Drucker D. Gut adaptation and the glucagon-like peptides. Gut 2002;50:428–35.

[79] Ding X, Saxena NK, Lin S, et al. Exendin-4, a glucagon-like protein 1 (GLP-1) receptor agonist, reverses hepatic steatosis in ob/ob mice. Hepatology 2006;43(1):173–81.

ELSEVIER
SAUNDERS

Endocrinol Metab Clin N Am
36 (2007) 1089–1105

ENDOCRINOLOGY
AND METABOLISM
CLINICS
OF NORTH AMERICA

Index

Note: Page numbers of article titles are in **boldface** type.

A

A Diabetic Outcome Progression Trial
(ADOPT), 884

Abscess, as pancreas transplant
complication, 1028

ACTH, deficiency of, hematopoietic stem
cell transplant causing, 986–987
stimulation of, prednisone effect on,
893

Adiponectin, thiazolidinediones impact on,
1073–1074

Adrenal function, glucocorticoids effect on,
893

Alanine aminotransferase (ALT), in
nonalcoholic fatty liver disease, 1070
metformin impact on, 1083
thiazolidinediones impact on,
1074–1079

Alendronate, for osteoporosis, 955–956

Allograft outcomes, in new onset diabetes
mellitus after transplant, 880–881

Allograft procurement, for pancreas
transplant, 1020–1021

Allograft selection, for pancreas transplant,
1019–1020

Alpha-glucosidase inhibitors, for
post-transplant diabetes mellitus, 916

American Diabetes Association (ADA),
diabetes mellitus diagnostic criteria of,
874–875
on pancreas transplant, 1018

Aminotransferases, metformin impact on,
1080–1083
thiazolidinediones impact on,
1074–1075, 1079

Anastomotic leak, as pancreas transplant
complication, 1027–1028

Angiography, of cardiac allograft
vasculopathy, 968, 970, 974

Angiotensin-converting enzyme (ACE)
inhibitors, for post-cardiac transplant
hypertension, 975

Antibodies, monoclonal versus polyclonal,
effect on glucose and lipid metabolism,
900
islet cell transplant and, 1009
thyroid, in interferon-induced
thyroiditis diagnosis, 1061

Antilymphocyte globulin, effect on glucose
and lipid metabolism, 900

Antirejection therapies, effect on glucose
and lipid metabolism, 900

Antithymocyte globulin, effect on glucose
and lipid metabolism, 900

Aspirin therapy, for post-transplant
diabetes mellitus complications, 918

Atherogenic triad, in insulin-resistance
syndrome, 971

Autoantibodies, thyroid, interferon-induced
thyroiditis associated with, 1052–1053
genetic predisposition to,
1058–1059
direct effects of, 1060
hepatitis C virus and,
1054–1055

Autoimmune thyroid diseases (AITD),
hematopoietic stem cell transplant
causing, 988
interferon-induced, epidemiology of,
1052–1053
genetic predisposition to,
1058–1059
direct effects of, 1060
hepatitis C virus role in,
1054–1055

Autonomic nervous system dysfunction,
diabetic, pancreas transplant and,
1032–1033

Avascular necrosis, following bone marrow
transplant, 945

United States Postal Service

Statement of Ownership, Management, and Circulation
(All Periodicals Publications Except Requestor Publications)

1. Publication Title	2. Publication Number	3. Filing Date
Endocrinology and Metabolism Clinics of North America	0 0 0 - 2 7 7 5	9/14/07

4. Issue Frequency	5. Number of Issues Published Annually	6. Annual Subscription Price
Mar, Jun, Sep, Dec	4	$193.00

7. Complete Mailing Address of Known Office of Publication (Not printer) (Street, city, county, state, and ZIP+4)

Elsevier Inc.
360 Park Avenue South
New York, NY 10010-1710

Contact Person
Stephen Bushing
Telephone (Include area code)
215-239-3688

8. Complete Mailing Address of Headquarters or General Business Office of Publisher (Not printer)

Elsevier Inc., 360 Park Avenue South, New York, NY 10010-1710

9. Full Names and Complete Mailing Addresses of Publisher, Editor, and Managing Editor (Do not leave blank)

Publisher (Name and complete mailing address)

John Schrefer, Elsevier, Inc., 1600 John F. Kennedy Blvd. Suite 1800, Philadelphia, PA 19103-2899

Editor (Name and complete mailing address)

Rachel Glover, Elsevier, Inc., 1600 John F. Kennedy Blvd. Suite 1800, Philadelphia, PA 19103-2899

Managing Editor (Name and complete mailing address)

Catherine Bewick, Elsevier, Inc., 1600 John F. Kennedy Blvd. Suite 1800, Philadelphia, PA 19103-2899

10. Owner (Do not leave blank. If the publication is owned by a corporation, give the name and address of the corporation immediately followed by the names and addresses of all stockholders owning or holding 1 percent or more of the total amount of stock. If not owned by a corporation, give the names and addresses of the individual owners. If owned by a partnership or other unincorporated firm, give its name and address as well as those of each individual owner. If the publication is published by a nonprofit organization, give its name and address.)

Full Name	Complete Mailing Address
Wholly owned subsidiary of	4520 East-West Highway
Reed/Elsevier, US holdings	Bethesda, MD 20814

11. Known Bondholders, Mortgagees, and Other Security Holders Owning or Holding 1 Percent or More of Total Amount of Bonds, Mortgages, or Other Securities. If none, check box. ☐ None

Full Name	Complete Mailing Address
N/A	

12. Tax Status (For completion by nonprofit organizations authorized to mail at nonprofit rates) (Check one)
The purpose, function, and nonprofit status of this organization and the exempt status for federal income tax purposes:
☐ Has Not Changed During Preceding 12 Months
☐ Has Changed During Preceding 12 Months (Publisher must submit explanation of change with this statement)

PS Form 3526, September 2006 (Page 1 of 3 (Instructions Page 3)) PSN 7530-01-000-9931 **PRIVACY NOTICE**: See our Privacy policy in www.usps.com

---

13. Publication Title	14. Issue Date for Circulation Data Below
Endocrinology and Metabolism Clinics of North America	September 2007

15.	Extent and Nature of Circulation	Average No. Copies Each Issue During Preceding 12 Months	No. Copies of Single Issue Published Nearest to Filing Date
a.	Total Number of Copies (Net press run)	3150	2900
b. Paid Circulation (By Mail and Outside the Mail)	(1) Mailed Outside-County Paid Subscriptions Stated on PS Form 3541. (Include paid distribution above nominal rate, advertiser's proof copies, and exchange copies)	1215	1156
	(2) Mailed In-County Paid Subscriptions Stated on PS Form 3541 (Include paid distribution above nominal rate, advertiser's proof copies, and exchange copies)		
	(3) Paid Distribution Outside the Mails Including Sales Through Dealers and Carriers, Street Vendors, Counter Sales, and Other Paid Distribution Outside USPS®	1100	1105
	(4) Paid Distribution by Other Classes Mailed Through the USPS (e.g. First-Class Mail®)		
c.	Total Paid Distribution (Sum of 15b (1), (2), (3), and (4))	2315	2261
d. Free or Nominal Rate Distribution (By Mail and Outside the Mail)	(1) Free or Nominal Rate Outside-County Copies Included on PS Form 3541	77	68
	(2) Free or Nominal Rate In-County Copies Included on PS Form 3541		
	(3) Free or Nominal Rate Copies Mailed at Other Classes Mailed Through the USPS (e.g. First-Class Mail)		
	(4) Free or Nominal Rate Distribution Outside the Mail (Carriers or other means)		
e.	Total Free or Nominal Rate Distribution (Sum of 15d (1), (2), (3) and (4))	77	68
f.	Total Distribution (Sum of 15c and 15e)	2392	2329
g.	Copies not Distributed (See instructions to publishers #4 (page #3))	758	571
h.	Total (Sum of 15f and g)	3150	2900
i.	Percent Paid (15c divided by 15f times 100)	96.78%	97.08%

16. Publication of Statement of Ownership

☐ If the publication is a general publication, publication of this statement is required. Will be printed in the **December 2007** issue of this publication. ☐ Publication not required

17. Signature and Title of Editor, Publisher, Business Manager, or Owner

[signature]
John Vassallo – Executive Director of Subscription Services

Date: September 14, 2007

I certify that all information furnished on this form is true and complete. I understand that anyone who furnishes false or misleading information on this form or who omits material or information requested on the form may be subject to criminal sanctions (including fines and imprisonment) and/or civil sanctions (including civil penalties).

PS Form 3526, September 2006 (Page 2 of 3)